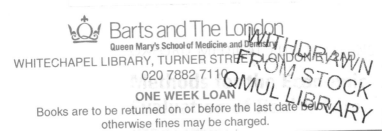

Methods for the Economic Evaluation of Health Care Programmes

THIRD EDITION

Michael F. Drummond
Professor and Director, Centre for Health Economics,
University of York, UK

Mark J. Sculpher
Professor, Centre for Health Economics,
University of York, UK

George W. Torrance
Professor Emeritus, Department of Clinical Epidemiology
and Biostatistics, McMaster University, Ontario, Canada

Bernie J. O'Brien
Director, Program for Assessment of Technology in Health,
Professor, Centre for Evaluation of Medicines,
Department of Clinical Epidemiology and Biostatistics,
McMaster University, Ontario, Canada

Greg L. Stoddart
Professor, Centre for Health Economics and Policy Analysis,
Department of Clinical Epidemiology and Biostatistics,
McMaster University, Ontario, Canada

OXFORD
UNIVERSITY PRESS

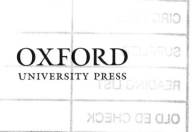

OXFORD
UNIVERSITY PRESS

Great Clarendon Street, Oxford OX2 6DP

Oxford University Press is a department of the University of Oxford.
It furthers the University's objective of excellence in research, scholarship,
and education by publishing worldwide in

Oxford New York

Auckland Cape Town Dar es Salaam Hong Kong Karachi
Kuala Lumpur Madrid Melbourne Mexico City Nairobi
New Delhi Shanghai Taipei Toronto

With offices in

Argentina Austria Brazil Chile Czech Republic France Greece
Guatemala Hungary Italy Japan Poland Portugal Singapore
South Korea Switzerland Thailand Turkey Ukraine Vietnam

Oxford is a registered trade mark of Oxford University Press
in the UK and in certain other countries

Published in the United States
by Oxford University Press Inc., New York

© Oxford University Press, 2005

The moral rights of the authors have been asserted
Database right Oxford University Press (maker)

First edition published 1987
Reprinted 1988 (twice), 1989, 1990, 1992, 1993, 1994 (twice), 1995, 1996
Second edition published 1997
Reprinted 1997, 1998, 2000, 2001, 2003, 2004
Third edition published 2005

British Library Cataloguing in Publication Data

Data available

Library of Congress Cataloging in Publication Data

Data available

Typeset by Newgen Imaging Systems (P) Ltd., Chennai, India
Printed in Great Britain
on acid-free paper by
Biddles Ltd, King's Lynn

ISBN 019–852945–7 (Pbk)   978–019–852945–3
ISBN 019–852944–9 (Hbk)   978–019–852944–6

10 9 8 7 6 5 4 3 2 1

In memory of our friend and colleague Bernie O'Brien

1959–2004

Tragically Bernie O'Brien passed away on 13th February 2004. He was 44 years old. At the time of his death we had already planned this edition and Bernie was looking forward to contributing to the revision, which the rest of us undertook during August 2004, when we were all together at McMaster.

After completing the MSc in Health Economics at the University of York, Bernie's career in health economics began in earnest when he became a research fellow in the Health Economics Research Group at Brunel University, London. His first project was the economic evaluation of the heart transplant programme in the UK, working alongside Professor Martin Buxton. Their report was widely acclaimed as one of the best health technology assessments of its time and helped to establish the importance of health economics in the minds of senior decision-makers in the UK.

After eight years, and several other projects at Brunel, Bernie sought new opportunities in Canada. The Department of Clinical Epidemiology and Biostatistics was the perfect place for Bernie to develop his talents, given his commitment to multidisciplinary working and interest in clinical research.

As well as undertaking a number of important empirical studies, Bernie made significant contributions to the development of the methodology of economic evaluation. Two in particular stand out. First, he produced several innovative papers concerning the application of statistical methods in cost-effectiveness studies. Secondly, Bernie had a strong interest in the valuation of health outcomes. He produced a number of conceptual papers on contingent valuation and its relationship with the more widely-used 'utility' approach. He also explored the difference between willingness-to-pay and willingness-to-accept in the context of health care.

When the time came to produce a second edition of *Methods for the Economic Evaluation of Health Care Programmes*, Bernie was an obvious fourth co-author. Not only was he primarily responsible for two chapters of the book, but he also had a substantial influence on the way in which issues were presented and discussed. This was no mean achievement faced, as he was, with three co-authors who thought they had got it right first time round!

A particular passion for Bernie was the development of young investigators. Therefore he invested considerable time and effort in attracting funding that would enable up-and-coming researchers to spend time working with him in the Centre for Evaluation of Medicines at McMaster. Several of these individuals have now developed into impressive researchers in their own right.

Although Bernie's scientific achievements were considerable, the lasting memory for those who worked with him will be his sense of humour. Teaching with Bernie was a joy and the hundreds of individuals who have passed through training programmes at McMaster will remember his skilful use of cartoons and anecdotes. Bernie was always looking for a humorous comment or joke that would help his students understand the concepts he was trying to convey.

Bernie will be greatly missed. He leaves a wife, Karen, and two daughters, Emma and Lucy. Our thoughts go out to them. We will miss a friend who was eternally cheerful and who hardly had a bad word to say about anyone.

Preface to the first edition

We regard this book as a truly joint effort arising from our common concern to improve the quality of economic evaluation in the health care field.

For a number of years we have been independently engaged in teaching, research, and consultancy in this area. In particular we have offered advice to colleagues from other disciplines and on many occasions have been part of multidisciplinary teams undertaking evaluations of programmes or treatments. These experiences have convinced us of the need for a book which discusses the methodological principles of economic evaluation in health care in a way that would benefit those who plan to undertake such studies.

The book has two particular roots. First, the MS737 course (Economic Analysis for the Evaluation of Health Services) in the Faculty of Health Sciences at McMaster University, which we all have instructed at some stage, attempts to provide a basic grounding in economic evaluation methodology. During the course, the students undertake an evaluation of a programme or health care treatment of their choice. The course assessment is based on the completion of the project.

Second, the Seminex Workshop Series, coordinated by the Faculty of Business at McMaster, has provided the impetus for us to polish our course materials and to make them more free-standing.

What you see here is the result of these roots. The material has been tried and tested both in graduate and continuing education settings. We hope that it meets the needs of the wide readership that is envisaged.

Birmingham, UK   M. F. D.
and Hamilton, Canada   G. L. S.
June 1986   G. W. T.

Preface to the second edition

Much has happened in economic evaluation in health care since the publication of the first edition of this book in 1987. There are now more empirical studies and there is greater acknowledgement of the usefulness of economic evaluation in healthcare decision making. In addition, there have been a number of methodological developments, particularly in cost–utility and cost–benefit analysis.

In producing this second edition our general aim has been to meet the need that the first edition was intended to meet 10 years ago; namely to serve as an introductory text for those contemplating undertaking, commissioning, or using an economic evaluation. As the field has moved on so, we hope, has the book. It is greatly enlarged and, in some places, more technical than the first edition.

We have been appreciative of the positive feedback to the first edition and have retained the critical appraisal framework, because this underpins many of the official guidelines to economic evaluation methodology that have been published in recent years. Also, we have added many new examples, whilst retaining some of the original ones that served us well.

Reactions to the writing style in the first edition have generally been favourable. However, we have tried to improve further the layout of the book, including boxes containing illustrations or points of particular interest. The prime mover in these changes was Bernie O'Brien, our new co-author, who had used our first edition with his own students. Bernie joined the faculty at McMaster a few years ago and has taught both on the graduate course in economic evaluation and on the two-day workshop for health care professionals, our informal 'prerequisite' for being a co-author.

The content of the book has changed in a number of ways, to reflect the advances in economic evaluation methodology. In Chapter 2 we have clarified the terminology and pointed out that there are many components, or building blocks, for an economic evaluation that can be assembled in a number of different ways. There have also been substantial changes to the chapters on cost-effectiveness, cost–utility and cost–benefit analysis. In particular, the chapters on cost–utility and cost–benefit analysis reflect the rapid expansion in the literature and the new approaches being proposed for the valuation of health outcomes.

We have also added completely new chapters. Chapter 8, on the collection and analysis of data, discusses the pros and cons of basing economic evaluation on trials versus models. It also discusses the application of statistical analysis in economic evaluation. Chapter 9, on the presentation and use of data, discusses issues in the comparison of economic evaluation results, in cost-effectiveness rankings or 'league-tables', and in the transferability or portability of economic data.

Another feature of the methodological debate over the past 10 years is that of whether or not economic evaluation should be solely based on the principles of welfare economics, or more particularly those of Paretian welfare economics. We have decided to adopt a broad-based approach, including discussion of methods that some would not wish to call 'economic evaluation'. This perspective is evident in our debate amongst three analysts in Chapters 2 and 9. Our general approach has been to outline the advantages and disadvantages of particular methodologies, rather than to prescribe one 'correct' methodology.

Finally, we were conscious from feedback received that many readers refer to the first edition as 'the little blue book'. Therefore we asked the publishers to retain the same colour scheme for the new edition. Perhaps this will be referred to as 'the big blue book' in the future! We hope you enjoy reading the new edition.

York, UK   M. F. D.
and Hamilton, Canada   B. J. O.
May 1997   G. L. S.
                                                                                                              G. W. T.

Preface to the third edition

In our view the second edition of *Methods for the Economic Evaluation of Health Care Programmes* was a great improvement on the first, reflecting the substantial advances in methodology that had taken place in the previous years. The second edition also embodied several improvements in the layout of the text, due primarily to Bernie O'Brien's influence.

Therefore, it was with some trepidation that we embarked on this third edition in the Summer of 2004. Would there be enough material? Could we further improve the general layout and style of the book?

As we embarked on our task, we were pleasantly surprised by the advances in the theory and practice of economic evaluation since 1997. These comprised developments in the measurement and valuation of health, including preference-based generic instruments and discrete choice experiments. Also, developments in the analysis of patient level data and in decision-analytic modelling meant that we now needed two chapters to cover issues such as cost-effectiveness acceptability curves, net benefit regression and the growing use of Bayesian Methods.

Furthermore, the increasing use of economic evaluation in decision-making meant that we needed to discuss cost-effectiveness thresholds, equity considerations and the new methods for generalising economic data from one setting to another. Rather than having too little new material, the problem was that we had too much!

The other big change from the second edition was the addition of Mark Sculpher as a fifth author. Just as Bernie O'Brien had done for the second edition, Mark questioned aspects of the work and provoked changes which otherwise may not have been made. We think it should be obligatory to add a new co-author every time a new edition is planned, although the authorship list for Samuelson's text might now be overly long!

We hope that you enjoy the third edition and, if you bought either of the first two, you consider it to be an improvement. We regret the fact that our friend Bernie O'Brien is not here to enjoy it with us.

York, UK   Mike Drummond
and Hamilton, Canada   Mark Sculpher
December 2004   Greg Stoddart
                                                    George Torrance

Acknowledgements

We are grateful to several individuals who commented on particular sections of the book. These include Andrew Briggs, Karl Claxton, Emma McIntosh and Andrea Manca. Of course, none of these individuals are in any way responsible for the final text.

We are also grateful to Christine Henderson, Jan Watson and all our academic colleagues at the Program for Assessment of Technology in Health (PATH) for being such excellent hosts and offering great support during the production of this edition, and to Stephanie Cooper for help with proof-reading.

Finally, special thanks are due to Vanessa Windass at the Centre for Health Economics, who coordinated the production of the final manuscript and acted as our *de facto* editorial assistant.

Contents

Chapter 1

How to use this book

There is a growing literature on economic evaluation in health care. Studies have been conducted by economists, medical researchers, clinicians, and multidisciplinary teams containing one or more of these parties. The studies go under a confusing range of labels, such as *cost-effectiveness analysis (CEA), cost–benefit analysis (CBA)*, and *cost–utility analysis (CUA)*. They also vary greatly in quality, as methodological critiques have shown (Drummond *et al.* 1986; Adams *et al.* 1992; Gerard 1992; Udvarhelyi *et al.* 1992; Donaldson and Shackley 1997; Neumann *et al.* 2005).

Several good introductions to economic evaluation in health care already exist (Weinstein 1981; Warner and Luce 1982; Luce and Elixhauser 1990; Kamlet 1992; Gold *et al.* 1996; Neumann 2005). All of these give the reader a basic appreciation of the nature of economic evaluation and its relevance to health care decision-making at all levels. This book is intended as a supplement to, and not a replacement for, such texts. It aims to take readers past the stage of general appreciation of the methodological steps involved, and towards preparing them for some *hands-on* experience in undertaking an evaluation, perhaps as part of a multidisciplinary team including economists, epidemiologists, and clinicians. We do not claim that we provide a comprehensive methodological 'cookbook', nor that after reading this book the uninitiated could work without support. Rather, we seek to provide a well-equipped 'tool kit' which, based on our own experience of undertaking economic evaluations, we believe will result in the reader being better prepared to meet most situations.

The next two chapters are concerned with equipping the reader to appraise the quality of the existing literature, an important precursor to one's own study. In Chapter 2, we establish a baseline by discussing the kinds of questions economic evaluations seek to answer, and the basic forms of evaluation. Then in Chapter 3, we present a check-list of questions to ask about any economic evaluation published in the literature. As well as providing a method of systematically appraising the quality of existing evidence, this chapter sets out, in an organized manner, the main methodological issues that would need to be resolved by anyone undertaking an economic evaluation in the health care field.

In Chapters 3, 5, and 6, this critical appraisal exercise is applied to published papers. It should be emphasized that it is not our intent to present the critical appraisals as our own expert assessment of the authors of published studies, nor to counsel perfection. Rather, these studies have been chosen because they demonstrate the complexity of economic evaluation and are generally extremely well-done pieces. (In including critical appraisals of some of our own work we have also demonstrated a willingness to swallow some of our own medicine!) There are a number of potential ways of

Table 1.1 Measurement of costs and consequences in economic evaluation

Type of study	Measurement/ valuation of costs in both alternatives	Identification of consequences	Measurement/ valuation of consequences
Cost analysis	Monetary units	None	None
Cost-effectiveness analysis	Monetary units	Single effect of interest, common to both alternatives, but achieved to different degrees	Natural units (e.g. life-years gained, disability-days saved, points of blood pressure reduction, etc.)
Cost–utility analysis	Monetary units	Single or multiple effects, not necessarily common to both alternatives	Healthy years (typically measured as quality-adjusted life-years)
Cost–benefit analysis	Monetary units	Single or multiple effects, not necessarily common to both alternatives	Monetary units

using the critical appraisal exercises, including self-study while reading this book, or as the basis for critical appraisal workshops for health care professionals (Chambers *et al.* 1983). The original articles are not reproduced here for copyright reasons. They should be easily accessible to the reader, however.

The remainder of the book gives exercises or examples dealing with the main methodological issues raised by the various forms of economic evaluation. In all forms the general approach is to compare the consequences of health care programmes with their costs. For purposes of exposition it is considered that there are four main forms of economic evaluation, each dealing with costs but differing in the way that the consequences of health care programmes are measured and valued (see Table 1.1).

The first form considered, *cost analysis*, is discussed in Chapter 4 and deals only with costs. Therefore this represents a partial form of economic appraisal, unless it can be independently shown that the consequences of the programmes or treatments being considered are broadly equivalent.

Chapter 5 examines *CEA*. In this form of economic evaluation the consequences of programmes are measured in the most appropriate natural effects or physical units, such as 'years of life gained' or 'cases correctly diagnosed'. No attempt is made to *value* the consequences, so implicitly it is assumed that the output concerned is in some sense 'worth having'. (It should be pointed out, however, that in estimating the costs of obtaining different amounts of the output in question, many cost-effectiveness studies do begin to raise this broader question.)

In its classical form, CEA considers a single measure of output, such as life-years gained. The results of studies are expressed in the form of a cost-effectiveness ratio (for example, $10 000 per life-year gained). However, some CEAs may present an array of output measures alongside cost and leave it to decision-makers to form their own view of the relative importance of these. Some analysts have used the term *cost–consequences analysis* for this variant of CEA (Canadian Coordinating Centre for Health Technology Assessment (CCOHTA) 1997; Mauskopf *et al.* 1998). The presentation of an array of output measures is a useful approach, even if the analyst then goes on to *value* the outcomes relative to one another (as discussed below).

Cost–utility analysis is discussed in Chapter 6. In this form of economic evaluation the consequences of programmes are adjusted by health state preference scores or *utility* weights; that is, states of health associated with the outcomes are valued relative to one another. In general terms this means that one can assess the quality of (for example) life-years gained, not just the crude number of years. This approach is particularly useful for those health treatments or programmes that extend life only at the expense of side-effects (for example, antihypertensive drug therapy or chemotherapy for certain types of cancer) or produce reductions in morbidity rather than mortality. The most common measure of consequences in CUAs is the quality-adjusted life-year (QALY).

Cost–utility analysis is therefore a broader form of analysis than CEA, but is a variant of that general approach. Some authors (Gold *et al.* 1996) prefer not to make a distinction between CEA and CUA, because they are so similar. We retain the two labels here for pedagogic reasons, because CUA involves additional analytic procedures that we discuss in Chapter 6. In particular, it incorporates *valuation* of the outcomes obtained.

Chapter 7 deals with *cost–benefit analysis*. In this form of economic evaluation attempts are made to value the consequences of programmes in money terms, so as to make them commensurate with the costs. Therefore, potentially this is the broadest form of analysis, where one can ascertain whether the beneficial consequences of a programme justify the costs. However, as will be seen, measurement problems often mean that the range of benefits valued in money terms is fairly limited. Thus, whilst in theory it is a broad form of evaluation, in practice many of the cost–benefit analyses published to date are more restricted than cost–utility or cost-effectiveness analyses and are limited to a comparison of those costs and consequences that can easily be expressed in money terms. This problem is being addressed by the developments in valuing the benefits of health care programmes in terms of individuals' willingness-to-pay, as discussed in Chapter 7.

An increasing number of studies in the literature calculate the *net benefit* of health care programmes by assuming a threshold value of the decision-maker's willingness-to-pay for a life-year or QALY (Phelps and Mushlin 1991; Stinnett and Mullahy 1998). However, these studies are not cost–benefit analyses, as all the consequences are not being valued. Rather, the assumed threshold value is being used to transform the cost-effectiveness ratio to a measure (net benefit) that has several analytic advantages. This approach is discussed further in Chapter 5.

It should be stressed that these clear distinctions among forms of analyses are made purely for pedagogic reasons. In real life the distinctions are often blurred, as evidenced by many of the examples we shall discuss. Certainly it is not always possible for analysts at the beginning of a study, to be clear on the most appropriate form of analysis to use. Sometimes they may decide to use more than one form. However, the main advantage of subdividing the material in this way is that in each chapter further methodological issues can be introduced in a logical, cumulative manner. Of course most, if not all, of the issues dealt with under cost analysis are also relevant to the other forms of economic evaluation discussed. The same applies to many of the issues first raised under CEA. Therefore *Chapters 4–7 are not free standing* and should not be read on that basis.

Chapters 8 and 9 discuss the two main approaches for data collection and analysis in economic evaluations. In Chapter 8 the collection and analysis of patient-level data are discussed. Such data would typically be collected alongside clinical trials and enable statistical analyses to be conducted. Chapter 9 discusses modelling studies, where data are drawn from a number of sources, including clinical trials, and synthesized by way of a decision analytic model.

Chapters 10 and 11 discuss various practical aspects of undertaking and using economic evaluations. Chapter 10 discusses the presentation and use of economic evaluation results, including issues surrounding the generalizability of findings and the interpretation of cost-effectiveness league tables. Chapter 11 concludes the book with some thoughts on how to take matters further. It contains some hints on issues to clarify before undertaking an economic evaluation (our 'survival guide') and some further sources on the more thorny methodological issues.

References

Adams, M. E., McCall, N. T., Gray, D. T., *et al.* (1992). Economic analysis in randomized control trials. *Medical Care*, **30**, 231–43.

Canadian Coordinating Centre for Health Technology Assessment (CCOHTA) (1997). *Guidelines for economic evaluation of pharmaceuticals: Canada.* CCOHTA, Ottawa.

Chambers, L. W., Stoddart, G. L., and Sullivan, B., (1983). Continuing education for health professionals and administrators: workshops on becoming a critical user of health care research. *Canadian Journal of Public Health*, **74**, 29–34.

Donaldson, C. and Shackley, P. (1997). Economic evaluation. In: *Oxford textbook of public health (third edition) Volume 2: the methods of public health* (ed. R. Detels, W. W. Holland, J. McEwen, and G. S. Omenn), pp. 949–71. Oxford University Press, Oxford.

Drummond, M. F., Ludbrook, A., Lowson, K. V., and Steele, A. (1986). *Studies in economic appraisal in health care (Volume 2).* Oxford University Press, Oxford.

Gerard, K. (1992). Cost–utility in practice: a policy maker's guide to the state of the art. *Health Policy*, **21**, 249–79.

Gold, M. R., Siegel, J. E., Russell, L. B., and Weinstein, M. C. (ed.) (1996). *Cost-effectiveness in health and medicine.* Oxford University Press, New York.

Kamlet, M. S. (1992). *The comparative benefits modeling project: a framework for cost–utility analysis of government health care programs.* US Department of Health and Human Services, Public Health Service, Washington DC.

Luce, B. and Elixhauser, A. (1990). *Standards for socioeconomic evaluation of health care products and services.* Springer, Berlin/Heidelberg.

Mauskopf, J. A., Paul, J. E., Grant, D. M., and Stergachis, A. (1998). The role of cost–consequence analysis in healthcare decision-making. *PharmacoEconomics*, **13**, 277–88.

Neumann, P. J. (2005). *Using cost-effectiveness analysis in health care.* Oxford University Press, New York.

Neumann, P. J., Greenberg, D., Olchanski, N. V., Stone, P. W., and Rosen, A. B. (2005). Growth and quality of the cost-utility literature, 1976–2001. *Value in Health*, **8(1)**, 3–9.

Phelps, C. E. and Mushlin, A. (1991). On the (near) equivalence of cost-effectiveness and cost–benefit analyses. *International Journal of Technology Assessment in Health Care*, 7, 12–21.

Stinnett, A. A. and Mullahy, J. (1998). Net health benefits: a new framework for the analysis of uncertainty in cost-effectiveness analysis. *Medical Decision Making*, **16**, 288–99.

Udvarhelyi, I. S., Colditz, G. A., Rai, A., and Epstein, A. M. (1992). Cost-effectiveness and cost–benefit analyses in the medical literature. Are methods being used correctly? *Annals of Internal Medicine*, **116**, 238–44.

Warner, K. E. and Luce, B. R. (1982). *Cost–benefit and cost-effectiveness in health care: principles, practice and potential*. Health Administration Press, Ann Arbor, Michigan.

Weinstein, M. C. (1981). Economic assessment of medical practices and technologies. *Medical Decision Making*, **1**, 309–30.

Chapter 2

Basic types of economic evaluation

Those who plan, provide, receive, or pay for health services face an incessant barrage of questions such as the following.

1 Should clinicians check the blood pressure of each adult who walks into their offices?

2 Should planners launch a scoliosis screening programme in secondary schools?

3 Should individuals be encouraged to request annual check-ups?

4 Should local health departments free scarce nursing personnel from well-baby clinics so that they can carry out home visits on lapsed hypertensives?

5 Should hospital administrators purchase each and every piece of new diagnostic equipment?

6 Should a new, expensive drug be listed on the formulary?

These are examples of general, recurring questions about who should do what to whom, with what health care resources, and with what relation to other health services.

The answers to these questions are most strongly influenced by our estimates of the relative merit or value of the alternative courses of action they pose. This book is concerned with the strategies and tactics whereby these estimates of relative value can be ascertained and interpreted; that is, with the evaluation of health services.

More specifically, the book focuses on one type of evaluation, sometimes referred to as *economic evaluation* or *efficiency evaluation* (the two terms are synonymous for our purposes). In this type of evaluation we are asking the following questions.

1 Is this health procedure, service, or programme worth doing compared with other things we could do with these same resources?

2 Are we satisfied that the health care resources (required to make the procedure, service, or programme available to those who could benefit from it) should be spent in this way rather than some other way?

It is imperative to note that although economic evaluation provides important information to decision-makers, it addresses only one dimension of health care programme decisions. Economic evaluation is most useful and appropriate when preceded by three other types of evaluation, each of which addresses a different question.

1 Can it work? Does the health procedure, service, or programme do more good than harm to people who fully comply with the associated recommendations or treatments? This type of evaluation is concerned with *efficacy*.

2 Does it work? Does the procedure, service, or programme do more good than harm to those people to whom it is offered? This form of health care evaluation, which considers both the efficacy of a service and its acceptance by those to whom it is offered, is the evaluation of *effectiveness* or usefulness.

3 Is it reaching those who need it? Is the procedure, service, or programme accessible to all people who could benefit from it? Evaluation of this type is concerned with *availability*.

Methodological criteria for assessing efficacy, effectiveness, and availability evaluations have been described elsewhere by Sackett (1980), from which the above questions have been drawn. These criteria will not be reviewed here. Those wishing to know more should consult Stevens *et al.* (2001) and Guyatt and Rennie (2002).

2.1. **Why is economic evaluation important?**

To put it simply, resources—people, time, facilities, equipment, and knowledge—are scarce. Choices must and will be made concerning their deployment, and methods such as 'what we did last time', 'gut feelings', and even 'educated guesses' are rarely better than organized consideration of the factors involved in a decision to commit resources to one use instead of another. This is true for at least three reasons.

1. *Without systematic analysis, it is difficult to identify clearly the relevant alternatives.* For example, in deciding to introduce a new programme (rehabilitation in a special centre for chronic lung disease), all too often little or no effort is made to describe existing activities (episodic care by family physicians in their offices) as an alternative 'programme' to which the new proposal must be compared. Furthermore, if the objective is, indeed, to reduce morbidity due to chronic lung disease then preventive programmes (for example, cessation of cigarette smoking) may represent a more efficient avenue and should be added to the set of programmes competing in the evaluation. Of course, in practice the range of alternative programmes compared may be restricted to those being compared in a given clinical study, or those that are the responsibility of a particular decision-maker (for example, a given decision-maker may be responsible for cancer treatment, but not cancer prevention). Also, if a new programme is compared to 'existing care', it is important to consider whether existing care is itself cost-effective. Current practice may itself be inefficient if there is an alternative, lower cost, programme that is just as effective. Although it is not possible to consider all conceivable alternatives in a given study, an important contribution of economic evaluation is to minimize the chances of an important alternative being excluded from consideration, or a new programme being compared to an inefficient baseline.

2. *The viewpoint assumed in an analysis is important.* A programme that looks unattractive from one viewpoint may look significantly better when other

viewpoints are considered. Analytic viewpoints may include any or all of the following: the individual patient, the specific institution, the target group for specific services, the Ministry of Health budget, the government's overall budget position (Ministry of Health plus other ministries), and the community or societal viewpoint.

3. *Without some attempt at measurement, the uncertainty surrounding orders of magnitude can be critical.* For example, when the American Cancer Society endorsed a protocol of six sequential stool tests for cancer of the large bowel, most analysts would have predicted that the extra cost per case detected would increase markedly with each test. But would they have guessed that it would reach $47 million for the sixth test, as Neuhauser and Lewicki (1975) have demonstrated? Admittedly, while this is an extreme example, it illustrates that without measurement and comparison of outputs and inputs we have little upon which to base any judgement about value for money. In fact, the real cost of any programme is not the number of dollars appearing on the programme budget, but rather the value of the benefits achievable in some other programme that has been forgone by committing the resources in question to the first programme. It is this 'opportunity cost' that economic evaluation seeks to estimate and to compare with programme benefits.

2.2. **What does economic evaluation mean?**

Two features characterize economic analysis, regardless of the activities (including health services) to which it is applied.

First, it deals with both the inputs and outputs, sometimes called *costs* and *consequences*, of activities. Few of us would be prepared to pay a specific price for a package whose contents were unknown. Conversely, few of us would accept a package, even if its contents were known and desired, until we knew the specific price being asked. In both cases, it is the linkage of costs and consequences that allows us to reach our decision.

Second, economic analysis concerns itself with choices. Resource scarcity, and our consequent inability to produce all desired outputs (even efficacious therapies!), necessitates that choices must, and will, be made in all areas of human activity. These choices are made on the basis of many criteria, sometimes explicit but often implicit. Economic analysis seeks to identify and to make explicit one set of criteria that may be useful in deciding among different uses for scarce resources.

These two characteristics of economic analysis lead us to define economic evaluation as *the comparative analysis of alternative courses of action in terms of both their costs and consequences.* Therefore, the basic tasks of any economic evaluation are to identify, measure, value, and compare the costs and consequences of the alternatives being considered. These tasks characterize all economic evaluations, including those concerned with health services (see Box 2.1).

In fact, these two characteristics of economic analysis may be employed to distinguish and label several evaluation situations commonly encountered in the health care evaluation literature. In Table 2.1, the answers to two questions—(1) Is

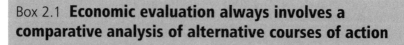

Box 2.1 **Economic evaluation always involves a comparative analysis of alternative courses of action**

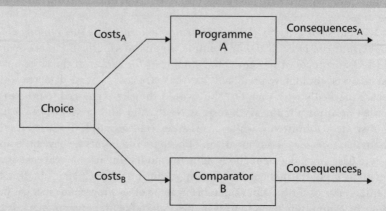

The diagram illustrates that an economic evaluation is usually formulated in terms of a choice between competing alternatives. Here we consider a choice between two alternatives, A and B. The comparator to Programme A, the programme of interest, does not have to be an active treatment. It could be doing nothing. Even when two active treatments are being compared, it may still be important to consider the baseline of doing nothing, or a low-cost option. This is because the comparator (Programme B) may itself be inefficient. (As mentioned earlier, it is important that the evaluation considers all relevant alternatives.)

The precise nature of the costs and consequences to be considered, and how they might be measured and valued, will be discussed in Section 2.4 below. However, the general rule when assessing programmes A and B is that the *difference* in costs is compared with the *difference* in consequences, in an incremental analysis.

there comparison of two or more alternatives? and (2) Are both costs (inputs) and consequences (outputs) of the alternatives examined?—define a six-cell matrix for evaluation situations.

In cells 1A, 1B, and 2 there is no comparison of alternatives (that is, a single service or programme is being evaluated). To put it more accurately, the service or programme is being *described*, because evaluation requires comparison. In cell 1A, only the consequences of the service or programme are examined, and thus the evaluation is labelled an *outcome description*. In cell 1B, because only costs are examined, it is called a *cost description*. The large literature on *cost of illness*, or *burden of illness*, falls into this category. These studies describe the cost of disease to society, but are not full economic evaluations because alternatives are not compared (Drummond 1992).

In cell 2, both outcomes and costs of a single service or programme are described and thus the evaluation is termed a *cost-outcome description*.

Table 2.1 Distinguishing characteristics of health care evaluation

Are both costs (inputs) and consequences (outputs) of the alternatives examined?

		No		Yes
		Examines only consequences	Examines only costs	
Is there comparison of two or more alternatives?	**No**	1A Partial evaluation 1B Outcome description	Cost description	2 Partial evaluation Cost-outcome description
	Yes	3A Partial evaluation 3B Efficacy or effectiveness evaluation	Cost analysis	4 Full economic evaluation Cost–effectiveness analysis Cost–utility analysis Cost–benefit analysis

An example of this type of study is that by Reynell and Reynell (1972) on coronary care units. They presented data on the costs of one such unit and gave an estimate of the likely number of lives saved. However, there was no explicit attempt to compare the costs and consequences of the coronary care unit with an alternative, or the *status quo*. Reynell and Reynell describe their study as 'cost–benefit analysis (CBA)'. As regular users of economic evaluation results may have recognized, and readers of this book will likely discover, the titles of published economic evaluations are not always accurate indicators of the type of evaluation actually performed!

Cells 3A and 3B contain evaluation situations in which two or more alternatives are compared, but in which the costs and consequences of each alternative are not examined simultaneously. In cell 3A, only the consequences of the alternatives are compared and thus we term these *efficacy* or *effectiveness evaluations*. This, of course, is the cell into which the large and important literature containing most randomized clinical trials falls. In cell 3B, only the costs of the alternatives are examined. In such situations the studies performed may be called *cost analyses*. An example of such a study is that by Lowson *et al.* (1981) on the comparative costs of three methods of providing long-term oxygen therapy in the home: oxygen cylinders, liquid oxygen, and the oxygen concentrator (a machine that extracts oxygen from air). The authors argued that a cost analysis was sufficient as the relative effectiveness of the three methods was not a contentious issue.

Note that none of the above-mentioned cells entirely fulfils both of the conditions for economic evaluation. For this reason they have all been designated *partial evaluations*. This does not imply that studies with these characteristics are unimportant, for they may represent important intermediate stages in our understanding of the costs and consequences of health services or programmes. However, the label *partial evaluation* does indicate that they will not allow us to answer efficiency questions. For this we need studies employing the techniques listed in cell 4 under *full economic evaluation*. We now turn to a consideration of these three techniques.

2.3. **Do all economic evaluations use the same techniques?**

The identification of various types of costs and their subsequent measurement in monetary units is similar across most economic evaluations; however, the nature of the consequences stemming from the alternatives being examined may differ considerably. Let us consider three examples to illustrate how the nature of consequences affects their measurement, valuation, and comparison to costs.

2.3.1. **Example 1: cost-effectiveness analysis**

Suppose that our interest is the prolongation of life after renal failure and that we are comparing the costs and consequences of hospital dialysis with kidney transplantation. In this case the outcome of interest—life-years gained—is common to both programmes; however, the programmes may have differential success in achieving this outcome, as well as differential costs. Consequently we would not automatically lean toward the least-cost programme unless, of course, it also resulted in a greater prolongation of life. In comparing these alternatives we would normally calculate this prolongation and compare cost per unit of effect (that is, cost per life-year gained). Such analyses, in which costs are related to a single, common effect that may differ in magnitude between the alternative programmes, are usually referred to as *cost-effectiveness analyses (CEAs)*. Note that the results of such comparisons may be stated either in terms of cost per unit of effect, as in this example, or in terms of effects per unit of cost (life-years gained per dollar spent). The latter is a particularly useful approach when working within a given budget constraint, as long as the alternatives under consideration are not of radically different scale (Donaldson and Shackley 1997*a*).

It is sometimes argued that if the two or more alternatives under consideration achieve the given outcome to the same extent, a *cost-minimization analysis* (CMA) can be performed. However, it is not appropriate to view CMA as a form of full economic evaluation (see Box 2.2).

Although the alternatives used in our example are similar in that both could be considered variants of an overall renal programme, it should be noted that CEA can be performed on any alternatives that have a common effect. Thus kidney transplantation could be compared to heart surgery (or even mandatory bicycle helmet legislation!) if the common effect of interest is life-years saved and these are independent programmes (that is, the costs and health effects in one patient group are not affected by the treatment alternative in any other patient group) (Tengs *et al.* 1995). Similarly, an influenza immunization programme could be compared to a home care programme (or even a community safety education programme!) if a common effect of interest, perhaps disability days avoided, could be identified.

There are many examples of CEA in the literature. Ludbrook (1981) provided an estimate of the cost-effectiveness of treatment options for chronic renal failure. In addition, a number of studies compare the cost-effectiveness of actions that do not produce health effects directly, but that achieve other clinical objectives that can be clearly linked to improvements in patient outcome. For example, Hull *et al.* (1981)

Box 2.2 **The death of cost-minimization analysis?**

Economic evaluations are sometimes referred to in the literature as *cost-minimization analyses (CMAs)*. Typically this is used to describe the situation where the consequences of two or more treatments or programmes are broadly equivalent, so the difference between them reduces to a comparison of costs.

It can be seen from the diagram that there are nine possible outcomes when one therapy is being compared with another. In two of the cases (boxes 4 and 6) it might be argued that the choice between the treatment and control depends on cost because the effectiveness of the two therapies is the same.

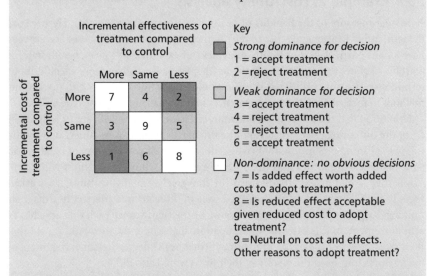

Incremental effectiveness of treatment compared to control

	More	Same	Less
More	7	4	2
Same	3	9	5
Less	1	6	8

Incremental cost of treatment compared to control

Key

Strong dominance for decision
1 = accept treatment
2 = reject treatment

Weak dominance for decision
3 = accept treatment
4 = reject treatment
5 = reject treatment
6 = accept treatment

Non-dominance: no obvious decisions
7 = Is added effect worth added cost to adopt treatment?
8 = Is reduced effect acceptable given reduced cost to adopt treatment?
9 = Neutral on cost and effects. Other reasons to adopt treatment?

However, Briggs and O'Brien (2001) point out that, because of the uncertainty around the estimates of costs and effects, the results of a given study rarely fit neatly into one of the nine squares shown in the diagram. Also, because of this uncertainty, CMA is not a unique study design that can be determined in advance.

The only possible application of CMA is in situations where a prior view has been taken, based on previous research or professional opinion, that the two options are equivalent in terms of effectiveness. However, here one might question the basis on which this view has been formed. It is likely only to be justifiable in situations where the two therapies embody a near-identical technology (for example, drugs of the same pharmacologic class).

compared diagnostic strategies for deep vein thrombosis in terms of the cost per case detected. Similarly, Logan *et al.* (1981) compared work-site and regular (physician office) care for hypertensives in terms of the cost per mm Hg drop in diastolic blood pressure obtained. Sculpher and Buxton (1993) compared treatments for asthma in terms of the cost per episode-free day.

Cost-effectiveness analysis is of most use in situations where a decision-maker, operating with a given budget, is considering a limited range of options within a given field. For example, a person with the responsibility for managing a hypertension treatment programme may consider blood pressure reduction to be a relevant outcome; a person managing a cancer screening programme may be interested in cases detected. However, even in these situations these outcomes may be insufficient. For example, the benefits from detecting a cancer will depend on the type of cancer and the stage of its development. Similarly, the benefits from reducing blood pressure by a given amount will depend on the patient's pre-treatment level.

2.3.2. Example 2: cost–utility analysis

A broader measure of the benefits of health care programmes is *utility*. Here we use the term utility in a general sense to refer to the preferences individuals or society may have for any particular set of health outcomes (for example, for a given health state, or a profile of states through time). Later, in Chapter 6, we shall be more specific about terminology, because utility has specific connotations in economics and the various methods to measure health state preferences may or may not estimate true utilities.

The notion that the utility of an outcome, effect, or level of health status is different from the outcome, effect, or level of health status itself can be illustrated by the following example. Suppose that twins, identical in all respects except occupation (one being a sign painter and the other a translator), both broke their right arm. While they would be equally disabled (or conversely, equally healthy), if we asked them to rank 'having a broken arm' on a scale of 0 (dead) to 1 (perfect health) their rankings might differ considerably because of the significance each one attaches to arm movement, in this case due to occupation. Consequently, we would expect that their assessments of the utility of treatment (that is, the degree to which treatment of the fractures improved the quality of their lives) would also differ.

Utility analysis is viewed as a particularly useful technique because it allows for health-related *quality of life* adjustments to a given set of treatment outcomes, while simultaneously providing a generic outcome measure for comparison of costs and outcomes in different programmes. The generic outcome, usually expressed as *quality-adjusted life-years (QALYs)*, is arrived at in each case by adjusting the length of time affected through the health outcome by the utility value (on a scale of 0 to 1) of the resulting level of health status (see Box 2.3). Other generic outcome measures, such as the *healthy years equivalent (HYE)* (Mehrez and Gafni 1989), the *disability-adjusted life-year (DALY)* (Tan-Torres Edejer *et al.* 2003), and the *saved-young-life equivalent* (Nord 1995), have been proposed as alternatives to the QALY. These are discussed further in Chapter 6.

Analyses that employ utilities as a measure of the value of programme effects are termed *cost–utility analyses (CUAs)*. The results of CUAs are typically expressed in terms of the cost per healthy year or cost per quality-adjusted life-year gained by undertaking one programme instead of another. Examples of CUAs include the study by Boyle *et al.* (1983) on neonatal intensive care for very-low-birth-weight infants, that by Oldridge *et al.* (1993) on a formal post-myocardial infarction rehabilitation programme, and that by Torrance *et al.* (2001) on the incorporation of a viscosupplementation product into the treatment of knee osteoarthritis.

Box 2.3 **QALYs gained from an intervention**

In the conventional approach to QALYs the quality-adjustment weight for each health state is multiplied by the time in the state (which may be discounted, as discussed in Chapter 5) and then summed to calculate the number of quality-adjusted life-years. The advantage of the QALY as a measure of health output is that it can simultaneously capture gains from reduced morbidity (quality gains) and reduced mortality (quantity gains), and integrate these into a single measure. A simple example is displayed in the figure below, in which outcomes are assumed to occur with certainty. Without the health intervention an individual's health-related quality of life would deteriorate according to the lower curve and the individual would die at time Death 1. With the health intervention the individual would deteriorate more slowly, live longer, and die at time Death 2. The area between the two curves is the number of QALYs gained by the intervention. For instruction purposes the area can be divided into two parts, A and B, as shown. Then part A is the amount of QALY gained due to quality improvements (that is, the quality gain during time that the person would have otherwise been alive anyhow), and part B is the amount of QALY gained due to quantity improvements (that is, the amount of life extension, but adjusted by the quality of that life extension).

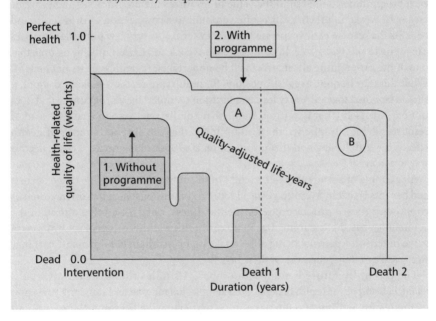

2.3.3. **Example 3: cost–benefit analysis**

Both CEAs and CUAs are techniques that relate to constrained maximization; that is, where a decision-maker is considering how best to allocate an existing budget. In this situation a decision to expand one programme, to increase the number of cancers detected or to increase the QALYs gained, has an opportunity cost in terms of benefits forgone in other programmes covered by the budget. However, what if we want to consider whether it is worthwhile expanding the budget?

In these situations, ideally we require a common denominator to facilitate comparison of outcomes; analysts frequently attempt to go beyond consideration of the specific effects themselves and to attach a generic measure of value to the set of effects resulting from a particular service or programme. The broadest measure of value is money, and the consequences of a service or programme could be expressed in terms of their monetary benefits in order to facilitate comparison to programme costs. This, of course, requires us to translate effects such as disability days avoided, life-years gained, medical complications avoided, or QALYs gained, into their monetary benefit. This is not always an easy task, but depending on the type of effect, it is sometimes both appropriate and feasible to attempt it. Analyses that measure both the costs and consequences of alternatives in monetary units are called *cost–benefit analyses*. The results of such analyses might be stated either in the form of a ratio of costs to benefits, or as a simple sum (possibly negative) representing the net benefit (loss) of one programme over another.

It is perhaps worth noting that (at least in theory) CBA provides information on the *absolute* benefit of programmes, in addition to information on their relative performance. That is, CBA provides an estimate of the value of resources used up by each programme compared to the value of resources the programme might save or create. However, in practice CBAs often amount to a comparison of those costs and benefits that can be easily expressed in money terms, so very few published analyses can aspire to this wider role. In contrast to CBA, CEA and CUA implicitly assume that one of the programme alternatives will be undertaken regardless of its net benefit. While this may be quite a realistic position for health care decision-makers to adopt, it should be noted that CEA may lead to a decision to undertake a programme that does not pay for itself (that is, a programme that entails a net resource cost instead of resource saving). Implicitly, the assumption is that the output, in terms of health effects, is worth having and the only question is to determine the most cost-effective way to achieve it. *Best value for lowest cost, it is a foregone conclusion that one action will be ...*

An example of a study that did attempt to quantify and value a wide range of costs and benefits is that by Weisbrod *et al.* (1980) on conventional hospital-oriented versus community-based programmes for mental illness. They found that although the community-based programme was more costly, this was more than offset by its extra value in terms of patients being able to take up or maintain employment (earnings were used as a dollar measure of these benefits).

The recent literature contains a number of studies that assess individuals' *willingness-to-pay* for health benefits. For example, Johanneson and Jönsson (1991) give estimates for willingness-to-pay for antihypertensive therapy, Neumann and Johanneson (1994) give them for *in vitro* fertilization, and O'Brien *et al.* (1995) give them for a new antidepressant. A comprehensive CBA of health care interventions would use this approach to value the health benefits. Paradoxically, although there has been considerable progress in willingness-to-pay methodology in recent years, very few CBAs incorporating these estimates have so far been published. See O'Byrne *et al.* (1996) for one example of such a study in the field of asthma.

In commenting on the different characteristics of the main types of economic evaluation, three further points warrant emphasis. First, the main purpose of classifying study types is to illustrate the different analytic characteristics of completed studies, not to prescribe a particular study type in advance. Often at the beginning of a study the analyst may not be able to predict what form the final analysis might take, as this may depend on the results of an associated clinical evaluation or the availability of other data. Second, the different approaches are sometimes used together to tackle a particularly thorny problem—Boyle *et al.* (1983) used all three of CEA, CUA, and CBA in their evaluation of neonatal intensive care, because each explores a different dimension of value. Third, in situations where the decision-maker clearly articulates their objectives, this will be the main driving force behind the choice of form of evaluation.

2.4. **What are the relevant costs and consequences in the economic evaluation of health care programmes?**

It was shown above that the different forms of economic evaluation measure and value the various costs and consequences to different extents. Which is the most appropriate form of analysis? The answer to this question depends not only on the problem being tackled, but also the institutional framework, the practical measurement challenges, and the perspective the analyst takes on the role of economic evaluation.

Box 2.4 contains a hypothetical debate among three analysts. This illustrates that there is more than one perspective on the role of economic evaluation in health care, each having its underlying rationale. For example, Analyst A has a strong theoretical perspective. Welfare economics, the branch of economics underpinning economic evaluation, places considerable emphasis on the values individuals place on outcomes, because individuals are considered to be the best judges of their own welfare (that is, a '*welfarist*' perspective). (We discuss this in more detail in Chapter 7.) Analyst B adopts a health sector budget perspective, which may be close to that adopted by many health care decision-makers (in the literature this is often referred to as an '*extrawelfarist*' perspective (Culyer 1989). Analyst C is clearly a pragmatist, but the pragmatism may be at the expense of having a clear underlying theory for this approach to economic evaluation (in the literature this has been referred to as the *decision-making* approach (Sugden and Williams 1979). Indeed, some economists feel that the term 'economic evaluation' ought to be reserved only for evaluations whose methods are consistent with the underlying principles of welfare economics (Birch and Gafni 1996). However, most economists use the term more broadly, to encompass all studies undertaking a systematic assessment of costs and consequences. (We return to this issue in Chapters 7 and 10.)

Because of these perspectives on economic evaluation, it is useful to view the various costs and consequences of health care programmes as building blocks that can be assembled in the evaluation in different ways. Figure 2.1 is an expansion of the diagram given in Box 2.1. Again we consider the costs and consequences of a health care programme (which is always evaluated in comparison with another programme,

Box 2.4 **The role of economic evaluation in health care: a conversation among three analysts**

Analyst A

I think the best way to undertake an economic evaluation is to ascertain the total amount that individuals would be willing to pay for the programme. This amount can then be directly compared with the costs in order to assess whether the programme is worthwhile. My approach is consistent with economic theory, and economic evaluation gives us the result we would have obtained from the market, had one been operating. (This is often referred to as the '*welfarist*' approach.)

Analyst B

In my mind the purpose of economic evaluation is to help us allocate the health care budget. Therefore, we should consider health care resources only and compare the resources consumed with the health improvement obtained. We might measure health improvements in natural units, or health effects, but health state preference scores would be better because this would allow us to make broader comparisons among programmes. I do not like willingness-to-pay valuations because these may be conditioned by individuals' ability to pay and may also reflect the non-health attributes of programmes, which I do not believe should be funded as part of the health care budget. (This is often referred to as the '*extrawelfarist*' approach.)

Analyst C

I think we should take a broad societal perspective, but some of the costs and consequences are easier to express in monetary terms than others. Also, like Analyst B, I am worried that willingness-to-pay valuations may reflect the prevailing income distribution, and in many countries ability to pay has been explicitly rejected as a method of allocating health care resources. Therefore, I think we should measure and value a wide range of costs and consequences and present them in a way that helps health care decision-makers form a better judgement. (This is often referred to as the '*decision-maker*' approach.)

or the *status quo*). However, here we give a more detailed breakdown of the costs and consequences and show, through the use of formulae, the possible alternative approaches to economic evaluation.

In Fig. 2.1 the resources consumed by the programme are considered to comprise four components. In each case their quantities (q) would be measured and the total cost calculated by multiplying the quantities by the relevant prices (p). The resource consumption in the health care sector is relatively straightforward and would consist of items such as drugs, equipment, hospitalization, physician visits, and so on. However, note that these include not only the costs of providing the initial programme

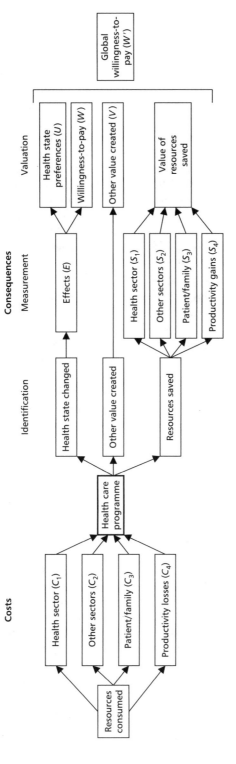

Fig. 2.1 Components of economic evaluation in health care.

(for example, a kidney transplant) but also all the continuing care costs (for example, immunosuppressive drugs, treatment of infections, and so on).

The resources consumed in other sectors are likely to depend on the nature of the health care programme being evaluated. For example, some programmes, such as those for the elderly or mentally ill, consume resources from other public agencies (for example, homemaker services or nursing home care). Also, many health care programmes rely on resource inputs from the voluntary sector.

The patient and family resources could consist of out-of-pocket expenses in travelling to hospital, various co-payments, and expenditure in the home (for example, adapting a room to accommodate a home dialysis machine). However, one of the most important patient and family resources consumed in treatment is *time*. This could be time of the patient in seeking and receiving care, or it could be the time of family members in providing informal nursing support at home. The time could either be from leisure activities or worktime, which would affect its valuation. (We discuss this further in Chapters 3 and 4.) To the extent to which treatments use up the worktime of the patient or family members, there may be associated productivity costs. The role of productivity costs in economic evaluation, and their estimation, have been debated widely. This is discussed further in Chapter 4.

Turning to the consequences, it can be seen that these consist of three main categories. First, the patient's health state will be changed (hopefully improved). This can be measured in terms of effects (E) (for example, life-years gained or disability days reduced), but also valued, either in terms of health state preferences (U) in a CUA, or in terms of willingness-to-pay (W) in a CBA.

Second, other value (V) can be created by health care programmes, not necessarily linked to the improvement in health state. This could include the value of information or reassurance about one's health. There is currently a debate about whether there is utility or value from the *process* of receiving care, independent of the outcome (Donaldson and Shackley 1997b). Whilst potentially a separate component of the value of health care programmes, V is usually incorporated in the measurement of U or W. (This is discussed further in Chapter 7.)

Third, resources can be saved by health care programmes. These savings (S_1 to S_4) mirror the costs (C_1 to C_4) and are measured and valued in a similar way. In fact, these savings (S_1 to S_4) are the costs (C_1 to C_4) not spent on the alternative programme. Indeed, all the assessments of consequences are comparative to an alternative.

Finally, the global willingness-to-pay (W') for the programme may be ascertained. This valuation could potentially include all the consequences identified in Fig. 2.1, depending on what the respondent(s) to the willingness-to-pay perceived to be important. The interesting feature of this approach, as opposed to the other approaches to valuation mentioned here, is that it could be applied on the population level, rather than on the level of the individual patient. For example, a representative sample of the population could be asked what additional amount they would be willing to pay in higher taxes for a new programme to be added to those already existing in a given country. (We discuss this approach further in Chapter 7 and distinguish among three approaches to willingness-to-pay assessment.)

Table 2.2 Possible formulations of economic evaluation

Cost-effectiveness analysis
$(C_1 - S_1)/E$
$[(C_1 + C_2 + C_3 + C_4) - (S_1 + S_2 + S_3 + S_4)]/E$
Cost–utility analysis
$(C_1 - S_1)/U$
$[(C_1 + C_2 + C_3 + C_4) - (S_1 + S_2 + S_3 + S_4)]/U$
*Cost–benefit analysis**
$(W') - (C_1 + C_2 + C_3 + C_4)$
$[(W + V + S_1 + S_2 + S_3 + S_4) - (C_1 + C_2 + C_3 + C_4)]$

* Cost–benefit analysis results can also be expressed as ratios, although this is not recommended (see Box 2.5). Please note that *E* and *U* represent *changes* in effectiveness or health status, compared to an alternative.

Thus there are a number of possible formulations of economic evaluation depending on the perspective adopted by analysts and the estimation methods they employ (see Table 2.2).

Considering again the three hypothetical analysts in Box 2.4, Analyst A is arguing for a CBA to be undertaken, with the formulation $(W') - (C_1 + C_2 + C_3 + C_4)$. If this approach were followed it would be important to make sure that W' did indeed capture the total value of all the consequences. However, in a country with a publicly financed health care system, individuals asked about their willingness-to-pay may not take account of the health care resource savings (S_1), resource savings in other sectors (S_2), or the productivity gains (S_4). Therefore, the appropriate formulation for the evaluation might be $(W' + S_1 + S_2 + S_4) - (C_1 + C_2 + C_3 + C_4)$, and the estimation procedure for W' would be designed so as to explicitly exclude S_1, S_2, and S_4 in order to avoid double counting.

Analyst B is clearly arguing for either a CEA, with the formulation $(C_1 - S_1)/E$, or a CUA, with the formulation $(C_1 - S_1)/U$. However, these are not the only possible formulations of CEA or CUA. Alternative formulations, assuming a societal viewpoint, would also consider C_2, C_3, C_4, S_2, S_3, and S_4 (see Table 2.2).

Analyst C, our pragmatist, does not appear to be set on a precise formulation for the analysis and might be satisfied by a display of all the costs and consequences, measured in the most appropriate units. (We called this a *cost–consequences analysis* in Chapter 1.) Alternatively, they may be happy with a CEA or CUA including a broad range of resource changes, for example, $(C_1 + C_2 + C_3 + C_4) - (S_1 + S_2 + S_3 + S_4)/U$. One potential problem here would be double counting. That is, the health state preference scores (U) might incorporate individuals' valuations of time savings to themselves or their family (for example, the ability to return to work and earn income). This was the view taken by the US Public Health Service Panel on Cost-Effectiveness in Health and Medicine (Gold *et al.* 1996). Therefore, if such a formulation were to be used, it would be important to ensure that the estimation of U was made so as to exclude the value of savings in patient and family time that is included in S_3 or S_4. The same double-counting problem could arise if willingness-to-pay was used to estimate the value of the change in health state (W) in money terms. Thus, the estimate would either have to be purged of the relevant components of S_3 and S_4, or these should be excluded from the formulation of the evaluation.

The three different analytical perspectives typified by Analysts A–C also imply differing views on the inclusion of the other value created (V). This could be, for example, the value to pregnant mothers of seeing an ultrasound image of their unborn baby (Berwick and Weinstein 1985), or the pleasure of being cared for even if one's health state was not changed. Whether or not these items are viewed as legitimate, or whether or not they are classified as health related, is for debate. However, it is clear that Analyst A would include them in an estimation of the global willingness-to-pay (W'), whereas Analyst B would definitely exclude them.

The purpose of this discussion is to illustrate that it is very difficult to outline one standard form of economic evaluation. First, there are different perspectives on the role of economic evaluation, as illustrated by Analysts A–C. Second, measurement difficulties may compromise any analytic approach. Finally, the institutional context may influence how the various 'building blocks' are assembled. For example, an

---

Box 2.5 **Be wary of ratios**

Suppose a health care programme had costs and consequences as follows:

Costs	*Consequences*
C_1 health care costs $1 000 000	health improvement
C_2 costs in other sectors $50 000	U (in preference scores) 10 QALYs
C_3 patient/family resources $5 000	W (in willingness-to-pay) $2 000 000
C_4 lost productivity $100 000	S_1 health care savings $25 000
	S_2 savings in other sectors $20 000
	S_3 savings in patient/family resources $12 000
	S_4 savings in productivity $100 000
	V (other value created) $0

The following ratios could be calculated:

(i) *Cost–utility ratio (health care resources only)*

$$\frac{(C_1 - S_1)}{U} = \$75\,000 \text{ per QALY}$$

(ii) *Cost–utility ratio (all resource use)*

$$\frac{(C_1 + C_2 + C_3 + C_4 - S_1 - S_2 - S_3 - S_4)}{U} = \$77\,300 \text{ per } QALY$$

(iii) *Benefit–cost ratio (including all consequences in the numerator as benefits)*

$$[(W + S_1 + S_2 + S_3 + S_4)/(C_1 + C_2 + C_3 + C_4)] = 2.163$$

(iv) *Benefit–cost ratio (treating resource savings as cost-offsets deducted from the denominator)*

$$[W/(C_1 + C_2 + C_3 + C_4 - S_1 - S_2 - S_3 - S_4)] = 2.587$$

analyst adopting the position of Analyst A may not attempt to capture all the benefits of the health care programme in the estimation of W' if they are operating in a setting where health care is provided free at the point of use. In such a case the element of value of the programme relating to savings in health care resources may best be handled separately. Therefore, the way in which each individual building block or component is measured may influence the measurement of others and also the way in which the various components are assembled in the analysis (Currie *et al.* 2002).

Two other points should be made about the alternative formulations for economic evaluation given in Fig. 2.1. First, because some of the formulations are presented as ratios, it is worth noting that the size of the ratio depends on what goes into the numerator and denominator respectively (see Box 2.5). Whereas this is not a problem within a particular study, providing the analysts are clear on what they have done, it can be a major problem if the ratios from two or more studies are subsequently compared (Birch and Donaldson 1987). (We return to this in Chapter 10.) This has led some to argue for a standard formulation of the cost-effectiveness ratio, known as a 'reference case' (Gold *et al.* 1996). (We discuss this further in Chapter 3.) Another option would be to assume a threshold value for U, thereby converting the cost-effectiveness ratio into an estimate of net benefit. (This is discussed further in Chapters 5 and 10.)

Second, in describing the various formulations of economic evaluation here, we have avoided using the terms *direct*, *indirect*, and *intangible* costs and benefits. Box 2.6 illustrates how these terms, which are common in the existing literature, relate to the terminology used here.

From the user's point of view the most important consideration is whether the complexity of the analysis matches the breadth of the question posed. Cost–benefit analyses and CUAs, because they address the issue of outcome valuation, enable us to assess broader choices than a simple CEA. Additionally, CBA can shed light on whether the treatments concerned are 'worthwhile' when compared to other uses of the same resources within and outside the health care sector. We would argue that to assess whether or not a particular evaluation has been appropriate to the question originally posed, the user needs to be aware of these analytic distinctions (see Box 2.7).

Second, the usefulness of these analytic techniques should not be overstated. None of the approaches is intended to be a magic formula for removal of judgement, responsibility, or risk from decision-making activities, though each is capable of improving the quality and consistency of decision-making.

At root, they are methods of critical thinking, of approaching choices, and often of placing difficult choices out in the open for discussion. While they generate quantitative statements about the value of programme costs and consequences, qualitatively they are simply frameworks for comprehensive identification and display of (economic) factors involved in decision-making. Whether factors covered by the economic analyses are, in fact, the dominant concerns in a specific decision and whether the limitations of economic evaluation (discussed in Chapter 3) restrict its usefulness in a specific situation, are judgements which quite properly remain the responsibility of the final decision-maker. In this sense, CEAs, CUAs, and CBAs may represent only a partial analysis of any specific choice. However, as Hutton and Brown (2002) point

Box 2.6 **New terms for old**

The existing literature in economic evaluation in health care, including the first edition of this book, classifies costs and benefits as *direct*, *indirect*, or *intangible*. For the reasons outlined below, we do not use the terms here.

Direct costs and benefits

These terms have been used in the past to denote the resources consumed (costs) or saved (benefits) by the programme, when compared to an alternative (which could be no programme). In the main these would be resources in the health care sector, but sometimes would include patient's out-of-pocket expenses and resources from other statutory agencies and voluntary bodies. However, use of the terms is not consistent across studies, which sometimes causes confusion.

Indirect costs and benefits

These terms have been used in the past to denote the time of patients (or their families) consumed or freed by the programme. In the main the focus has been on worktime, and indirect costs and benefits have been synonymous with productivity gains and losses. The term 'indirect costs' has often caused confusion as it is used by the accountancy profession to denote overhead costs.

Intangible costs and benefits

These terms have been used in the past to denote those consequences that are difficult to measure and value, such as the value of improved health *per se*, or the pain and suffering associated with treatment. However, the latter are not costs (that is, resources denied other uses) and in any case these items are not strictly intangible as they are often measured and valued, through the utility or willingness-to-pay approach.

Box 2.7 **The key distinctions between CBA and CEA/CUA**

CBA
- ◆ Grounded in welfare economic theory
- ◆ Can assess whether a programme is worthwhile, without reference to any external standard
- ◆ Can assess whether the budget should be expanded to accommodate the new programme

CEA/CUA
- ◆ Assumes that the decision-maker seeks to maximize achievement of a defined objective by using a given budget
- ◆ Assessments of whether a programme is worthwhile have to be made by reference to an external standard (for example, a budget constraint or threshold cost-effectiveness ratio)
- ◆ Decisions on the expansion of the budget require consideration of the opportunity cost that is likely to fall outside the health care sector

out, if decision-makers are not satisfied with the economic decision framework, it is incumbent upon them to explain why and to be explicit about any alternative decision-making framework. We discuss this further in Chapter 10.

In this chapter, we have attempted to provide the reader with an introduction to the nature of economic evaluation itself, and the distinguishing characteristics of the principal types of economic evaluation which may be encountered. Of course, identifying an evaluation is one thing; deciding whether it has been soundly executed (and then whether it is potentially useful for a particular decision) is quite another! Therefore, in Chapter 3 we outline the elements common to sound economic evaluations.

References

Berwick, D. M. and Weinstein, M. C. (1985). What do patients value? Willingness-to-pay for ultrasound in normal pregnancy. *Medical Care*, **23**, 881–93.

Birch, S. and Donaldson, C. (1987). Applications of cost benefit analysis to health care: departures from welfare economic theory. *Journal of Health Economics*, **6**, 211–25.

Birch, S. and Gafni, A. (1996). Cost-effectiveness and cost utility analysis: methods for the non-economic evaluation of health care programmes and how we can do better. In: *Managing technology in health care* (ed. E. Geilser and O. Heller), pp. 51–68. Kluwer, Norwell, Massachusetts.

Boyle, M. H., Torrance, G. W., Sinclair, J. C., and Horwood, S. P. (1983). Economic evaluation of neonatal intensive care of very-low-birth-weight infants. *New England Journal of Medicine*, **308**, 1330–7.

Briggs, A. H. and O'Brien, B. J. (2001). The death of cost-minimisation analysis? *Health Economics*, **10**, 179–84.

Culyer, A. J. (1989). The normative economics of health care finance and provision. *Oxford Review of Economic Policy*, **5**, 34–58.

Currie, G. R., Donaldson, C., O'Brien, B. J., Stoddart, G. L., Torrance, G. W., and Drummond, M. F. (2002). Willingness-to-pay for what? A note on alternative definitions of healthcare program benefits for contingent valuation studies. *Medical Decision Making*, **22**, 493–7.

Donaldson, C. and Shackley, P. (1997a). Economic evaluation. In: *Oxford textbook of public health (third edition) Volume 2: the methods of public health* (ed. R. Detels, W. W. Holland, J. McEwen, and G. S. Omenn), pp. 949–71. Oxford University Press, Oxford.

Donaldson, C. and Shackley, P. (1997b). Does 'process utility' exist? A case study of willingness to pay for laparoscopic cholecystectomy. *Social Science and Medicine*, **44**, 699–707.

Drummond, M.F. (1992). Cost of illness studies: a major headache? *PharmacoEconomics*, **2**, 1–4.

Gold, M. R., Siegel, J. E., Russell, L. B., and Weinstein, M. C. (ed.) (1996). *Cost-effectiveness in health and medicine*. Oxford University Press, New York.

Guyatt, G. and Rennie, D. (ed.) (2002). *Users' guides to the medical literature: a manual for evidence-based clinical practice*. AMA, Chicago.

Hull, R., Hirsh, J., Sackett, D. L., and Stoddart, G. L. (1981). Cost-effectiveness of clinical diagnosis, venography and non-invasive testing in patients with symptomatic deep-vein thrombosis. *New England Journal of Medicine*, **304**, 1561–7.

Hutton, J. and Brown, R. E. (2002). Use of economic evaluation in decision making: what needs to change? *Value in Health*, **5**, 65–6.

Johannesson, M. and Jönsson, B. (1991). Economic evaluation in health care: is there a role for cost–benefit analysis? *Health Policy*, **17**, 1–23.

Logan, A. G., Milne, B. J., Achber, C., Campbell, W. P., and Haynes, R. B. (1981). Cost-effectiveness of a work-site hypertension treatment programme. *Hypertension*, **3**, 211–18.

Lowson, K. V., Drummond, M. F., and Bishop, J. M. (1981). Costing new services: long-term domiciliary oxygen therapy. *Lancet*, **ii**, 1146–9.

Ludbrook, A. (1981). A cost-effectiveness analysis of the treatment of chronic renal failure. *Applied Economics*, **13**, 337–50.

Mehrez, A. and Gafni, A. (1989). Quality-adjusted life-years, utility theory and health years equivalents. *Medical Decision Making*, **9**, 142–9.

Neuhauser, D. and Lewicki, A. M. (1975). What do we gain from the sixth stool guaiac? *New England Journal of Medicine*, **293**, 226–8.

Neumann, P. and Johannesson, M. (1994). The willingness to pay for *in vitro* fertilization: a pilot study using contingent valuation. *Medical Care*, **32**, 686–699.

Nord, E. (1995). The person-trade-off approach to valuing health care programs. *Medical Decision Making*, **15**, 201–8.

O'Brien, B. J., Novosel, S., Torrance, G., and Streiner, D. (1995). Assessing the economic value of a new antidepressant: a willingness-to-pay approach. *PharmacoEconomics*, **8**, 34–5.

O'Byrne, P., Cuddy, L., Taylor, D. W., Birch, S., Morris, J., and Syrotuik, J. (1996). Efficacy and cost–benefit of inhaled corticosteroids in patients considered to have mild asthma in primary care practice. *Canadian Respirology Journal*, **3**, 169–75.

Oldridge, N., Furlong, W., Feeny, D., *et al.* (1993). Economic evaluation of cardiac rehabilitation soon after acute myocardial infarction. *American Journal of Cardiology*, **72**, 154–61.

Reynell, P. C. and Reynell, M. C. (1972). The cost–benefit analysis of a coronary care unit. *British Heart Journal*, **34**, 897–900.

Sackett, D. L. (1980). Evaluation of health services. In: *Health and preventive medicine* (ed. J. M. Last), pp. 1800–23. Appleton-Century Crofts, New York.

Sculpher, M. J. and Buxton, M. J. (1993). The episode-free day as a composite measure of effectiveness. *PharmacoEconomics*, **4**, 345–52.

Stevens, A., Abrams, K., Brazier, R., Fitzpatrick, R., and Lilford, R. (ed.) (2001). *The advanced handbook of methods in evidence-based healthcare*. Sage, London.

Sugden, R. and Williams, A. H. (1979). *The principles of practical cost-benefit analysis*. Oxford University Press, Oxford.

Tan-Torres Edejer, T., Baltussen, R., Adam, T., *et al.* (2003). *WHO guide to cost-effectiveness analysis*. World Health Organization, Geneva.

Tengs, T. O., Adams, M. E., Pliskin, J. S., *et al.* (1995). Five-hundred life-saving interventions and their cost-effectiveness. *Risk Analysis*, **15**, 369–90.

Torrance, G. W., Raynauld, J. P., Walker, V., *et al.* (2001). A prospective, randomised, pragmatic, health outcomes trial evaluating the incorporation of hylan G-F 20 into the treatment paradigm for patients with knee osteoarthritis (Part 2 of 2): economic results. *Osteoarthritis and Cartilage*, **10**, 518–27.

Weisbrod, B. A., Test, M. A., and Stein, L. I. (1980). Alternatives to mental hospital treatment: economic cost–benefit analysis. *Archives of General Psychiatry*, **37**, 400–5.

Chapter 3

Critical assessment of economic evaluation

Those who receive or read an economic evaluation are often faced with the difficult task of assessing study results. The question that readers of evaluations are most likely to ask themselves is '*Are these results useful to me in my setting?*' The answer to this question is determined by the answers to the following specific questions.

1 Is the methodology employed in the study appropriate and are the results valid?

2 If the results are valid, would they apply to my setting?

This chapter concentrates on question (1), and is designed to assist users of economic evaluation in assessing the validity of the results they encounter.

When assessing the validity of evidence, whether pertaining to efficacy, effectiveness, availability, or efficiency, we normally proceed by examining closely the methods employed to produce the evidence. Often it is helpful to separate the various elements of a methodology so that each can be scrutinized more closely. In this chapter we identify the key elements of any economic evaluation and discuss methodological characteristics that users may expect to find in well-executed studies. A brief summary of relevant questions to ask about an economic evaluation is provided in Box 3.1, and this critical appraisal check-list is then applied to a published article.

Of course, it is unrealistic to expect every study to satisfy all of the points; however, the systematic application of these points will allow readers to identify and assess the strengths and weaknesses of individual studies.

3.1. Elements of a sound economic evaluation

1. Was a well-defined question posed in answerable form?

Such a question will clearly identify the alternatives being compared and the viewpoint(s) from which the comparison is to be made. Questions such as, '*Is a chronic home care programme worth it?*' and, '*Will a community hypertension screening programme do any good?*' solicit the issues of *to whom and compared to what*. Similarly, questions such as, '*How much does it cost to run our intensive care unit?*', and '*What are the costs and outcomes of adolescent counselling by social workers?*' are not efficiency questions because they fail to specify the alternatives for comparison. (See Chapter 2 for a review of the basic types of economic evaluation.) This is not to say that the questions do not provide important accounting or management information; they may do so, but the answers to them do not by themselves qualify as efficiency statements.

Box 3.1 **A check-list for assessing economic evaluations**

1. **Was a well-defined question posed in answerable form?**
   1.1. Did the study examine both costs and effects of the service(s) or programme(s)?
   1.2. Did the study involve a comparison of alternatives?
   1.3. Was a viewpoint for the analysis stated and was the study placed in any particular decision-making context?

2. **Was a comprehensive description of the competing alternatives given? (that is, can you tell who did what to whom, where, and how often?)**
   2.1. Were any relevant alternatives omitted?
   2.2. Was (Should) a *do-nothing* alternative (be) considered?

3. **Was the effectiveness of the programmes or services established?**
   3.1. Was this done through a randomized, controlled clinical trial? If so, did the trial protocol reflect what would happen in regular practice?
   3.2. Were effectiveness data collected and summarized through a systematic overview of clinical studies? If so, were the search strategy and rules for inclusion or exclusion outlined?
   3.3. Were observational data or assumptions used to establish effectiveness? If so, what are the potential biases in results?

4. **Were all the important and relevant costs and consequences for each alternative identified?**
   4.1. Was the range wide enough for the research question at hand?
   4.2. Did it cover all relevant viewpoints? (Possible viewpoints include the community or social viewpoint, and those of patients and third-party payers. Other viewpoints may also be relevant depending upon the particular analysis.)
   4.3. Were capital costs, as well as operating costs, included?

5. **Were costs and consequences measured accurately in appropriate physical units (for example, hours of nursing time, number of physician visits, lost work-days, gained life-years)?**
   5.1. Were the sources of resource utilization described and justified?
   5.2. Were any of the identified items omitted from measurement? If so, does this mean that they carried no weight in the subsequent analysis?
   5.3. Were there any special circumstances (for example, joint use of resources) that made measurement difficult? Were these circumstances handled appropriately?

6. **Were costs and consequences valued credibly?**
   6.1. Were the sources of all values clearly identified? (Possible sources include market values, patient or client preferences and views, policy-makers' views, and health professionals' judgements.)
   6.2 Were market values employed for changes involving resources gained or depleted?

Box 3.1 **A check-list for assessing economic evaluations** (*continued*)

6.3. Where market values were absent (for example, volunteer labour), or market values did not reflect actual values (such as clinic space donated at a reduced rate), were adjustments made to approximate market values?

6.4. Was the valuation of consequences appropriate for the question posed (that is, has the appropriate type or types of analysis—cost-effectiveness, cost–utility, cost–benefit—been selected)?

7. **Were costs and consequences adjusted for differential timing?**
   7.1. Were costs and consequences that occur in the future 'discounted' to their present values?
   7.2. Was any justification given for the discount rate used?

8. **Was an incremental analysis of costs and consequences of alternatives performed?**
   8.1. Were the additional (incremental) costs generated by one alternative over another compared to the additional effects, benefits, or utilities generated?

9. **Was allowance made for uncertainty in the estimates of costs and consequences?**
   9.1. If patient-level data on costs or consequences were available, were appropriate statistical analyses performed?
   9.2. If a sensitivity analysis was employed, was justification provided for the ranges or distributions of values (for key study parameters), and the form of sensitivity analysis used?
   9.3. Were the conclusions of the study sensitive to the uncertainty in the results, as quantified by the statistical and/or sensitivity analysis?

10. **Did the presentation and discussion of study results include all issues of concern to users?**
    10.1. Were the conclusions of the analysis based on some overall index or ratio of costs to consequences (for example, cost-effectiveness ratio)? If so, was the index interpreted intelligently or in a mechanistic fashion?
    10.2. Were the results compared with those of others who have investigated the same question? If so, were allowances made for potential differences in study methodology?
    10.3. Did the study discuss the generalizability of the results to other settings and patient/client groups?
    10.4. Did the study allude to, or take account of, other important factors in the choice or decision under consideration (for example, distribution of costs and consequences, or relevant ethical issues)?
    10.5. Did the study discuss issues of implementation, such as the feasibility of adopting the 'preferred' programme given existing financial or other constraints, and whether any freed resources could be redeployed to other worthwhile programmes?

A well-specified question, for example, might look as follows: '*From the viewpoint of (a) both the Ministry of Health and the Ministry of Community and Social Services budgets, and (b) patients incurring out-of-pocket costs, is a chronic home care programme preferable to the existing programme of institutionalized, extended care in designated wards of general hospitals?*' Note that the viewpoint for an analysis may be that of a specific provider or providing institution, the patient or groups of patients, a third-party payer (public or private), or society (that is, all costs and consequences to whomsoever they accrue). Sometimes it may be specified by a decision-maker when requesting a study.

Obviously it is difficult for the analyst to consider every single cost and consequence of a health care programme to all members of society. Indeed, the 'ripple effects' of some programmes may be far reaching and consideration of some items may have to be excluded for practical reasons. However, it is important to recognize that in considering the use of the community's scarce resources, the viewpoint of the providing institution may often be too restrictive and a broader viewpoint should also be considered. For example, it may be that a programme is preferable from the societal viewpoint, but not from the viewpoint of the providing institution. In such a case the Ministry of Health may wish to consider giving an incentive to the providing institution to ensure that the socially preferred programme goes ahead. The existence of different viewpoints was highlighted by Weisbrod *et al.* (1980) in their study of community-oriented and hospital-based treatments for mental illness.

2. Was a comprehensive description of the competing alternatives given?

A clear and specific statement of the primary objective of each alternative programme, treatment, or service is critical in selecting cost-effectiveness analysis, cost–utility analysis, or cost–benefit analysis (CEA, CUA, and CBA, respectively) as the type of evaluation to be undertaken. A full description of the competing alternatives is essential for three further reasons.

1 Readers must be able to judge the applicability of the programmes to their own settings.

2 Readers should be able to assess for themselves whether any costs or consequences may have been omitted in the analysis.

3 Readers may wish to replicate the programme procedures being described.

Therefore, readers should be provided with information allowing an identification of costs (Who does what to whom, where, and how often?) and consequences. (What are the results?)

For many treatments and programmes, the capacity to benefit will differ for patients with differing characteristics. Therefore, apart from considering the main treatment alternatives, it may be relevant to consider alternative patient subgroups and to present data on costs and consequences for each. For example, Mark *et al.* (1995) presented data on the incremental cost-effectiveness of tissue plasminogen activator (t-PA) (compared with streptokinase (SK)) for patients of different age groups and type of myocardial infarction. Other relevant alternatives, within a given treatment or programme, could include intensity (that is, dosage) and length of treatment. For example, Sculpher *et al.* (2000) compared low and high doses of an angiotensin-converting enzyme inhibitor in patients with chronic heart failure. Finally, the alternatives could consist of various sequences of care or clinical care pathways. (This issue is discussed in more detail in Chapters 5 and 9.)

As mentioned in Chapter 2, an important contribution of economic analysis is to minimize the risk of important, relevant alternatives being excluded from consideration. Therefore the analyst should consider (1) whether a 'do-nothing' alternative is a feasible option and (2) whether the formulation of the decision-making problem is being unduly constrained by the existing effectiveness evidence base or by the professional or managerial responsibilities of the person commissioning the study. This is explored further in Chapter 9.

3. Was the effectiveness of the programmes or services established?

We are not interested in the efficient provision of ineffective services, that is, those services which have been shown to do no more good than harm (by themselves, or compared with no treatment). In fact, we are not interested in the provision of such services under any conditions, efficient or otherwise. *If something is not worth doing, it is not worth doing well!* Therefore, if the economic evaluation assumes effectiveness, some indication of the validation of effectiveness should be given. Thus, economic evaluations using decision-analytic modelling (Chapter 9) typically take estimates of treatment effect from randomized clinical trials. It is also possible that the efficiency evaluation may have been conducted simultaneously with the evaluation of efficacy or effectiveness. This is the case in many randomized trials of therapies that also include a comparison of the costs of the experimental programme and a control, which may be a placebo or the currently existing programme. Note, however, that efficiency evaluations, by themselves, are incapable of establishing effectiveness. Precedent or simultaneous evidence of effectiveness is required. After all, there are efficient methods of worsening health-related quality of life as well as improving it! (Those wishing to know more about the methods of establishing whether a therapy does more good than harm should consult Sackett *et al.* (1991) or Guyatt and Rennie (2002).)

Evidence on effectiveness may come from a single study, especially when the economic evaluation is carried out alongside a clinical study. Alternatively it can come from a systematic overview of several clinical studies. In the former case it is important to consider whether the estimate of treatment effect from that particular trial is representative of the whole body of evidence for the treatments concerned. In the latter case it is important that the reasons for inclusion or exclusion of studies from the overview are given, so that the reader can assess whether or not a biased subset of the available clinical evidence has been used. For more details of the methodology of systematic reviews see Khan *et al.* (2001).

4. Were all the important and relevant costs and consequences for each alternative identified?

Even though it may not be possible or necessary to measure and value all of the costs and consequences of the alternatives under comparison, a full identification of the important and relevant ones should be provided. The combination of information contained in the viewpoint statement and programme description should allow

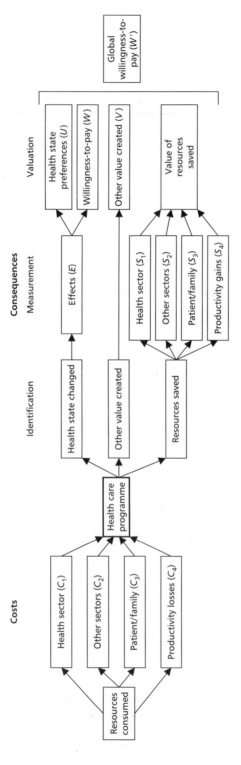

Fig. 3.1 Components of economic evaluation in health care.

judgement of what specific costs and consequences or outcomes it is appropriate to include in the analysis.

An overview of the categories of costs and consequences that are relevant to an economic evaluation of health services and programmes was given in Fig. 2.1. (This is presented again here as Fig. 3.1.) Four categories of cost are identified. The health care resources consumed consist of the costs of organizing and operating the programme, including dealing with the adverse events caused by the programme. The identification of these costs often amounts to listing the *ingredients* of the programme—both variable costs (such as the time of health professionals or supplies) and fixed or overhead costs (such as light, heat, rent, or capital costs). The ways of measuring and valuing these items are discussed in more detail in Chapter 4.

The patient and family resources consumed include any out-of-pocket expenses incurred by patients or family members as well as the value of any resources that they contribute to the treatment process. When patients or family members lose time from work while seeking treatment or participating in a health care programme there could be associated productivity losses. (The measurement and valuation of these is also discussed in Chapter 4.)

While the above three categories of costs cover most of the cost items relevant to economic evaluations of health services, a fourth category, resources consumed in other sectors, also warrants mention. As mentioned in Chapter 2, some programmes, such as those for the care of the elderly, consume resources from other public agencies or the voluntary sector. Occasionally it may also be the case that the operation of a health service or programme changes the resource use in the broader economy. Examples of situations where these factors may be important are given below.

1 An occupational health and safety programme (perhaps legislated by government) that changes the production process in an automobile manufacturing plant, thereby using up more resources, perhaps in a more labour-intensive way. These costs are passed on in the increased price of cars and are borne by the purchasers of cars, who are likely not the workers for whom the programme was initiated.

2 A 55-mile-per-hour speed limit policy, which reduces morbidity and mortality due to accidents, but increases the price of, for example, fruit which now takes longer to arrive (that is, a higher wage bill for the truck driver).

In principle, these factors should be considered in the economic evaluation, though for many health care programmes they may be insignificant. (In practice, few economic analyses of alternative health care programmes take them into account.)

Three categories of consequences of health services or programmes are also shown in Fig. 3.1. The changes in health state relate to changes in the physical, social, or emotional functioning of individuals. In principle, such changes can be measured objectively, and refer only to an individual's ability to function and not to the significance, preference, or value attached to this ability by the individual, or by others. However, as indicated in Fig. 3.1 and discussed later, values can be attached either by health state preference scores or willingness-to-pay.

In addition, other value may be created by the programme (for example, reduction in anxiety) and resources may be freed. For example, a vaccination programme may free resources if fewer individuals contract the disease and thus require treatment. This was discussed in Chapter 2.

Given the wide range of costs and consequences indicated above, it may be unrealistic to expect all relevant items to be measured and valued in the analysis, due to their small size or influence relative to the effort required to measure or value them accurately; however, it is helpful to users to identify as many relevant items as possible. It is particularly important that the outcomes of interest be identified clearly enough for a reader to judge the appropriateness of the type (or types) of economic evaluation chosen; that is, it should be apparent

1 whether a single outcome is of primary interest as opposed to a set of outcomes;

2 whether the outcomes are common to both alternatives under comparison;

3 to what degree each programme is successful in achieving each outcome of interest.

Similarly, it is important to know whether the consequences of primary interest are the therapeutic effects themselves (thus implying CEA if possible), the change in the health-related quality of life of patients and their families (CUA), or the overall value created (CBA). Primarily this is determined by the audience(s) for the study and their objectives, as discussed in Chapter 2.

5. Were costs and consequences measured accurately in appropriate physical units?
While identification, measurement, and valuation often occur simultaneously in analyses, it is a good practice for users of evaluation results to view each as a separate phase of analysis. Once the important and relevant costs and consequences have been identified, they must be measured in appropriate physical and natural units. For example, measurement of the operating costs of a particular screening programme may yield a partial list of *ingredients* such as 500 physical examinations performed by physicians, 10 weeks of salaried nursing time, 10 weeks of a 1000-square-foot clinic, 20 hours of medical research librarian time from an adjoining hospital, and so on. Similarly, costs borne by patients may be measured, for instance, by the amount of medication purchased, the number of times travel was required for treatment, or the time lost from work while being treated.

Notice that situations in which resources are jointly used by one or more programmes present a particular challenge to accurate measurement. How much resource use should be allocated to each programme? And on what basis? A common example of this is found in every hospital, where numerous clinical services and programmes share common overhead services (for example, electric power, cleaning, and administration), provided centrally. In general, there is no non-arbitrary solution to the measurement problem; however, users of results should satisfy themselves that *reasonable* criteria (number of square feet, number of employees, number of cases, and so on) have been used to distribute the common costs. Users should definitely ascertain that such shared costs have been allocated, in fact, to participating services or programmes, as this is a common omission in evaluations! Clinical service directors often argue that small changes in the size of their programmes (up or down) do not affect the consumption of central services. Sometimes it is even argued that overhead costs are unaffected by the service itself. However, though this argument may be intuitively appealing from the viewpoint of a particular programme or service director, the extension of this method to each service in the hospital would imply that the totality of services could be operated without light, heat, power, and secretaries! (The allocation of overhead costs is discussed further in Chapter 4.)

With respect to the measurement of consequences, if the identification of outcomes of interest has been clearly performed, then selection of appropriate units of measurement for programme effects should be relatively straightforward. For example, effects might relate to mortality and be measured in life-years gained or deaths averted; they might relate to morbidity and be measured, for example, in reductions in disability days or improvements on some index of health status measuring physical, social, or emotional functioning; they may be even more specific, depending upon the alternatives under consideration. Thus, percentage increase in weight-bearing ability may be an appropriate natural measurement unit for an evaluation of a physiotherapy programme, while the number of correctly diagnosed cases may be appropriate for a comparison of venography with leg scanning in the diagnosis of deep-vein thrombosis (DVT).

In some cases the measurement of consequences will be based directly on the clinical evidence used in the economic evaluation. For example, the evaluation may use data from clinical trials estimating the number of cases detected or life-years gained. However, it is much more common for trials to estimate the number of patients surviving at the end of a follow-up period (that is, 1 year), or the progression of disease over a fixed period of time. The choice of time horizon is an important methodological consideration in economic evaluations. It should be long enough to capture the major health and economic consequences, both intended effects and unintended side-effects. Thus, for many economic evaluations the relevant time horizon is the patient's lifetime.

Therefore the measurement of consequences for the economic evaluation may require extrapolation of effectiveness over time. This is particularly true for economic evaluations measuring consequences in terms of life-years or quality-adjusted life-years (QALYs) gained. Extrapolation of effects beyond the end of the trial requires additional data (from long-term observational studies) and may also require several assumptions, such as the likely progression of disease in patients who discontinue therapy. There may be no unambiguously right way to make such extrapolations, but at least the methods used should be transparent. Extrapolation is a central feature of economic evaluations using a decision-analytic modelling approach. Therefore, it is discussed in more detail in Chapter 9.

Changes in resource use resulting from the effects will be measured in physical units similar to those employed for costs. Thus the changes in utilization resulting from any particular programme will likely be recorded in numbers of procedures, or amounts of time, space, or equipment. Changes in the resource use by patients will continue to be measured in amounts of medication purchased, trips taken for treatment, and so forth.

While the nature of changes in health-related quality of life may be described, this is one case where measurement in objective, physical, or natural units is difficult, although the consequence of some surgical interventions may be quantified in number of complications. However, the adjustment of effects for health-related quality of life is usually a matter of valuation, although we also discuss the use of quality of life scales in CEA in Chapter 5.

6. Were costs and consequences valued credibly?

The sources and methods of valuation of costs, benefits, and utilities should be clearly stated in an economic evaluation. Costs are normally valued in units of local currency, based on prevailing *prices* of, for example, personnel, commodities, and services, and can often be taken directly from programme budgets. All current and future programme costs are normally valued in constant dollars of some base year (usually the present), in order to remove the effects of inflation from the analysis.

It should be remembered that the objective in valuing costs is to obtain an estimate of the worth of resources depleted by the programme. This may necessitate adjustments to some apparent programme costs (for example, the case of subsidized services or volunteer labour received by one programme instead of another). In addition, valuation of the cost of a day of institutional care for a specific condition is particularly troublesome in that the use of an average cost per day (the widely quoted *per diem*), calculated on the basis of the institution's entire annual case-load, is almost certainly an overestimate or underestimate of the actual cost for any specific condition, sometimes by quite a large amount.

In principle and (with great effort) in practice, it is possible to identify, measure, and value each depleted resource (for example, drugs, nursing time, light, food, and so on) in treating a specific patient or group of patients. While this yields a relatively accurate cost estimate, the detailed monitoring and data collection are usually prohibitively expensive. The other broad alternative costing strategy is to start with the institution's total costs for a particular period and then to improve upon the method of simply dividing by the total patient-days to produce an average cost per day. Quite sophisticated methods of cost allocation to individual hospital departments or wards have been developed, as illustrated by Boyle *et al.* (1982) with respect to neonatal intensive care. An intermediate method involves acceptance of the components of the general *per diem* relating to *hotel* costs (as these are relatively invariant across patients) combined with more precise calculation of the medical treatment costs associated with the specific patients in question. For an example of this intermediate approach see Hull *et al.* (1982). Of course, the effort devoted to accurate *per diem* estimates depends upon their overall importance in the study; however, unthinking use of *per diems* or average costs should be guarded against. (This is discussed further in Chapter 4.)

In valuation of preferences or utilities, we are basically attempting to ascertain how much better the quality of life is in one health situation or 'state' compared with another (for example, dialysis at home with help from a spouse or friend versus dialysis in hospital). Several techniques are available for making the comparison; the important thing to note is that each will produce an adjustment factor with which to increase or decrease the value of time spent in health situations or 'states', resulting from the alternative in question relative to some baseline. The results of these analyses are usually expressed in *healthy years* or *QALYs* gained, as a result of the programmes being evaluated.

In recent years many more economic evaluations have employed one of the generic preference-based health measures, such as the EuroQoL EQ-5D or the Health Utilities Index (EuroQoL Group 1990; Feeny *et al.* 1995). These measures employ a questionnaire, administered to patients in the study, to classify them into one of a pre-determined set of health states. The health state preference values, or utilities, are then available from a scoring formula (or tariff) that accompanies the measure. Typically the source of values is the general public.

Because the measurement of preferences in health is still a relatively new field, there are many unresolved issues, which readers of CUAs should note. Users of such analyses will probably want to know, at minimum, *whose* preferences were used to construct the adjustment factor—the patient's, the provider's, the taxpayer's or the decision-maker's? If patients' preferences have not been employed, we may want to assure ourselves further that the persons whose preferences did count clearly understood the characteristics of the health state, either through personal experience or through a description of the state presented to them. These issues are taken up in Chapter 6.

Many of the same issues arise when estimating willingness-to-pay, either for a change in health state or for the overall impact of the programme in question. These issues are taken up in Chapter 7.

One of the important consequences of health care programmes is the creation of healthy time. The valuation of this item poses difficulties. Indeed, its categorization, under changes in health state or patient and family resources freed, is uncertain. The reasons for this are as follows.

The value of healthy time can manifest itself in a number of ways. First, living in a better health state has a value to the individual in its own right (e.g. less pain, better health-related quality of life). Secondly, healthy time can be used in leisure. Thirdly, healthy time can be used for work, which generates income for the individual and productive output for society.

In a CEA, the measurement of the effects (E) does not capture the value of healthy time. Therefore, if it is to be included it would have to be estimated separately, as an element of the patient and family resources freed. In a CUA or CBA, where we are attempting to *value* the consequences of the programme, we might expect that the value of living in a better health state is captured in the preference score (U), or the willingness-to-pay (W). The value of healthy time in leisure is probably also captured in U or W, as it is closely linked with improved health-related quality of life.

Whether or not the value of using healthy time for work is also included in U or W probably depends on how the scenario (used for valuation) is written. It may be possible, for example, to ask individuals to imagine that their income would not be affected by their health state, as this is covered by unemployment insurance. In such a case, an analyst undertaking an evaluation from a societal viewpoint may wish to include a separate estimate of productivity gains to society if a person's health state is improved. If so, it would be important to ensure that the person did *not* include this in their own valuation, so as to avoid double counting.

Of course, healthy time can also be consumed by a programme if it requires the individual to spend time seeking or undergoing treatment, perhaps in hospital. In a CEA, the value of healthy time lost would have to be estimated separately.

In a CUA or CBA, the way forward would again depend on how the health state scenario is described. If the description contained elements of the process of undergoing care (for example, 'you will be admitted to hospital for seven days for treatment'), this may be reflected in the U or W. Otherwise, the value of healthy time lost in therapy may have to be estimated separately.

Therefore, we have another example of where the assembly of components (building blocks) in the analysis is partly dependent on how they are measured and valued. In conducting an economic evaluation from a societal perspective, it is important to avoid both zero counting and double counting. Of course, the estimation of global willingness-to-pay (W') avoids the problem of categorizing the value of healthy time, either as a component of the change in health state or as a component of patient and family resources freed. Rather, the challenge of this approach is to ensure that individuals appreciate *all* the elements of value created and resources consumed by a health care programme, so that this is reflected in their valuation (W').

7. Were costs and consequences adjusted for differential timing?

Because comparison of programmes or services must be made at one point in time (usually the present), the timing of programme costs and consequences that do not occur entirely in the present must be taken into account. Different programmes may have different time profiles of costs and consequences. For example, the primary benefits of an influenza immunization programme are immediate while those of hypertension screening occur well into the future. The time profile of costs and consequences may also differ within a single programme; the costs of the hypertension screening programme would be incurred in the present. Therefore, future dollar cost and benefit streams are reduced or 'discounted' to reflect the fact that dollars spent or saved in the future should not weigh as heavily in programme decisions as dollars spent or saved today. This is primarily due to the existence of *time preference*. That is, individually and as a society we prefer to have dollars or resources now, as opposed to later, because we can benefit from them in the interim. This is evidenced by the existence of interest rates (as well as the popular wisdom about 'a bird in the hand'). Moreover because *time preference* is not exclusively a financial concept, discounting of consequences should also be considered in cost-effectiveness and cost–utility studies. The mechanics of discounting and the choice of discount rate are discussed in Chapter 4.

8. Was an incremental analysis of costs and consequences of alternatives performed?

For meaningful comparison, it is necessary to examine the additional costs that one service or programme imposes over another, compared with the additional effects, benefits, or utilities it delivers. This *incremental* approach to analysis of costs and consequences can be illustrated by reference to one of the examples cited in Chapter 2, namely strategies for the diagnosis of DVT (Hull *et al.* 1981).

Table 3.1 shows the costs and outcomes (in terms of correct diagnoses) generated by two alternative strategies: impedance plethysmography (IPG) alone versus IPG

Table 3.1 Economic evaluation of alternative diagnostic strategies for 516 patients with clinically suspected deep-vein thrombosis

Programme	Cost (US$)	Outcome (number of correct diagnoses)	Ratio of cost to outcome (US$ per correct diagnosis)
1. IPG (alone)	321 488	142	2264
2. IPG plus out-patient venography if IPG negative	603 552	201	3003
3. Increment (of Programme 2 over Programme 1)	282 064	59	4781

IPG, impedance plethysmography.

Data drawn from Table 1, Hull *et al.* (1981), by permission.

plus out-patient venography if impedance plethysmography is negative. (IPG is a non-invasive strategy, whereas venography, the diagnostic 'gold standard' for DVT, can cause pain and other unpleasant side-effects.) Although one could compare the simple ratios of costs to outcomes for the two alternatives, the correct comparison is the one of incremental costs over incremental outcomes, because this tells us how much we are paying (for each extra correct diagnosis) in adding the extra diagnostic test. In this case the relevant figure is therefore $4781 per correct diagnosis, not the average figure for the second programme, $3003 per correct diagnosis. It may be decided that $4781 is still a price worth paying; however, it is important to be clear on the principle because earlier (in Chapter 2) we pointed out that, in the case of screening for cancer of the colon, there was a big difference between the average cost (per case detected) of a protocol of six sequential tests and the incremental cost of performing a sixth test, having already done five (Neuhauser and Lewicki 1975).

Similar incremental analyses could be performed if the effects were in years of life or healthy years. These can be illustrated graphically on a four quadrant diagram known as the cost-effectiveness plane. (Black 1990). (See Box 3.2.)

In practice the impact of most interventions falls in quadrant I. That is, they add to cost but increase effectiveness, certainly when compared with no intervention. Let us therefore plot the data given in Table 3.1 (see Fig. 3.2). Here we only show quadrant I and the slopes of the lines from the origin give the average cost-effectiveness ratios for the two programmes, which are $2264 and $3003 per case detected for A and B respectively. The incremental cost-effectiveness ratio ($4781 per case detected) is given by the slope of the line joining points A and B. (The interpretation of incremental cost-effectiveness ratios is discussed further in Chapter 5.)

9. Was allowance made for uncertainty in the estimates of costs and consequences?
Every evaluation will contain some degree of uncertainty, imprecision, or methodological controversy. What if the compliance rate for influenza vaccination was 10% higher than considered for the analysis? What if the *per diem* hospital cost still understated the true resource cost of a treatment programme by $100? What if a discount rate of 6% had been used instead of 3%? Or what if productivity changes had been excluded from

Box 3.2 **The cost-effectiveness plane**

In the diagram, the horizontal axis represents the difference in effect between the intervention of interest (A) and the relevant alternative (O), and the vertical axis represents the difference in cost. The alternative (O) could be the status quo or a competing programme.

If point A is in quadrants II or IV the choice between the programmes is clear. In quadrant II the intervention of interest is both more effective and less costly than the alternative. That is, it *dominates* the alternative. In quadrant IV the opposite is true. In quadrants I and III the choice depends on the maximum cost-effectiveness ratio one is willing to accept. The slope of the line OA gives the cost-effectiveness ratio.

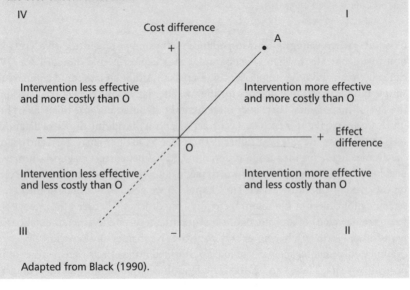

Adapted from Black (1990).

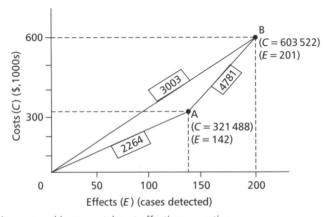

Fig. 3.2 Average and incremental cost-effectiveness ratios.

the analysis? Users of efficiency studies will often ask these and similar questions; therefore, careful analysts will identify critical methodological assumptions or areas of uncertainty.

Briggs (2001) distinguishes among several different types or sources of uncertainty, relating to the data used in the analysis, the main methodological assumptions, and the desire to extrapolate the data or generalize results to other settings. The methods for handling uncertainty differ according to its source and the type of economic evaluation being performed (see Box 3.3).

For example, in an economic evaluation conducted concurrently with a clinical trial, data (say) on length of hospital stay will be stochastic (that is, have a mean

Box 3.3 **Methods for handling different types of uncertainty**

Uncertainty in economic evaluations can arise because of

- methodological disagreement among analysis
- the data requirements of the study
- the need to extrapolate results over time, or from intermediate to final health outcomes
- the desire to generalize the results of the study to another setting (Briggs *et al.* 1994).

Briggs (2001) argues that the preferred method for handling uncertainty depends on the source. It also depends on whether the economic evaluation is a patient level analysis with stochastic data, or a decision analytic modelling study. In both cases methodological uncertainty can only be handled by sensitivity analysis, or by the development of methodological standards (that is, a 'reference case') (Gold *et al.* 1996).

Methods for handling uncertainty in patient-level analyses

Type of uncertainty	Handling uncertainty
Methodological	Reference case/sensitivity analysis
Sampling variation	Statistical analysis
Extrapolation	Modelling methods
Generalizability/transferability	Sensitivity analysis

Methods for handling uncertainty in decision-analytic modelling studies

Type of uncertainty	Handling uncertainty
Methodological	Reference case/sensitivity analysis
Parameter uncertainty	Probabilistic sensitivity analysis
Modelling uncertainty	
• structure	Sensitivity analysis
• process	No established method
Generalizability/transferability	Sensitivity analysis

and variance). Therefore in the analysis of *patient level data* it is possible to conduct statistical analyses (see Chapter 8). In the case of studies employing decision-analytic modelling, data on key model parameters are drawn from a number of sources. Here the approach for dealing with parameter uncertainty is called *sensitivity analysis* (Briggs *et al.* 1994). (Here the various parameters in the model are varied in order to assess how this impacts upon study results.) Sensitivity analysis is also used to handle other types of uncertainty, such as that relating to methodological assumptions. (This will be discussed further in Chapter 9.)

Sensitivity analysis is an important feature of economic evaluations and study results can be sensitive to the values taken by key parameters. In a review of 70 CUAs, Schackman *et al.* (2004) found that quantitatively important changes in results were obtained in 31% of sensitivity analyses of health-related quality of life estimates, 20% of those of cost estimates, and 15% of those using different discount rates.

In judging the quality of a sensitivity analysis conducted in an economic evaluation, readers should consider (1) how the uncertain parameters were identified, (2) how the plausible ranges for the variables were specified, and (3) whether an appropriate form of sensitivity analysis was used (Briggs and Sculpher 1995).

1. *Identifying the uncertain parameters.* It is difficult to specify firm guidelines for this step, beyond the fact that, in principle, all variables in the analysis are potential candidates for sensitivity analysis. One approach might be for the analyst to give the reasons why particular variables had *not* been included. Possible reasons for exclusion could be that parameter estimates are known with absolute certainty, or that a preliminary analysis shows that, even if the variable is allowed to vary over a wide range, this has a minimal impact on the overall study results.

2. *Specifying the plausible range.* A frequent weakness in published economic evaluations is that, while they include a sensitivity analysis, the reasons for specifying the plausible ranges for the variables are not given. Frequently estimates are doubled or halved with no justification. A plausible range could be determined by

- reviewing the literature
- consulting expert opinion
- using a specified confidence interval around the mean (for stochastic data).

When judging published studies the user should assess the justification given for plausible ranges, in conjunction with the statements authors make about their analyses. Sometimes the author's conclusion is that the result is very robust, although the ranges chosen for varying key estimates are unjustifiably small. The moral appears to be that if you do not shake your study too hard it is unlikely to fall apart!

Instead of taking point estimates for the base case (best guess) estimate and the upper and lower bound, an alternative approach is to apply probability distributions to the specified ranges (see below).

3. *Deciding on the form of sensitivity analysis.* The simplest form of sensitivity analysis is to undertake a *one-way analysis*. Here estimates for each parameter are varied one at a time in order to investigate the impact on study results. Although this

is one of the most common forms of sensitivity analysis in the literature, it is not now regarded as a satisfactory approach for handling parameter uncertainty, because the overall uncertainty in the cost-effectiveness ratio depends on the *combined* variability in several factors. It may still suffice for handling methodological uncertainty.

A more sophisticated approach is to undertake a *multiway analysis*. This recognizes that more than one parameter is uncertain and that each could vary within its specified range. Overall, this approach is more realistic but, unless there are only a few uncertain parameters, the number of potential combinations becomes very large. In this case the principles of experimental design can be applied to select the particular combinations to be included (Goldsmith *et al.* 1987).

Another approach is to use *scenario analysis*. Here a series of scenarios is constructed representing a subset of the potential multiway analyses. Typically, the scenarios will include a base case (best guess) scenario and the most optimistic (best case) and most pessimistic (worst case) scenarios. Alternatively they may include scenarios that the analyst or user of the study feel could probably apply.

Yet another approach is to undertake a *threshold analysis*. Here the critical value(s) of a parameter or parameters central to the decision are identified. For example, a decision-maker might specify an increase in cost, or an incremental cost-effectiveness ratio, above which the programme would not be acceptable. Then the analyst could assess which combinations of parameter estimates could cause the threshold to be exceeded. Alternatively, the threshold values for key parameters that would cause the programme to be too costly or not cost-effective could be defined. The decision-makers could then make a judgement about whether particular thresholds were likely to be breached or not (see Box 3.4).

A final form of sensitivity analysis, *probabilistic sensitivity analysis*, is now becoming widely used in decision-analytic modelling studies. Here probability distributions are applied to the specified ranges for the key parameters and samples drawn at random from these distributions to generate an empirical distribution of the cost-effectiveness ratio (see Chapter 9 for a full discussion).

10. Did the presentation and discussion of study results include all issues of concern to users?

It will be clear from the foregoing discussion that the economic analyst has to make many methodological judgements when undertaking a study. Faced with users who may be mainly interested in the 'bottom line'—for example, 'Should we buy a computed tomography scanner'—how should the analyst present the results?

Decision indices such as cost-effectiveness and cost–benefit ratios are a useful way of summarizing study results. However, they should be used with care, as in interpreting them, the user may not be completely clear on what has gone into their construction. Some analysts give a range of results. For example, in their economic evaluation of neonatal intensive care for very-low-birth-weight infants, Boyle *et al.* (1983) compare the results for infants below 1000 g and from 1000 to 1500 g in terms of costs to hospital discharge, costs and consequences to age 15, and costs

Box 3.4 **Cost-effectiveness of hip prostheses: a two-way threshold analysis**

The newer hip prostheses are more expensive than the existing, well-established ones. However, they may offer several advantages, one of which is a lower rate of revision (that is, re-operation) due to failure of the prosthesis. Whilst new prostheses may require fewer revisions, this reduction is now known with certainty. Therefore, in their economic evaluation, Briggs *et al.* (1988) conducted a two-way threshold analysis, on price and revision rate. This is shown in the figure below.

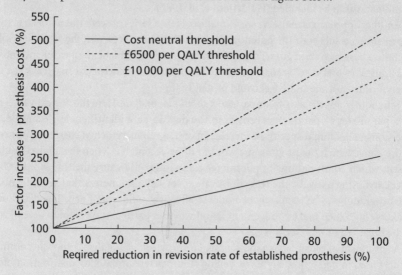

The interpretation is as follows. If, as a decision-maker, your requirement was neutrality in overall treatment costs, a prosthesis cost of 150% (of the cost of existing prostheses) would be justified if the reduction in the revision rate was round 35%. If, on the other hand, you also valued the increased benefits, in QALYs, that new prostheses may confer (in improved quality of life or reduced mortality from the re-operations), a prosthesis cost of around 230% (of existing prostheses) would be justified at a willingness-to-pay threshold of £10,000 per QALY.

and consequences for lifetime (Table 3.2). They leave it to the users of the study to decide on which index (or indices) neonatal intensive care should be judged, because the different measures incorporate different value judgements and varying amounts of precision. (For example, the index of 'net economic benefit' includes production gains/losses, and the index of 'cost per QALY' incorporates the preferences for health states of a sample of the local population.) This leads to another general point, namely it is important for analysts to be as explicit as possible about the various judgements they have made in carrying out the study. A good

Table 3.2 Measures of economic evaluation of neonatal intensive care according to birth-weight class (5% discount rate)

Period	Birth-weight class	
	1000–1499 g ($)	500–999 g ($)
To hospital discharge*		
Cost/additional survivor at hospital discharge	59 500	102 500
To age 15 (projected)		
Cost/life-year gained	6 100	12 200
Cost/QALY gained	7 700	40 100
To death (projected)		
Cost/life-year gained	2 900	9 300
Cost/QALY gained	3 200	22 400
Net economic benefit		
(Loss)/live birth	(2 600)	(16 100)
Net economic cost/life-year gained	900	7 300
Net economic cost/QALY gained	1 000	17 500

QALY, quality-adjusted life-year.

Values are expressed in 1978 Canadian dollars. Multiply by 0.877 to calculate equivalent 1978 US dollars.

* All costs and effects occurred in year one.

From Boyle *et al.* (1983), by permission.

study should leave the user more (rather than less!) aware of the various technical and value judgements necessary to arrive at resource allocation decisions in health care.

Finally, a good study should begin to help users interpret the results in the context of their own particular situation. This can be done by being explicit about the viewpoint for the analysis (an earlier point) and by indicating how particular costs and benefits might vary by location. For example, the costs of instituting day-care surgery may vary, depending on whether a purpose-built day-care unit already exists or whether wards have to be converted. Similarly, the benefits of day-care surgery may vary depending on whether, in a particular location, there is pressure on beds and whether beds will be closed or left empty. Obviously it is impossible for the analyst to anticipate every possibility in every location, but one limitation of economic evaluation techniques (discussed in Section 3.2) is that they assume that freed resources will be put to other beneficial uses.

The presentation, interpretation, and use of economic evaluation results raise a number of practical issues. For example, can the results (for example, cost-effectiveness ratios) from different studies be meaningfully compared? Can results of studies be generalized from one setting, or country, to another? Can guidelines for good practice in the presentation of results be specified (see Box 3.5)? These issues will be explored further in Chapters 9 and 10.

Box 3.5 **Developing guidelines for the presentation of results: specifying a 'reference case'**

The notion of a 'reference case' was first proposed by the Public Health Service Panel on Cost-Effectiveness in Health and Medicine (Gold *et al.* 1996). In considering the methodology and practice of economic evaluation in health care, the panel recognized that many methodological issues were unresolved. On the other hand, they recognized the need to develop a standardized approach for the conduct and reporting of studies, so that the results from different studies could be compared.

Therefore, the 'reference case' is a preferred set of methodological principles that should be used for the 'base case' analysis. Then, if the analyst prefers, they can also report other results, applying different methods. However, if the reference case analysis is always reported, reliable comparisons of studies can be made.

The reference case proposed by the panel embodied most of the good methodological principles of economic evaluation existing at the time. The main features were as follows

(1) the societal perspective should be adopted;

(2) effectiveness estimates should incorporate benefits and harms;

(3) mortality and morbidity consequences should be combined using QALYs;

(4) effectiveness estimates from best-designed and least-biased sources should be used;

(5) costs should include health care services, patient and caregiver time and costs of non-health impacts;

(6) comparison should be made with existing practice and (if necessary) a viable low-cost alternative;

(7) discounting of costs and health outcomes should be undertaken at a real rate of 3% per annum (plus 5% for comparison with existing studies);

(8) one-way and multi-way sensitivity analysis (for important parameters) should be undertaken;

(9) comparison of the incremental cost-effectiveness ratio should be made with those for other relevant interventions.

3.2. **Limitations of economic evaluation techniques**

Our main purpose in this chapter is to make the user of economic evaluation results more aware of the methodological judgements involved in undertaking an economic evaluation in the health care field. In Box 3.1 we have consolidated the points made in this chapter into a suggested check-list of questions to ask when critically assessing economic evaluation results. In addition, there are several other limitations of which users should be aware.

Of primary concern from a policy viewpoint is the fact that economic evaluations do not usually incorporate the importance of the distribution, of costs and consequences, among different patient or population groups, into the analysis. Yet, in some cases, the identity of the recipient group (for example, the poor, the elderly, working mothers, or a geographically remote community) may be an important factor in assessing the social desirability of a service or programme. Indeed, it may be the motivation for the programme in the first place. Although it is sometimes suggested that differential weights be attached to the value of outcomes accruing to special recipient groups, this is not normally done within an economic evaluation. Rather, an equitable distribution of costs and consequences across socioeconomic or other defined groups in society is viewed as a competing dimension upon which decisions are made, in addition to that of efficient deployment of resources.

A more subtle, yet important, point is that the various forms of analysis discussed above embody different equity criteria. For example, CBA values health outcomes in terms of individuals' willingness-to-pay. Sometimes willingness-to-pay may be constrained by ability to pay and therefore valuations are dependent on the existing income distribution. On the other hand the simple aggregation of QALYs in a CUA implies that a QALY is being valued the same no matter to whom it accrues. Therefore, in reality it is difficult to divorce equity considerations from the economic evaluation and analysts should be aware of this when selecting a particular analytic technique.

It should also be noted that economic evaluation techniques assume that resources freed or saved by preferred programmes will not in fact be wasted but will be employed in alternative worthwhile programmes. This assumption warrants careful scrutiny, for if the freed resources are consumed by other ineffective or unevaluated programmes, then not only is there no saving, but overall health system costs will actually increase without any assurance of additional improvements in the health status of the population.

Finally, evaluation of any sort is in itself a costly activity. Bearing in mind that *even economic evaluations should be subject to economic evaluation*, it seems reasonable to suggest that economic evaluation techniques will prove most useful in situations where programme objectives require clarification, the competing alternatives are significantly different in nature, or large resource commitments are under consideration. The uses and limitations of economic evaluation are discussed further in Chapter 10.

3.3. Conclusions

In these introductory chapters, we have tried to assist users of economic evaluations in interpreting evaluation studies and assessing their usefulness for health care decisions, or for planning further analyses. The rationale for economic evaluation, its fundamental characteristics, and the basic types of economic evaluation were described in Chapter 2. In Chapter 3 we have identified and discussed 10 questions that readers of economic evaluations can ask in order to critically assess a particular study; a check-list of these questions is given in Box 3.1.

Our intent in offering a check-list is not to create hypercritical users who will be satisfied only by superlative studies. It is important to realize, as emphasized at the outset, that for a variety of reasons it is unlikely that every study will satisfy all criteria.

However, the use of these criteria as screening devices should help users of economic evaluations to identify quickly the strengths and weaknesses of studies. Moreover, in assessing any particular study, users should ask themselves one final question, '*How does this evaluation compare with our normal basis for decision-making?*' They may find that the method of organizing thoughts embodied in the evaluation compares well with alternative approaches, even bearing in mind the possible deficiencies in the study.

3.4. **Critical appraisal of a published article**

Reference: Mark D. B., Hlatky, M. A., Califf, R. M., *et al.* (1995). Cost-effectiveness of thrombolytic therapy with tissue plasminogen activator as compared with streptokinase for acute myocardial infarction. *New England Journal of Medicine*, **332**, 1418–24.

1. Was a well-defined question posed in an answerable form?

X YES _____NO _____CAN'T TELL

The authors explain the context of their study, which is that some observers have questioned whether the improved survival rates observed in the GUSTO study (a multicentre, randomized clinical trial, comparing t-PA with SK) are worth the substantial additional cost (p. 1418).

The authors state that they conducted a CEA to compare the value of t-PA treatment with that of SK (p. 1418).

They state that they used a social perspective to identify relevant costs, although indirect costs (for example, time lost from work) and non-medical costs were not included (p. 1419). The reasons for exclusion of some relevant costs are not given. The reader would have to assess whether the exclusion of some costs biases the results.

2. Was a comprehensive description of the competing alternatives given (that is, can you tell who did what, to whom, where, and how often)?

X YES _____NO _____CAN'T TELL

Details are given of the GUSTO study, which compared four different regimens: accelerated t-PA, SK with intravenous heparin, SK with subcutaneous heparin, and a combination of t-PA and SK. Accelerated is defined as the administration of t-PA over a period of 1.5 hours, rather than the conventional period of 3 hours (p. 1418). The alternatives for the economic study are accelerated t-PA and SK.

For further details the reader would have to consult the GUSTO clinical study. However, one can infer a hospital setting as SK can only be administered in hospital. One important factor is the period of time after acute myocardial infarction before patients receive thrombolytic therapy. This has been shown to be important in previous studies, but no details are given here.

In addition, some subgroup analyses are performed, by age of patient and location of infarction. Implicitly these represent additional alternatives for economic analysis, although they are not the major alternatives being examined.

The alternatives considered in the economic study are constrained by those being compared in the clinical trial. Therefore, the reader would need to consider whether there are any other relevant alternatives. These could include other drugs, or non-pharmacological interventions such as angioplasty. In principle the alternative of 'doing nothing' could be relevant but, because prior clinical studies have found that SK is efficacious, it could be considered unethical to offer no therapy at all, although it would also be important to establish that SK therapy was itself cost-effective.

3. Was there evidence that the programme's effectiveness had been established?

X YES_____ NO _____CAN'T TELL

The primary clinical endpoint, survival to 1 year, was estimated in the randomized controlled trial, representing the strongest form of evidence. One year after enrolment, patients who received t-PA had a higher survival rate (an increase of 1.1%, or 11 per 1000 patients treated) than SK-treated patients.

However, in order to calculate the life-years gained, the denominator in the cost-effectiveness ratio, it was necessary to extrapolate beyond 1 year. This was done by (1) a Cox proportional-hazards model based on the experience of 4379 patients in the Duke Cardiovascular Disease Database (giving an extrapolation from 1 to 15 years) and (2) a statistical extrapolation for the tail of the survival curve (beyond 15 years) (p. 1419).

A number of assumptions were necessary for the extrapolation, the main one being that the hazard of death after 1 year did not depend on the thrombolytic agent received (that is, that the survival curves of the two treatment groups were parallel).

4. Were all the important and relevant costs and consequences for each alternative identified?

_____YES _____NO X CAN'T TELL

As mentioned above, changes in productive output and non-medical costs were excluded. This probably makes no substantial difference to the cost-effectiveness ratio, but it is hard to tell.

One area where these costs could be important is in disabling, non-fatal stroke. In the first 30 days after treatment in the GUSTO study, t-PA produced a net increase of one disabling non-fatal stroke per 1000 patients treated, as compared with the rate with SK. The authors investigate the impact of stroke on medical costs and overall reduction in the life expectancy for the t-PA group in a sensitivity analysis (see below). This has a modest impact on the cost-effectiveness ratio for t-PA. The impact could be greater if the excluded costs were considered.

5. Were costs and consequences measured accurately in appropriate physical units?

X YES _____NO _____CAN'T TELL

The use of medical resources during the initial hospitalization was measured for all the US participants (23 105) in the GUSTO study. Resource use up to 1 year was estimated for a random sample (2600) of the surviving members of the cohort. This was done by telephone survey. (These data are given in Table 2, p.1420.)

Many of the data presented in Table 2 are medians. This is appropriate for testing statistically, as the data are positively skewed. However, for descriptive purposes, means are more informative, as in planning (say) hospital bed provision, it is important to know about the tail of the distribution. However, the resource consumption in the first year was generally similar for the two groups, so did not enter in the incremental cost-effectiveness ratio.

Resource use beyond 1 year was assumed to be the same for both groups. Although telephone surveys may not be the ideal method of determining resource use, practical considerations would seriously limit other methods. Overall, the authors provide an accurate measurement of resource use.

The main consequence of therapy (life-years gained) was estimated by the methods described above.

6. Were costs and consequences valued credibly?

(for costs)   (for consequences)

X YES _____NO X CAN'T TELL

Health state preference values were measured in structured telephone interviews 1 year after treatment by the time trade-off method (p. 1419). Thus, the quality of life impact of some morbidity, particularly that caused by strokes, may have been missed if these patients were unable to complete the interview. However, it would be unlikely to have a major impact on the result of the study.

The unit costs (prices) used in the analysis are given in Table 1 of the paper. These were a mixture of costs (from Duke University Hospital) and charges (Medicare Diagnosis Related Group (DRG) reimbursement rates). Two approaches were used to estimate the costs of the thrombolytic drugs, because these had a major impact on the results.

7. Were costs and consequences adjusted for differential timing?

X YES _____NO _____CAN'T TELL

Both survival and costs were discounted at an annual rate of 5% (p. 1419). The authors state that this is consistent with conventional practice.

8. Was an incremental analysis of costs and consequences of alternatives performed?

X YES _____NO _____CAN'T TELL

All the cost-effectiveness ratios presented in the paper are incremental of t-PA relative to SK. The primary analysis gave an incremental cost per year of life saved of $32 678.

9. Was allowance made for uncertainty in the estimates of costs and consequences?

X YES _____NO _____CAN'T TELL

A number of one-way sensitivity analyses were performed. These included varying survival and costs in both the short- and the long-term for the t-PA group, such as

(1) taking the 95% confidence interval for the 1.1% increase in 1-year survival, as estimated in the clinical trial;

(2) reducing life expectancy or assuming that the survival curves converge after 1 year;

(3) assuming that the (non-significant) increase in 1-year costs of t-PA (excluding the cost of the drug) did truly exist;

(4) assuming that the non-significant increase in costs was maintained beyond 1 year;

(5) assuming that the price for t-PA was much lower (for example, the same as a typical European price).

In addition, sensitivity analyses were conducted on the impact of disabling strokes, and leaving costs and consequences undiscounted.

Finally, the quality of life adjustment is presented as a sensitivity analysis on the cost-effectiveness ratio. The incremental cost-effectiveness ratio changes from $32 678 per life-year gained to $36 402 per QALY.

In general, the authors highlight the changes in assumptions that would cause the incremental cost-effectiveness ratio to rise above a threshold of $50 000 per life-year gained.

10. Did the presentation and discussion of study results include all issues of concern to users?

___ YES _____ NO X CAN'T TELL

The authors include a fairly full discussion of the results. They introduce the notion that the upper limit for an acceptable cost-effectiveness ratio remains controversial, but values of more than $100 000 per year of life saved are generally considered too high (p. 1422). Most estimates of the incremental ratio are less than $100 000.

The authors state that their subgroup analyses should be interpreted cautiously. A major finding is that the incremental cost-effectiveness ratios for treatment by t-PA are more favourable for the older patients (especially those above 60 years old). This is because, although the younger patients have potentially the greatest number of life-years to gain, they also have the lowest 1-year mortality rates and the smallest increases in survival due to treatment with t-PA. The clinical and social implications of this finding are not explored.

Another issue, not explored in the paper, is whether the findings are generalizable beyond the trial and transferable to other settings. For example, the accelerated use of t-PA may not be achievable in some hospitals. In addition, other papers commenting on the GUSTO study have pointed out that the US patients (56% of total recruitment) were managed differently from the non-US patients in a number of ways, including greater use of invasive revascularization such as percutaneous transluminal coronary angioplasty and coronary artery bypass grafting, and greater use of non-protocol medications (van der Werf *et al.* 1995).

This could lead to differences in costs and, in addition, the mortality reduction with t-PA was greater in the USA (1.2% absolute decrease versus 0.7% elsewhere). However, the test for treatment-by-country interaction was not significant.

Finally, the costs of resources could vary from place to place, so it may not be wise to assume that similar results would be found in other locations.

References

Black, W. C. (1990). The cost-effectiveness plane: a graphic representation of cost-effectiveness. *Medical Decision Making*, **10**, 212–15.

Boyle, M. H., Torrance, G. W., Horwood, S. P., and Sinclair, J. C. (1982). *A cost analysis of providing neonatal intensive care to 500–1499-gram birth-weight infants*, Research Report No. 51, Programme for Quantitative Studies in Economics and Population. McMaster University, Hamilton, Ontario.

Boyle, M. H., Torrance, G. W., Sinclair, J. C., and Horwood, S. P. (1983). Economic evaluation of neonatal intensive care of very-low-birth-weight infants. *New England Journal of Medicine*, **308**, 1330–7.

Briggs, A. H. (2001). Handling uncertainty in economic evaluation. In: *Economic evaluation in health care: merging theory with practice* (ed. M. F. Drummond and A. McGuire), pp. 172–214. Oxford University Press, Oxford.

Briggs, A. H. and Sculpher, M. J. (1995). Sensitivity analysis in economic evaluation: a review of published studies. *Health Economics*, **4**, 355–71.

Briggs, A. H., Sculpher, M. J., Britton, A., Murray, D., Fitzpatrick, R. (1988). The costs and benefits of primary total hip replacement. *International Journal of Technology Assessment in Health Care*, **14**, 743–61.

Briggs, A. H., Sculpher, M. J., and Buxton, M. J. (1994). Uncertainty in the economic evaluation of health care technologies: the role of sensitivity analysis. *Health Economics*, **3**, 95–104.

Drummond, M. F. (1981). Welfare economics and cost–benefit analysis in health care. *Scottish Political Economy*, **28**, 125–45.

EuroQoL Group (1990). EuroQoL—a new facility for the measurement of health-related quality of life. *Health Policy*, **16**, 199–208.

Feeny, D., Furlong, W., Boyle, M., and Torrance, G. (1995). Multi-attribute health status classifications systems: health utilities index. *PharmacoEconomics*, **7**, 490–502.

Gold, M. R., Siegel, J. E., Russell, L. B., and Weinstein, M. (ed.) (1996). *Cost-effectiveness in health and medicine*. Oxford University Press, New York.

Goldsmith, C. H., Gafni, A., Drummond, M. F., Torrance, G. W., and Stoddart, G. L. (1987). Sensitivity analysis and experimental design: the case for economic evaluation of health care programmes. In: *Proceedings of the Third Canadian Conference on Health Economics 1986* (ed. J. M. Horn), pp. 129–48. Department of Social and Preventive Medicine, University of Manitoba, Winnipeg.

Guyatt, G. and Rennie, D. (ed.) (2002). *Users' guides to the medical literature: a manual for evidence-based clinical practice*. AMA, Chicago.

Hull, R., Hirsh, J., Sackett, D. L., and Stoddart, G. L. (1981). Cost-effectiveness of clinical diagnosis, venography and non-invasive testing in patients with symptomatic deep-vein thrombosis. *New England Journal of Medicine*, **304**, 1561–7.

Hull, R., Hirsh, J., Sackett, D. L., and Stoddart, G. L. (1982). Cost-effectiveness of primary and secondary prevention of pulmonary embolism in high-risk surgical patients. *Canadian Medical Association Journal*, **127**, 990–5.

Khan, K. S., ter Riet, G., Glanville, J., Sowden, A. J., and Kleijnen, J. (ed.) (2001). *Undertaking systematic reviews of research on effectiveness*, CRD Report Number 4 (2nd edn). Centre for Reviews and Dissemination, University of York, York.

Mark D. B., Hlatky, M. A., Califf, R. M., *et al.* (1995). Cost-effectiveness of thrombolytic therapy with tissue plasminogen activator as compared with streptokinase for acute myocardial infarction. *New England Journal of Medicine*, **332**, 1418–24.

Neuhauser, D. and Lewicki, A. M. (1975). What do we gain from the sixth stool guaiac? *New England Journal of Medicine*, **293**, 226–8.

Sackett, D. L., Haynes, R. B., Guyatt, G. H., and Tugwell, P. (1991). *Clinical epidemiology: a basic science for clinical medicine* (2nd edn). Little Brown, Boston, Massachusetts.

Schackman, B. R., Taffet Gold, H., Stone, P. W., and Neumann, P. J. (2004). How often do sensitivity analyses for economic parameters change cost–utility analysis conclusions? *PharmacoEconomics*, **22**, 293–300.

Sculpher, M. J., Poole, L., Cleland, J., *et al.* (2000). Low doses versus high doses of angiotensin converting enzyme inhibitor lisinopril in chronic heart failure: a cost-effectiveness analysis based on the Assessment of Treatment with Lisinopril and Survival Analysis (ATLAS) study. *European Journal of Heart Failure*, **2**, 447–54.

van der Werf, F., Topol, E. J., Lee, K. L., *et al.* (1995). Variations in patient management and outcomes for acute myocardial infarction in the United States and other countries. *Journal of the American Medical Association*, **273**, 1586–91.

Weisbrod, B. A., Test, M. A., and Stein, L. I. (1980). Alternatives to mental hospital treatment, II. Economic benefit–cost analysis. *Archives of General Psychiatry*, **37**, 400–5.

Chapter 4

Cost analysis

4.1. **Some basics**

The analysis of the comparative costs of alternative treatments or health care programmes is common to all forms of economic evaluation and therefore most of the methodological issues discussed in this chapter are likely to be of relevance to all analyses. Although many of the issues surrounding costing are context specific and the analyst's options are often limited by the availability of data, it is possible to give some general guidance. Three particularly thorny issues, the treatment of overhead costs (techniques for allocating shared overhead costs to individual projects), the allowance for differential timing of costs (the techniques of discounting and annuitization of capital expenditure), and the role and estimation of productivity costs will be discussed in some detail. However, the chapter begins by covering some of the basic questions that an evaluator might have when embarking on a costing study in the health field.

4.1.1. **Which costs should be considered?**

The main categories of costs of health care programmes or treatments were identified in Fig. 3.1 of Chapter 3; these are the costs arising from the use of resources within the health sector, the resource use by patients and their families, the resource use in other sectors, and productivity changes. The particular range of costs included in a given study is likely to be decided upon as a result of considering the following four points.

1. What is the viewpoint for the analysis?
It is essential to specify the viewpoint because an item may be a cost from one point of view, but not a cost from another (see Box 4.1). For example, patients' travel costs are a cost from the patient's point of view and from society's point of view, but not a cost from the Ministry of Health's point of view. Workers compensation payments are a cost to the paying government, a gain to the patient (recipient), and neither a cost nor a gain to society. (These money transfers, which do not reflect resource consumption, are called *transfer payments* by economists; costs are involved in their administration, but these are not measured by the amounts themselves.)

Possible points of view include those of society, the Ministry of Health, other government ministries, the government in general, the patient, the employer, and the agency providing the programme. If the evaluation is being commissioned by a given body, this may give a clue to the relevant point(s) of view. However, when in doubt the analyst should always adopt the societal point of view, which is the broadest one and is always relevant.

Box 4.1 **The influence of viewpoint on study results**

The study by Weisbrod *et al.* (1980) shows how a different answer can be obtained depending upon the viewpoint adopted. It can be seen from the table that a community-oriented programme for mental illness patients looks expensive from the viewpoint of the agency providing the programme, compared with a traditional hospital-based programme (an extra $1700 per annum).

However, when costs falling on other health care agencies and those involved in law enforcement are considered, the cost difference is reduced. Finally, when broader societal costs and benefits are considered, such as the provision of food and shelter and the differences in productivity resulting from patients' ability to work, the community-oriented programme has a lower net cost ($400 per annum lower).

Item	Community-oriented programme ($ per annum)	Hospital-based programme ($ per annum)	Difference in programmes ($ per annum)
Costs (C)			
Primary treatment costs	4800	3100	1700
Other treatment costs (e.g. social services)	1800	2100	
Wider social costs (e.g. law enforcement, food, shelter)	1420	2020	
Benefits (B)			
Patient earnings	2400	1200	
Net economic cost (B–C)	5620	6020	400

Adapted from Weisbrod *et al.* (1980).

2. Is the comparison restricted to the two or more programmes immediately under study?

If the comparison is restricted to the programmes or treatments immediately under study, costs common to both need not be considered as they will not affect the choice between the given programmes. (Elimination of such costs can save the evaluator a considerable amount of work.) However, if it is thought that at some later stage a broader comparison may be contemplated, including other alternatives not yet specified, it might be prudent to consider all the costs of the programmes.

3. Are some costs merely likely to confirm a result that would be obtained by consideration of a narrower range of costs?

Sometimes the consideration of patients' costs merely confirms a result that might be obtained from, say, consideration of only operating costs within the health sector. Therefore, if consideration of patients' costs requires extra effort and the choice of programme is very unlikely to be changed, it may not be worthwhile to complicate the analysis unnecessarily. However, some justification for such an exclusion of a cost category should be given.

4. What is the relative order of magnitude of costs?

It is not worth investing a great deal of time and effort considering costs that, because they are small, are unlikely to make any difference to the study result. However, some justification should be given for the elimination of such costs, perhaps based on previous empirical work. It is still worthwhile identifying such cost categories in any event, although the estimation of them might not be pursued in any great detail.

Above all, the main point to remember when embarking on a costing study is that, to an economist, cost refers to the sacrifice (of benefits) made when a given resource is consumed in a programme or treatment. Therefore, it is important not to confine one's attention to expenditures, but to consider also other resources, the consumption of which is not adequately reflected in market prices, for example, volunteer time, patients' leisure time, and donated clinic space.

4.1.2. **How should costs be estimated?**

Once the relevant range of costs has been identified, the individual items must be measured and valued. That is, costing has two elements: measurement of the *quantities* of resource use (q) and the assignment of unit costs or *prices* (p). The measurement of resource quantities often depends on the context for the economic evaluation. For example, if an economic study is being conducted alongside a clinical trial, data on the resource quantities may be collected on the case report forms. On the other hand, if the economic study is free standing, resource quantities may be estimated by a review of patients charts (case notes) or from routine data systems, such as hospital records. The quantities of some resources, such as domiciliary nursing visits, may only be estimated by asking patients, or by having them keep a diary.

Market prices will be available for many of the resource items. Although the theoretical proper price for a resource is its opportunity cost (that is, the value of the forgone benefits because the resource is not available for its best alternative use), the pragmatic approach to costing is to take existing market prices unless there is some particular reason to do otherwise (for example, the price of some resources may be subsidized by a third party such as a charitable institution). This is discussed further below.

Although the costing of most resource items is relatively unambiguous, the following issues commonly arise in costing studies.

1. How are values imputed for non-market items?

The major non-market resource inputs to health care programmes are volunteer time and patient/family leisure time. One approach to the valuation of these would be to use market wage rates (for example, for volunteer time one might use unskilled wage rates). The market value of leisure time is harder to assess. One can argue for a value of lost leisure time of anything from zero, through average earnings, to average overtime earnings (time and a half or double time). The argument for the overtime rate is that this is the price that an employer must pay, at the margin, to buy some of the worker's leisure time. Brouwer *et al.* (2001) argue that the valuation of informal care (for example, provided by relatives or volunteers) should depend on what time is being sacrificed (for example, paid work, unpaid work, or leisure time). The most common practice in the literature is to value leisure time at zero in the base case (or primary) analysis. This reflects the fact that often the viewpoint specified by the decision-maker or person commissioning the study excludes consideration of patient or family costs. However, patients' time costs in obtaining care are a relevant considera-tion in an economic evaluation undertaken from a societal perspective (Gold *et al.* 1996). Therefore they should at least be pointed out to the decision-maker, even if they are not included in the primary analysis.

A slightly different approach is to identify and measure units of (say) volunteer, family, or patient time input and to document these alongside the other costs when reporting results. This would enable the decision-maker to note those programmes relying heavily on volunteer or family support. It would then be up to the programme director (or advocate of the programme or therapy) to demonstrate that such an input could be obtained without an opportunity cost to other programmes arising from the diversion of volunteer or family time to the new programme.

2. When should existing market prices be adjusted?

It has long been recognized that, owing to the imperfections in health care markets, market prices may not reflect opportunity costs. For example, hospital charges may deviate from costs if a hospital has a local monopoly or seeks to cross-subsidize one activity from another (Finkler 1982). Physician fees may not accurately reflect the relative skill level and time required for different procedures. Drug prices may be set in negoti-ations between a pharmaceutical company and the government, where the company's commitment to research and provision of employment might be taken into account, as well as the costs of discovery, production, and distribution of the drug in question.

Having said that, it is by no means clear when an analyst should attempt to adjust observed market prices to reflect true opportunity costs. As mentioned above, most studies use market prices unadjusted and it has often been remarked that health economists recognize that market imperfections exist in health care, unless they are undertaking an economic evaluation!

In order for analysts to attempt to adjust market prices, they should be convinced that

1 to leave prices unadjusted would introduce substantial biases into the study;

2 there is a clear and objective way of making the adjustments.

These issues have been explored most extensively in the context of hospital charges in the USA. For example, Cohen *et al.* (1993) found that charges for cardiac procedures were substantially different from costs, although the relationships between the four procedures were largely unchanged (see Box 4.2). In a more recent study Taira *et al.* (2003) compared four methods of estimating costs in three trials involving percutaneous coronary revascularization: (1) hospital charges; (2) hospital charges converted to costs by use of hospital-level cost-to-charge ratios; (3) hospital charges converted to costs by use of department-level cost-to-charge ratios; and (4) itemized laboratory costs with non-procedural hospital costs generated from department-level cost-to-charge ratios.

Their findings were similar to those of Cohen *et al.* (1993), in that, while there were big differences in the magnitude of the estimates obtained by the various methods,

Box 4.2 **Costs or charges: does it make a difference?**

An analysis was undertaken by Cohen *et al.* (1993) of in-hospital charges from the itemized hospital accounts of 3000 patients at Boston's Beth Israel Hospital (1990 and 1991). Costs were then derived by adjusting for department-specific cost/charge ratios by using data on actual resource consumption. Comparison of estimates showed the following.

	Standard hospital charges (SD)	Costs (SD)
PTCA	$8369 ($3885)	$5396($2829)
Atherectomy	$8391($2299)	$5726 ($2716)
Stent	$12670 ($5247)	$7828 ($3270)
CABG	$27739($7051)	$20927 ($6048)

It can be seen that whilst the ordering (in expense) of the procedures remains the same, the absolute differences change. From Cohen *et al.* (1993).

the method used to approximate costs did not affect the main results of the economic comparisons for any of the trials. They also concluded that conversion of hospital charges to costs on the basis of department-level cost-to-charge ratios appears to represent a reasonable compromise between accuracy and ease of implementation.

The methodology employed by Cohen *et al.*, and many other studies in the USA, was to derive costs by adjusting for department-specific cost-to-charge ratios. (These are generally in the public domain.) This is probably an improvement on the uncritical use of charges, but it is still dependent upon the quality of the accountancy study that generated the costs in the first place. Often this is difficult to assess. Nevertheless, adjustments by cost-to-charge ratios are becoming more commonplace in studies undertaken in the USA. For example, Nigrovic and Chiang (2000) calculated costs from charges 'using a standard cost-to-charge ratio of 0.65'. Zupancic *et al.* (2003) converted charges to costs 'using cost center-specific Medicare ratios of costs to charges for the Brigham and Women's Hospital for 1991'.

If the results of studies are relatively insensitive to the method used to approximate costs, should we be concerned about this issue? Only to the extent that, when costs or cost-effectiveness ratios for treatments are compared across studies, the differences observed may be partly dependent on the precise type of cost-to-charge adjustments.

In general, there is probably no substitute for a well-conducted original costing study. In most countries, where hospital charges are not as detailed as in the USA, this is often the analyst's only alternative to using a general *per diem* or average hospital cost. However, comparisons across studies could still be problematic due to the range of costing methods used. In a recent review, Adam *et al.* (2003) identified considerable variations in the costing methods used. In their view this raises questions about the validity of study results and makes it difficult to compare the results of different studies.

Furthermore, in multicountry studies the availability of financial data and the variations in accounting practices can impact upon results, even if attempts are made to standardize costing methodology. Schulman *et al.* (1998) attempted to cost procedures used in the treatment of subarachnoid haemorrhage in seven countries. The results are shown in Table 4.1. It can be seen that there are considerable variations in estimates across countries, many of which do not appear to be systematic. Also, approximately 30% of the estimates had to be imputed because they were not available in the countries concerned.

Finally, we should note that if the economic study is being undertaken from the viewpoint of the third party payer, the actual charges may be more relevant than the costs, although often the third party does not pay the full amount billed.

Table 4.1 Reported procedure and *per diem* costs for study countries

	Costs (US$)						
	Germany	**Italy**	**France**	**Sweden**	**UK**	**Australia**	**Spain**
Procedure Costs							
Burr holes	130	77	216	*372*	365	711	72
Chest tubes	87	210	*150*	175	*201*	120	93
Central nervous system shunt	1148	1749	617	371	357	699	*526*
Craniofacial procedures	*350*	*471*	*628*	693	*843*	888	*673*
Cranioplasty	*590*	794	*1059*	*1557*	1420	*1197*	*1134*
Debridement of brain	824	357	740	1386	2247	717	552
Dialysis	*153*	206	*275*	*404*	*368*	*310*	294
Elevation of skull fracture	367	357	483	693	377	*505*	336
Evacuation of lesion	506	357	493	1386	476	*722*	705
Filtration for renal failure	*248*	*334*	*441*	*655*	597	759	234
Gastroscopy	*106*	245	63	347	256	156	*204*
Gastrostomy (procedure)	79	*148*	361	*290*	*264*	*223*	95
Humeral shaft fracture	*287*	*386*	106	*757*	1904	*582*	21
Intracranial drainage	273	432	*340*	175	365	389	259
Laparotomy (exploratory)	130	209	301	866	462	573	492
Lobectomy	*544*	830	*977*	1040	569	2251	705
Peritoneal lavage	*38*	117	*69*	*102*	*93*	23	34
Removal of bone flap	506	357	411	175	408	1650	332
Replacement of bone flap	809	604	524	*1203*	526	1308	616
Shunt placement	*642*	1749	*1152*	260	2087	*1302*	580
Spine operation	*1125*	1515	*2019*	*2970*	2708	*2283*	2164
Splenectomy	249	389	*483*	*711*	648	*547*	*518*
Swan-Ganz monitor	*207*	335	*371*	*546*	498	420	317
Superficial laceration	16	31	20	175	154	*68*	36
Tracheostomy	151	120	301	347	256	1105	132
Per diem costs							
Daily intensive care unit	445	601	774	1231	1159	945	876
Daily intermediate care unit	*169*	304	301	573	315	207	*324*
Daily routine care unit	134	187	350	267	173	159	236
Daily rehabilitation unit	140	324	210	336	*384*	186	464

Actual costs are in plain text; market-basket imputed costs are in italic text.

From Schulman *et al.* (1998).

3. For how long should costs be tracked?

It can be seen from Fig. 4.1 that not only does the analyst have a choice about whose costs to consider but also a choice of time period. In assessing how long costs should be tracked, the main objective should be to avoid misleading the decision-maker or user. For example, a comparison of the costs of coronary artery bypass grafting (CABG) versus percutaneous transluminal coronary angioplasty (PTCA) to hospital discharge has shown CABG to be substantially more expensive ($9138 versus $22 711) (Black *et al.* 1988). However, there is a possibility that patients receiving PTCA may require additional treatment subsequently, including CABG. In a costing study undertaken alongside a randomized controlled trial, Sculpher *et al.* (1993) showed that by 24 months after randomization, the cost difference between patients randomized to the alternative therapies had reduced substantially. After 72 months the cumulative costs were virtually indistinguishable, with overlapping confidence intervals (Henderson *et al.* 1998) (see Fig. 4.2).

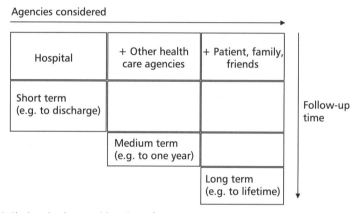

Fig. 4.1 Choices in the consideration of costs.

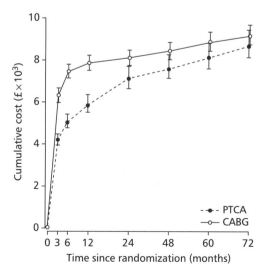

Fig. 4.2 Cumulative costs of percutaneous transluminal coronary angioplasty (PTCA) and coronary artery bypass grafting (CABG) over time (confidence intervals indicated by the bars) (from Henderson *et al.* 1998).

There is fairly broad agreement amongst analysts that in the case of *therapy-specific* or *disease-specific* costs, the choice of follow-up period should not bias the analysis in favour of one intervention over another. In some cases this may involve tracking costs for lifetime, although the quantitative impact of costs (on the analysis) far into the future will be reduced by discounting to present values (see Section 4.2). Nevertheless, most analysts feel that all *related* health care costs should be included.

Another issue related to the costing period is that of learning curves (Brouwer *et al.* 2001). That is, because health professionals learn how to become more efficient in the use of new health technologies, the costs in the early stages of use may not be a good predictor of costs in the long run. Examples include the dosage, administration and wastage of drugs, the time taken to perform surgical procedures, and the monitoring of adverse events. Therefore, when costing new or emerging technologies it may be prudent to anticipate that learning effects may occur, although of course the timing of the economic evaluation will often be determined by the need to make a decision about the appropriate use of the new technology. In particular, in costing a new procedure over time it may be worthwhile checking whether the costs towards the end of the period are similar to those in the early months.

4. Should health care costs unrelated to the programme or intervention under study be included?

The question of whether *unrelated* health care costs in the future should be included is much more open to debate. On the one hand, health care costs in later years of life are a clear consequence of keeping individuals alive. On the other hand, it does not seem totally fair to assign these costs to a prevention programme (for example, hypertension screening), when they result from therapeutic decisions (for example, to give cancer chemotherapy for advanced stages of disease) that should be considered on their own merits. Nevertheless, it is common in evaluations of prevention programmes to assign all the credit for life extension, or gains in QALYs, to the programme concerned. Therefore, it would make sense to assign all costs if a generic measure of outcome is being used.

In considering this issue it has to be remembered that all the forms of economic evaluation discussed in this book are what economists call partial equilibrium analyses. That is, whilst it is recognized that any change in economic activity (such as investment in health programmes) includes many ripples throughout the economy, it is argued that such investments can be assessed against a background of all else remaining constant. Therefore, an artificial boundary is always being drawn around analyses.

There is no agreement amongst economic analysts about whether unrelated health care costs in later years of life should be included (Gold *et al.* 1996). However, two considerations may guide our decision about the importance of trying to estimate them. These are

(1) the extent to which the provision of additional care in added years of life is a necessary consequence of the programme being evaluated;

(2) the availability of data.

Taking the first consideration, if we were evaluating a new drug for treatment of septic shock in intensive care, it would be reasonable to assume that patients surviving an episode of septic shock were likely to have treatment for their underlying morbid condition. Therefore, these costs would be a direct consequence of giving the drug therapy (Schulman *et al.* 1991). The same would be true of the costs of diagnosing and treating cases of disease identified by a screening programme. These costs are very closely linked and it would make sense to evaluate the costs and consequences of screening, diagnosis, and treatment as a single package.

On the other hand, if we were evaluating a new drug for treatment of hypercholes-terolaemia, the added years of life, through reduction in the incidence of coronary heart disease, may be in the distant future. Treatment of unrelated disease (for example, cancer) is not a necessary consequence of treatment of hypercholesterolaemia and may be determined by protocols that have not yet been defined. Few analysts attempt to track all these costs and consequences, although it is clear that additional costs will be incurred if individuals live longer. However, the fact that such costs and consequences are more distant is not the only consideration that leads to their frequent exclusion from economic evaluations. (Indeed it could be argued that the costs of treating the coronary heart disease events are themselves distant, but most analysts would include these in an evaluation of drugs for hypercholesterolaemia.) In commenting on this debate, Weinstein and Manning (1997) argue that, in order to be consistent in the practice of including only 'related' costs, we would have to tease out which costs were truly 'related' and which were not.

The other consideration relates to the availability of data. Ideally, in projecting to the future we would like data on the likely health care costs of those individuals whose lives would be extended by drug therapy for hypercholesterolaemia. Often it is very difficult to be more precise than an average annual per capita health expenditure, perhaps age related. Therefore, one approach would be to include an estimate of age-related per capita health expenditure on the cost side of the equation for every year of life added by the intervention. This amount could either be included as a gross amount, or net of medical expenses that were already being included for treatment of the individual's main condition. Depending on the importance the analyst attaches to costs in added years of life, these could either be included in the primary analysis or a sensitivity analysis.

When estimates such as these have been included in economic evaluation of health care programmes they sometimes do not alter cost-effectiveness ratios by very much. For example, Drummond *et al.* (1993) found that adding an average expenditure figure for costs in added years of life only changed their estimate of the cost per life-year gained from treatment for hypercholesterolaemia by 2%. However, when Daly *et al.* (1992) added costs in extra years of life to their evaluation of hormone replacement therapy, this increased total programme costs, and the cost per life-year gained, by around 10%.

The small quantitative impact in the examples given is partly due to the fact that costs in added years of life are often heavily discounted and, in the words of one analyst, 'may amount to no more than a hill of beans' (Bush 1973). Therefore, in many instances it may be that unrelated health care costs in added years of life can be ignored without seriously biasing the analysis. However, the quantitative importance of costs in added years of life may vary from one evaluation to another and requires more empirical investigation.

A much broader issue is that of whether related and unrelated *non-health care* costs should be included. Meltzer (1997) makes a strong case for considering *all* future costs in economic evaluations, including the impacts that treatments have on individuals' production and consumption. Studies have shown that this analytic judgement does make a difference to the results. Johannesson *et al.* (1997) found that, relative to other health care interventions, including unrelated non-health care costs improves the cost-effectiveness of life-saving programmes among younger individuals.

Weinstein and Manning (1997) argue that, from a 'welfarist perspective', the inclusion of future non-health care costs is technically correct, 'but will give some practitioners pause to accepting the welfare-theoretical foundation of CEA'. This is clearly an issue on which our three fictitious analysts, introduced in Chapter 2, would take different views. Analyst A would definitely include non-health care costs in added years of life, whereas Analyst B would definitely exclude them. Analyst C might adopt a position similar to that of Olsen and Richardson (1999), who argue that in collectively financed health care systems there is a strong preference for 'equal access for equal need'. This suggests that some production gains should be disregarded. The 'socially relevant' part of the production gains depends on differences in patients' potential contributions to the rest of society and the strength of preferences for equity. In particular, society may be interested in production gains to the extent that these increase the resources available for health care. Therefore analysts should indicate clearly the stance that they take on these issues and perhaps consider a sensitivity analysis of the inclusion and exclusion of costs in added years of life.

5. How should capital outlays (on equipment, buildings, and land) be handled?
Capital costs are the costs to purchase the major capital assets required by the programme; generally equipment, buildings, and land. Capital costs differ from operating costs in a number of ways. First, they represent investments at a single point in time, often at the beginning of the programme, rather than annual sums like operating costs. Frequently, the capital costs are often not listed in the accounts or budgets of the organization because they have been funded in advance, perhaps by a one-time grant, while the budgets and accounts represent operating expenses only. Sometimes, the annual budgets and accounts contain an item called depreciation, which relates to capital costs, as explained below.

Capital costs represent an investment in an asset that is used over time. Most assets, such as equipment and buildings, wear out or depreciate with time. On the other hand, land is a non-depreciable asset because it maintains its value. There are two components of capital cost. One is the opportunity cost of the funds tied up in the capital asset. This is clearly seen in the case of land. Although an investment in non-depreciable land will return the original capital sum when sold, there is still a 'cost'. This cost is the lost opportunity to invest the sum in some other venture yielding positive benefits. It is usually valued by applying an interest rate (equal to the discount rate used in the study) to the amount of capital invested. (Discounting is discussed below.)

The second component of a capital cost represents the depreciation over time of the asset itself. Various accounting procedures (straight line, declining balance, double declining balance, and so on) are available for use in the accounts of the organization. Often, accounting practices relate more to the company tax laws governing the depreciation of assets than to the real change in the value of the asset.

There are several methods of measuring and valuing capital costs in an economic evaluation. The best method is to annuitize the initial capital outlay over the useful life of the asset; that is, to calculate the 'equivalent annual cost'. This method and its advantages are discussed in more detail by Richardson and Gafni (1983). The method automatically incorporates both the depreciation aspect and the opportunity cost aspect of the capital cost. It is our preferred approach and will be described in Section 4.2. An alternative but less exact method is to determine the depreciation cost each year using an accounting method and to determine the opportunity cost on the undepreciated balance for each year (see Levin 1975; Boyle *et al.* 1982). Where market rates exist for the rental of buildings or lease of equipment, these may be used to estimate capital costs. This method also incorporates both the depreciation and the opportunity components of the cost.

If capital outlays relate to resources that are used by more than one programme they may require allocation in a similar fashion to 'overhead' costs. See the discussion of this point below.

6. What is the significance of the average cost-marginal cost distinction?

Economists tend to emphasize this point, and the example of the sixth stool guaiac in Chapter 2 illustrated the pitfalls in making decisions based on average cost. In fact, marginal cost and average cost are but two concepts relating costs to quantity (Horngren 1994). (See Boxes 4.3 and 4.4.)

The major significance of the average cost/marginal cost distinction to the evaluator is as follows. First, when making a comparison of two or more programmes it is worth asking independently of each, 'What would be the costs (and consequences) of having a little more or a little less?' (For example, suppose Neuhauser and Lewicki (1975) had been comparing the six-stool protocol for detecting colonic cancer with

---

Box 4.3 **Various definitions of cost**

Total cost (TC)	= cost of producing a particular quantity of output
Fixed cost (FC)	= costs which do not vary with the quantity of output in the short run (about 1 year), for example, rent, equipment lease payments, some wages and salaries. That is, costs which vary with time, rather than quantity
Variable cost (VC)	= costs which vary with the level of output, for example, supplies, food, fees for service
Cost function (TC)	= $f(Q)$, total cost as a function of quantity
Average cost (AC)	= TC/Q, the average cost per unit of output
Marginal cost (MC)	= (TC of $x + 1$ units) − (TC of x units)
	= d(TC)/dQ evaluated at x
	= the *extra* cost of producing *one* extra unit of output

Box 4.4 **Is it marginal or incremental?**

The terms 'marginal' and 'incremental' are often used interchangeably in the literature. They both refer to a change in the scale of an activity. Strictly speaking, the *marginal cost* relates to the cost of producing *one extra* unit of output. However, it is often used to refer to the cost of producing the *next logical batch* of output, for example, in expanding a screening programme from high-risk people only to the whole population.

The term 'incremental' is sometimes also used to refer to such a change, but is more often used to refer to the difference, in cost or effect, between the two or more programmes being compared in the evaluation.

In the figure below, MC_A, Q_1 is the marginal cost of programme A evaluated at quantity (scale of activity) Q_1. MC_B, Q_1 is the equivalent estimate for programme B. The incremental cost, of programme A over programme B, evaluated at Q_1, is IC_{A-B}, Q_1.

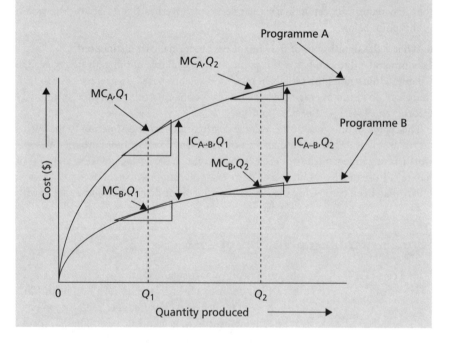

another diagnostic test. Perhaps the question of six- versus five-tests may never have been asked!) Second, when examining the effects (on cost) of small changes in output, it is likely that these will differ from average costs. For example, the extra cost of keeping patients in hospital for another day at the end of their treatment might be less than the average daily cost for the whole stay. (In fact, this issue usually arises in the opposite sense—the savings from a reduction of one day's stay are usually lower than the average daily cost (see Box 4.5).)

Box 4.5 **Estimating the cost savings associated with reductions in hospital in-patient stay**

Hospital cost can be considered to consist of two elements: the hotel cost, which is broadly constant over the length of stay, and the treatment cost, which may peak just after admission but then tail off in the later days of the stay (see the figure below).

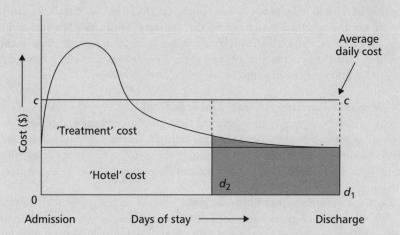

If the length of stay is reduced from d_1 to d_2, use of the average daily cost (c) would give an estimate of the saving of $c(d_1 - d_2)$. However, this would overestimate the actual saving, the shaded area on the diagram. Saving in this case means the value of the resources freed for alternative uses. Whether they *will* be usefully redeployed, or actual expenditure saved, also needs to be investigated.

In practice, whereas it is important to acknowledge the difference between marginal and average costs (or savings), this issue can only really be explored in the context of specific locations or situations. For example, the extent to which costs can be saved when hospital stay is shortened depends on the flexibility available locally and the time period over which the change is made.

Therefore, in some studies analysts turn their attention to issues of marginal costs or savings in the discussion, after presenting average results as the primary analysis. For example, in a study investigating the costs and benefits of shortening time to discharge from a coronary intensive care unit by use of a more expensive sedative agent, Sherry *et al.* (1996) investigated the impact on nurse staffing requirements through fewer patients requiring intensive care during the night. It turned out that the hospital concerned had access to a bank of agency nurse staff that could be called in as required; so it was possible to realize potential savings from fewer patients requiring care. In another hospital, with different nurse staffing arrangements, the outcome could be quite different.

The study by Sherry *et al.* (1996) illustrates that costs, and cost savings, depend greatly on the local context. Very rarely do analysts undertake a 'costing in context'. It was mentioned in Chapter 3 that economic evaluations tacitly assume that freed resources will be redeployed efficiently. Clearly this is not always the case and it is the responsibility of analysts to at least point this out, even if they do not explore the implications in great detail.

The recent report of the United States Public Health Service Panel on *Cost-effectiveness in health and medicine* (Gold *et al.* 1996), recommends that when information on capacity utilization in hospitals or other health care facilities is not available, analysts should use the benchmark assumption that capacity is utilized at the rate of 80%, under a long-run perspective. However, the prime motivation for this was to encourage some consistency in study reporting and the 80% figure is not etched in stone. It is very unlikely to apply in all settings or all health care systems.

7. How should shared (or overhead) costs be handled?

The term '*overhead costs*' is an accounting term for those resources that serve many different departments and programmes, for example, general hospital administration, central laundry, medical records, cleaning, porters, power, and so on. If individual programmes are to be costed, these shared costs may need to be attributed to programmes.

The main point to note at the outset is that there is no unambiguously *right* way to apportion such costs. The approach that is favoured by economists is to employ marginal analysis. That is, to see which (if any) of such costs would change if a given programme were added to, or subtracted from, the overall activity. Whilst this is fine up to a point, the most common situation is that the choice is not such an addition or subtraction, but one between two programmes, each of which would consume the given central services (perhaps because they are competitors for the same space in the hospital). For example, suppose the question concerned space in the hospital that could be used either for anticoagulant therapy for pulmonary embolism, or for renal dialysis. If the economic evaluation concerned a choice between these two programmes then there would be no methodological problem; the costs associated with use of the space would be common to both and could be excluded from the analysis. However, typically the comparison might be between the anticoagulant therapy and another programme in the same field. This could be a programme of more definitive diagnosis of pulmonary embolism, which would avert some hospitalization. In such an instance it would be relevant to obtain an estimate of the value of the freed resources (for example, hospital floor space) that could be diverted to other uses.

A number of methods can be used to determine a more accurate cost of a programme in a hospital or other setting where shared (or overhead) costs are involved. The methods are illustrated below in terms of a hospital setting. The basic idea is to determine the quantities of service consumed by the patient (days of stay in ward A, B, or C, number of laboratory tests of each type, number of radiological procedures, number of operations, and so on), to determine a full cost (including the proper share of overhead, capital, and so on) for a unit of each type of service, and to multiply these together and sum up the results. The allocation methods described below are different ways to determine the cost per unit for each type of service. In these methods the overhead costs (for example, housekeeping) are allocated to other departments (for example, radiology) on the basis of some measure, called an *allocation basis*, judged to be related to usage of the overhead item (for example, square feet of floor space in the radiology department might be used to allocate housekeeping costs to radiology).

In deciding which of the following approaches to use, the comments made in Section 4.1.1 should be borne in mind. That is, the more important the cost item is for the analysis, the greater the effort that should be made to estimate it accurately. There may conceivably be evaluations for which simple *per diem*, or average daily costs will suffice, because the result is unlikely to change irrespective of the figure assumed for the cost of hospital care. However, we suspect that such situations are in the minority, given the relative order of magnitude of hospital costs compared with other elements of health care expenditures.

Alternatively, the intermediate approach suggested by Hull *et al.* (1982) may suffice. Here the *per diem* cost is purged of any items relating to medical care costs, leaving just the 'hotel' component of hospital expenditure. It is then assumed that all patients are 'average' in respect of their hotel costs and that this expenditure can therefore be apportioned on the basis of patient-days. Thus, the hotel cost can be calculated for the patients in the programme of interest and combined with the medical care costs attributable to those patients to give the total costs of the programme. (The medical care costs would be estimated separately, using data specifically relating to the patients in the programme.)

If a more detailed consideration of costs is required, various methods for allocating shared (or overhead) costs are available, namely the following.

1 *Direct allocation (ignores interaction of overhead departments)*. Each overhead cost (for example, central administration or housekeeping) is allocated directly to final cost centres (for example, programmes like day surgery, or departments like wards or radiology). Therefore, a given ward's share of central administration would be equal to the total cost of central administration, multiplied by the ward's share (or proportion) of the allocation basis (say, paid hours for staff). Note that the ward's share is its paid hours divided by total paid hours of all final cost centres, not total paid hours for the whole organization. The latter method would underestimate the costs in all final cost centres.

2 *Step-down allocation (partial adjustments for interaction of overhead departments)*. The overhead departments are allocated in a step-wise fashion to all of the remaining overhead departments and to the final cost centres.

3 *Step-down allocation with iterations (full adjustment for interaction of overhead departments)*. The overhead departments are allocated in a step-wise fashion to all of the other overhead departments and to the final cost centres. The procedure is repeated a number of times (about three) to eliminate residual unallocated amounts.

4 *Simultaneous allocation (full adjustment for interaction of overhead departments)*. This method uses the same data as (2) or (3) but it solves a set of simultaneous linear equations to give the allocations. It gives the same answer as method (3) but involves less work. (The method is shown diagrammatically in Fig. 4.3.)

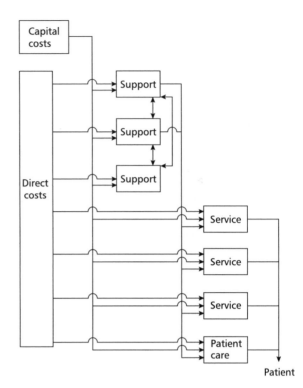

Fig. 4.3 Schematic illustration of cost allocations (from Boyle *et al.* 1982).

An example showing the different approaches to the allocation of overhead costs is presented in Section 4.3. Further details are available in Horngren (1994), Clements (1974), Kaplan (1973), and Boyle *et al.* (1982).

The effort that one would put into overhead cost allocation would depend on the likely importance of overhead costs (in quantitative terms) for the whole analysis. A much simpler, but cruder, approach is to do the following.

1 Identify those hospital costs unambiguously attributable to the treatment or programme in question (for example, physicians' fees, laboratory tests, and drugs). (These are known as the directly allocatable costs.) Allocate these directly and immediately to the programme.

2 Deduct, from total hospital operating expenses, the cost of departments already allocated above and departments known not to service the programme being costed.

3 Allocate the remainder of hospital operating expenses on the basis of number of patient-days, for example,

$$\text{Hospital cost of the programme} = \text{Directly allocatable costs} + \frac{\text{Net hospital expenditure}}{\text{Total number of hospital patient-days}} \times \text{Hospital patient-days attributable to the programme}$$

4 Finally, undertake a sensitivity analysis.

Whilst there is nothing to suppose that this method is anything but crude, if the choice between programmes is fairly insensitive to the value derived it may suffice.

There is now a growing literature on *activity-based costing* for hospitals (Ramsey 1994). This does not refer to a separate allocation methodology, but instead emphasizes the importance of identifying the activities/inputs that drive the final cost of a product or service. Activity-based costing is implicitly shown in the allocation example in Section 4.3. In this example the costs of overhead departments (for example, administration, housekeeping, or laundry) are allocated to service departments based on the activities/inputs that drive them (for example, paid hours for administration, square footage for housekeeping), instead of using a more generic allocation basis for all overhead departments, such as direct costs.

4.1.3. Overall, how accurate does costing have to be?

Costing can take considerable time and effort and it is not possible to do a perfect job every time. However, it is important not to make the perfect the enemy of the merely good. Therefore, analysts need to form a judgement on how accurate (or precise) cost estimates need to be within a given study.

Box 4.6 indicates the different levels of precision in costing for hospital costs. The least precise estimates are likely to be based on average *per diems* (or daily costs); the most precise estimates are likely to be based on micro-costing.

The guidance for deciding on the accuracy of costing is similar to that for deciding on the inclusion or exclusion of costs discussed earlier. Clearly a major factor is the likely

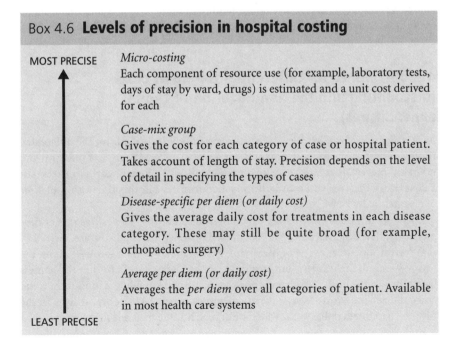

Box 4.6 **Levels of precision in hospital costing**

MOST PRECISE

Micro-costing
Each component of resource use (for example, laboratory tests, days of stay by ward, drugs) is estimated and a unit cost derived for each

Case-mix group
Gives the cost for each category of case or hospital patient. Takes account of length of stay. Precision depends on the level of detail in specifying the types of cases

Disease-specific per diem (or daily cost)
Gives the average daily cost for treatments in each disease category. These may still be quite broad (for example, orthopaedic surgery)

Average per diem (or daily cost)
Averages the *per diem* over all categories of patient. Available in most health care systems

LEAST PRECISE

quantitative importance of each cost category in the evaluation. For example, in an evaluation comparing two drug therapies it is likely that the study result will be sensitive to the costs of the drugs themselves. Therefore, it will be important to record dosages and routes of administration carefully, to facilitate micro-costing. On the other hand, if the drugs concerned have side-effects that may infrequently cause hospitalizations, it may suffice to use a *per diem* or case-mix group cost for these, if one is available.

Similarly, even if it has been decided to follow a micro-costing approach, different levels of accuracy can be applied to different cost items. For example, it is well known that many laboratory tests cost only a few cents each. Therefore, it does not make sense to invest considerable effort in costing these accurately. An average laboratory charge may suffice. On the other hand, nursing costs are often a major component of overall hospital costs. Therefore, it may be important to record the numbers and grades of nursing staff in the ward where the patients of interest are being cared for.

In using routinely available cost data, such as hospital *per diems*, or case-mix group costs (for example, diagnosis-related groups), it is important to pose the following questions. First, how was the cost estimate derived? Namely, what categories of costs are included? Second, how up to date is the cost estimate? Simple adjustments for inflation will not suffice if recent technological advances have dramatically changed the costs of the treatment concerned (for example, the introduction of drug-eliciting stents in coronary care).

Finally, it is worth bearing in mind that the calculation of total cost requires the quantities of resources to be multiplied by the prices (unit costs) of those resources. Therefore, when deciding on the level of precision in the estimation of resource quantities, it is worthwhile considering what degree of detail will be available on the costs, or vice versa. For example, it may not be worthwhile collecting considerable detail on the resource quantities if, for example, only average *per diem* costs are available in a given setting.

4.2. **Allowance for differential timing of costs (discounting and the annuitization of capital expenditures)**

As was mentioned in Chapter 3, some allowance needs to be made for the differential timing of costs and consequences. That is, even in a world with zero inflation and no bank interest, it would be an advantage to receive a benefit earlier or to incur a cost later—it gives you more options. Economists call this the notion of *time preference*.

There are a number of reasons why individuals may have a *positive rate of time preference*; that is, a preference for benefits today rather than in the future. First, they may have a short-term view of life; living for today rather than thinking about the future. Second, the future is uncertain, so, as the saying goes, a bird in the hand is worth two in the bush. Third, with positive economic growth, the long-term trend since the Second World War, individuals might expect to be more wealthy in the future. Therefore, a dollar today would be of higher value than one in the future when you are richer. Finally, since most individuals appear to have a positive rate of time preference, one can usually obtain a positive return when making a riskless investment.

However, it should be noted that the notion of preferring benefits today, or wanting to postpone costs, extends beyond money transactions and could extend to goods and services that could not easily be traded. It is of most significance for those economic evaluations that compare programmes or interventions with different time profiles. For example, if two options for dealing with heart disease were (1) expanding funding for CABG, and (2) a health education campaign to influence diet and lifestyle, we might expect option (1) to deliver benefits earlier. Therefore, if a positive rate of time preference were acknowledged, it would look more attractive, compared with the preventive option, than would otherwise be the case.

Typically, economic evaluation texts discuss the situation where the costs of the alternative programmes A and B can be identified by the year in which they occur.

Year	Cost of Programme A ($000s)	Cost of Programme B ($000s)
1	5	15
2	10	10
3	15	4

In this example, B might be a preventive programme that requires more outlay in Year 1 with the promise of lower cost in Year 3. The crude addition of the two cost streams shows B to be of lower cost (29 000 versus 30 000), but the outlays under A occur more in the later years.

A comparison of A and B (adjusted for the differential timing of resource outlays) would be made by discounting future costs to present values. The calculation is performed as follows. If P = present value, F_n = future cost at year n, and r = annual interest (discount) rate (for example, 0.05 or 5%), then

$$P = \sum_{n=1}^{3} F_n (1 + r)^{-n} = \frac{F_1}{(1 + r)} + \frac{F_2}{(1 + r)^2} + \frac{F_3}{(1 + r)^3}$$

$$= \frac{F_1}{(1.05)} + \frac{F_2}{(1.05)^2} + \frac{F_3}{(1.05)^3}$$

In our example this gives the following: present value of cost of A = 26.79; present value of cost of B = 26.81.

This assumes that the costs all occur at the end of each year. An alternative assumption that is commonly used is to assume that the costs all occur at the beginning of each year. Then, Year 1 costs need not be discounted, Year 2 costs should be discounted by 1 year, and so on. Calculated in this way, the previous example is

$$P = \sum_{n=0}^{2} F_n (1 + r)^{-n} = F_0 + \frac{F_1}{(1 + r)} + \frac{F_2}{(1 + r)^2}$$

The present value of A = 28.13 and the present value of B = 28.15.

The factor $(1 + r)^{-n}$ is known as the *discount factor* and can be obtained for a given n and r from Table 1 in Annex 4.2. For example, the discount factor for three periods (years) at a discount rate of 5% is 0.8638.

While this approach is the most convenient for many programme comparisons, a more common situation is that where most of the costs are easily expressed on an annual recurring basis and it is only capital costs which differ from year to year (typically these will be at the beginning of the programme, or Year O). Here it might be more convenient to express all the costs on an annual basis, obtaining an *equivalent annual cost (E)* for the capital outlay by an amortization or annuitization procedure. This works as follows:

If the capital outlay is K, we need to find the annual sum E which over a period of n years (the life of the facility), at an interest rate of r, will be equivalent to K.

This is expressed by the following formula:

$$K = \frac{E_1}{(1 + r)} + \frac{E}{(1 + r)^2} + \cdots + \frac{E}{(1 + r)^n}$$

$$K = E \frac{1 - (1 + r)^{-n}}{r}$$

$$K = E \,[\text{Annuity factor, } n \text{ period, interest } r]$$

As before, the annuity factor is easily obtainable from Table 2 in Annex 4.2. For example, in the cost analysis of providing long-term oxygen therapy, Lowson *et al.* (1981) found the total capital (set up) costs (K) to be £2153. Therefore, applying the formula given above,

$$2153 = \frac{E}{(1 + r)} + \frac{E}{(1 + r)^2} + \frac{E}{(1 + r)^3} + \frac{E}{(1 + r)^4} + \frac{E}{(1 + r)^5}$$

$$2153 = E \,(\text{annuity factor, 5 years, interest rate 7\%})$$
$$2153 = E \,(4.1002) \,(\text{from Table 2 in Annex 4.2})$$
$$E = £525 \,(\text{as shown in Table III of Lowson } et\ al.\ (1981).$$

Note that Lowson *et al.* (1981) assumed that the annuity was in arrears, that is, due at the end of the year. It might be argued that a more realistic assumption would be that it were payable in advance. This is equivalent to the formula

$$2153 = E + \frac{E}{(1 + r)} + \frac{E}{(1 + r)^2} + \frac{E}{(1 + r)^3} + \frac{E}{(1 + r)^4}$$

The value for E can still be obtained from Table 2 by taking one less period and adding 1.000. This gives a lower value for $E = £491$. This is logical because the repayments are being made earlier (at the beginning of each year) rather than in arrears.

This approach can be generalized to handle the situation where the equipment or buildings have a resale value at the end of the programme. If

S = the resale value,
n = the useful life of the equipment,
r = discount (interest rate),
$A(n, r)$ = the annuity factor (n years at interest rate r),
K = purchase price/initial outlay, and
E = equivalent annual cost,

then,

$$E = \frac{K - (S/(1 + r)^n)}{A(n, r)}$$

The method described above is unambiguous for new equipment. For old equipment, there are two choices.

Choice 1. Use the replacement cost of the equipment or the original cost indexed to current dollars and a full life.

Choice 2. Use the current market value of the old machine and its remaining useful life.

Choice 1 is usually better as the results are more generalizable—less situational. Note that using the undepreciated balance from the accounts of the organization is never a method of choice.

It can be seen that the equivalent annual cost of buildings or equipment to a given programme depends on the values of n, r, and S, all of which must be assumed at the time of evaluation. Practical points that evaluators might care to note are given below.

1 *Useful life and resale value (n and S).* It is important to make a distinction between the physical life of a piece of equipment and its useful clinical life. The latter is highly dependent on technological change. Obviously one can undertake a sensitivity analysis using different values for n, but in general it is best to be conservative and assume short lives (say, around 5 years) for clinical equipment.

2 *Choice of discount rate (r).* Traditionally there have been *two competing theories* regarding the proper measure for the discount rate for public projects (the social discount rate):

   (a) r = the real rate of return (to society) forgone in the private sector (known as the social opportunity cost approach)—this can be estimated empirically, although not without controversy;

   (b) r = the social rate of time preference.

The basic notion behind the social opportunity cost approach is that public investments can displace or crowd out private investments or consumption. Thus the discount rate is constructed as a weighted average of discount rates applicable to the various sectors of the economy contributing resources to the programmes under evaluation.

The social rate of time preference is a measure of society's willingness collectively, to forgo consumption (gratification) today in order to have greater consumption (gratification) tomorrow. Frequently it is argued that the interest rate on a risk-free investment (for example, long-term government bonds) represents the individual investor's willingness to forgo the present for the future, and that this rate is the individual's rate of time preference. Then if society's collective rate of time preference is simply the aggregate of the individual rates (a controversial assumption), the required rate is simply given by the real (adjusted for inflation) rate of return on long-term government bonds. In the absence of such assumptions, the practical difficulty in using an extra market process for determining the social discount rate is the absence of a well-defined political process or other mechanism for determining the rate.

The Panel on Cost-effectiveness in Health and Medicine recommended the shadow price of capital (SPC) approach, which they argued was conceptually superior (Gold *et al.* 1996). The SPC approach uses the social rate of time preference to discount costs and benefits, once they have been transformed. The stream of programme costs is transformed into the corresponding stream of consumption losses that would be induced by the forgone investment and consumption opportunities. The stream of programme benefits is transformed into the corresponding stream of consumption gains. The basic premise is that the ultimate purpose of all private investment (and economic activity in general) is consumption; thus, the proper measure of the opportunity cost of a public programme, in terms of forgone private activities, is the present value of the consumption that would be given up.

In practice, analysts have followed one of two conventions in choosing a discount rate. First, in jurisdictions (like the UK), where the government announces a common discount rate for all public sector projects, the advised rate is used. Alternatively, where there is no announced rate, the convention has been to use a rate consistent with the existing literature. A 5% rate was used by a number of analysts publishing articles in the *New England Journal of Medicine* in the late 1970s and early 1980s, and this became the *de facto* convention for economic evaluations in the health care field.

The prevalence of a 5% rate in the existing literature has the advantage that different studies are comparable, at least on this methodological dimension. However, Krahn and Gafni (1993) point out that the conventional practice of discounting all health care programmes at a rate of 5% may not consistently reflect societal or individual preferences. They recommend, among other things, that a consensus approach, with political participation, offers a flexible, pragmatic, and explicit way of synthesizing the empirical, normative, and ethical considerations that underlie choice of a discount rate.

In the UK the choice of a public sector discount rate had its origins in the social opportunity cost approach, but it has increasingly been viewed as a general statement about social time preference. That is, the discount rate is a societal value judgement about intergenerational equity; namely to what extent should we, as a community, postpone our own gratification for the sake of future generations?

As mentioned above, the US Public Health Service Panel on Cost-Effectiveness in Health and Medicine (Gold *et al.* 1996) revisited the issue of the discount rate for health programmes. They argued that costs and consequences should be discounted at a rate consistent with the shadow-price-of-capital approach to evaluating public investments. At the time they estimated that 3% would be the most appropriate real (riskless) discount rate for economic evaluations. However, they recognized that, given the large pool of existing studies using 5%, it would also be useful to continue using this rate for a number of years.

Therefore, the best current advice would be the following:

(a) to present costs and consequences in their undiscounted form, so that others can investigate the implications, for the evaluation, of employing different discount rates;

(b) to undertake a base case analysis using either the announced rate in the jurisdiction concerned, or the rates of 3% and 5% currently recommended by analysts;

(c) to undertake a sensitivity analysis, making sure that this includes 0%, 3%, and 5%;

(d) to alert decision-makers to the importance of the choice of discount rate, in those situations where it has a substantial impact on the study result. (Given that the choice of discount rate is a value judgement, as opposed to a technical judgement, this is probably the most important point.)

Finally, we should note that the discussion here has focused primarily on the discounting of costs. The discounting of consequences raises additional issues, which will be discussed further in Chapter 5.

3 *How to handle inflation.* If it is assumed that all the items of cost in the programme will inflate at the same rate and that this will be the same rate as inflation in general, there are two equivalent choices:

(a) inflate all future costs by this predicted inflation rate and then use a larger discount rate that allows for the effect of general inflation (the inflation adjusted discount rate*);

(b) do not inflate any future costs (that is, use constant dollars) and use a smaller discount rate that does not allow for inflation (the real discount rate). (All the announced rates, and the rates recommended by analysts, are real rates.)

Method (b) is the simpler and preferred approach.

If it is assumed that different items of cost in the programme will inflate at different rates, there are also two equivalent choices:

(a) inflate all future costs by their particular predicted inflation rates and then use a larger discount rate that allows for the effect of general inflation (the inflation adjusted discount rate*);

(b) do not inflate any future costs (that is, use constant dollars) and use a smaller discount rate that does not allow for inflation (the real discount rate), but adjust the discount rate for each item to account for the differential inflation rate between this item and the 'general' rate of inflation, for example, if general inflation is 8%, this item is expected to inflate by 10%, and the real r is equal to 4%, then r adjusted for this item is

$$r = 1.04 \times \frac{1.08}{1.10} = 1.021, \text{ i.e. 2.1per cent}$$

....

* Calculation of inflation-adjusted discount rate: if the real discount rate is 5% and general inflation is 8%, then the inflation-adjusted $r = (1.05)(1.08) = 1.134$ or 13.4%.

Method (b) is again the preferred approach. In general, however, most studies perform the whole analysis in constant price terms and use a single discount rate. (See Annex 4.1 for a tutorial on methods of measuring and valuing capital costs.)

4.3. **Allocation of overhead costs: example**

The following example demonstrates the various methods of handling overhead costs discussed in Section 4.1.2(7). Suppose we wish to determine the cost of neonatal intensive care for a specific group of patients. For each patient we have data on the length of stay in the neonatal intensive care unit (NICU) and data on the number and type of laboratory tests performed. For simplicity, let us assume that these were the only services received by the patients—that is, the patients had no operations, no radiological or nuclear medicine investigations, no social work, and so on. Furthermore, let us assume that there are only three overhead departments that serve the laboratory and the NICU: administration, housekeeping, and laundry. (In principle it would be possible to consider other overhead departments, like plant operations and maintenance, bioengineering, and materials management.)

The first task is to determine a unit of output for those departments that directly serve patients. We will be determining a cost per unit of output, and multiplying this cost by the usage of each patient to determine the cost per patient. Thus, the unit of output must be as homogeneous as possible with respect to cost, and yet be available in the data for each patient. We have selected a *patient-day* as the unit of output of the NICU, and a *workload measurement unit* for the laboratory. Each laboratory test is assigned a pre-determined number of workload measurement units according to the amount of work needed to perform the test.

An allocation basis must be determined for each overhead department. For example, square feet of floor space has been selected for housekeeping. This means that housekeeping costs will be allocated to departments receiving housekeeping services in proportion to the square footage of floor space in the department. Similarly, paid hours has been selected as the allocation basis for administration costs, and pounds of laundry for the laundry costs.

The data for this simplified example are given in Table 4.2. The calculations, as performed by the different methods, are given in Tables 4.3–4.8.

4.4. **The role and estimation of productivity changes**

This is a particularly thorny issue in economic evaluation, which surfaced briefly during the discussion of unrelated health care costs above. In cost analysis the relevant productivity changes are those arising from the patient or family member taking time off work in order to receive health care. In practice these costs may not be very substantial because the patient may already be off work because of their health condition. In addition, many patients are elderly and not in full-time employment. However, there may be some programmes for which these costs are substantial, such as screening programmes.

Rather, the major debate about the role and estimation of productivity changes relates to their consideration as a major consequence of health care programmes.

Table 4.2 Cost allocation data

	Annual direct cost ($)*	Annual units of output †	Direct cost per unit ($)	Allocation basis	Annual paid hours	ft²	Annual laundry (lb)
			Overhead departments				
Administration	2 000 000			pd-hrs	200 000	30 000	0
Housekeeping	1 500 000			ft²	300 000	4 000	80 000
Laundry	1 300 000			Lbs	200 000	8 000	0
Other	10 200 000				300 000	158 000	120 000
Subtotal	*15 000 000*				*1 000 000*	*200 000*	*200 000*
			Final departments (patient service)				
Laboratory	4 000 000	8 000 000	0.50/WMU		250 000	30 000	25 000
NICU	500 000	5 000	100/pt.-day		50 000	8 000	75 000
Other	30 500 000				1 700 000	562 000	1 200 000
Subtotal	*35 000 000*				*2 000 000*	*600 000*	*1 300 000*
Hospital total	50 000 000				3 000 000	800 000	1 500 000

* Direct cost consists of salaries plus supplies.

† Laboratory output is in workload measurement units (WMUs) and neonatal intensive care unit (NICU) output is in patient-days.

Table 4.3 Method 1—ignore overhead

Laboratory cost/WMU = $4 000 000/8 000 000 = $0.50/WMU

NICU cost/patient-day = $500 000/5 000 = $100/patient-day

WMU, workload measurement unit; NICU, neonatal intensive care unit.

Table 4.4 Method 2—direct allocation of overhead*

Laboratory cost = direct cost + laboratory's share of administration + laboratory's share of housekeeping + laboratory's share of laundry

$$= 4\,000\,000 + \frac{250\,000}{2\,000\,000}(2\,000\,000) + \frac{30\,000}{600\,000}(1\,500\,000) + \frac{25000}{1\,300\,000}(1\,300\,000)$$

$$= 4\,000\,000 + 250\,000 + 75\,000 + 25\,000 = 4\,350\,000$$

Laboratory cost/WMU = 4 350 000/8 000 000 = $0.54/WMU

NICU cost = direct cost + share of administration + share of housekeeping + share of laundry

$$= 500\,000 + \frac{50\,000}{2\,000\,000}(2\,000\,000) + \frac{8\,000}{600\,000}(1\,500\,000) + \frac{75\,000}{1\,300\,000}(1\,300\,000)$$

$$= 500\,000 + 50\,000 + 20\,000 + 75\,000 = 645\,000$$

NICU cost/patient-day = 645 000/5 000 = $129/patient-day

WMU, workload measurement unit; NICU, neonatal intensive care unit.

* Allocation denominator = sum of 'final' department.

Table 4.5 Method 3—step down allocation of overhead*

	Administration	Housekeeping	Laundry	Other	Laboratory	NICU	Other	
Direct cost	2 000 000	1 500 000	1 300 000	10 200 000	4 000 000	500 000	30 500 000	50 m
Allocate administration	2 000 000 →	$\frac{3}{28} = 214\,286$	$\frac{2}{28} = 142\,857$	$\frac{3}{28} = 214\,286$	$\frac{2.5}{28} = 178\,571$	$\frac{0.5}{28} = 35\,174$	$\frac{17}{28} = 1\,214\,286$	
Allocate housekeeping		1 714 286 →	$\frac{8}{766} = 17\,904$	$\frac{158}{766} = 353\,599$	$\frac{30}{766} = 67\,139$	$\frac{8}{766} = 17\,904$	$\frac{562}{766} = 1\,257\,740$	
Allocate laundry			1 460 761 →	$\frac{120}{1420} = 123\,445$	$\frac{25}{1420} = 25\,718$	$\frac{75}{1420} = 77\,153$	$\frac{1200}{1420} = 1\,234\,446$	
Total cost				10 891 330	4 271 428	630 771	34 206 472	50 m
Units					÷8 000 000	÷5 000		
Cost/unit					$0.53/WMU	$126.15/patient-day		

NICU, neonatal intensive care unit; WMU, workload measurement unit.

* Allocation denominator = sum of remaining departments in the step-down sequence.

Table 4.6 Method 4—step down with iterations*

	Administration	Housekeeping	Laundry	Other	Laboratory	NICU	Other	50 m
Iteration 1								
Direct cost	*2 000 000*	1 500 000	1 300 000	10 200 000	4 000 000	500 000	30 500 000	50 m
Allocate administration	2 000 000 →	$\frac{3}{28} = 214\,286$	$\frac{2}{28} = 142\,857$	$\frac{3}{28} = 214\,286$	$\frac{2.5}{28} = 178\,571$	$\frac{0.5}{28} = 35\,714$	$\frac{17}{28} = 1\,214\,286$	
Allocate housekeeping	$\frac{30}{796} = 64\,609$ ←	1 714 286 →	$\frac{8}{796} = 17\,229$	$\frac{158}{796} = 340\,273$	$\frac{30}{796} = 64\,609$	$\frac{8}{796} = 17\,229$	$\frac{562}{796} = 1\,210\,338$	
Allocate laundry	$\frac{0}{1500} = 0$	$\frac{80}{1500} = 77\,871$ ←	1 460 086 ←	$\frac{120}{1500} = 116\,807$	$\frac{25}{1500} = 24\,335$	$\frac{75}{1500} = 73\,004$	$\frac{1200}{1500} = 1\,168\,069$	
New totals	*64 609*	77 871	0	10 871 366	4 267 515	625 947	34 092 693	50 m
Iteration 2								
Allocate administration	64 609	$\frac{2}{28} = 6\,922$	$\frac{2}{28} = 4\,615$	$\frac{3}{28} = 6\,922$	$\frac{2.5}{28} = 5\,769$	$\frac{0.5}{28} = 1\,154$	$\frac{17}{28} = 39\,227$	
Allocate housekeeping	$\frac{30}{796} = 3\,196$ ←	84 793 →	$\frac{8}{796} = 852$	$\frac{158}{796} = 16\,831$	$\frac{30}{796} = 3\,196$	$\frac{8}{796} = 852$	$\frac{562}{796} = 59\,866$	
Allocate laundry	$\frac{0}{1500} = 0$	$\frac{80}{1500} = 292$ ←	5467 →	$\frac{120}{1500} = 437$	$\frac{25}{1500} = 91$	$\frac{75}{1500} = 273$	$\frac{1200}{1500} = 4\,374$	
New totals	*3 196*	292	0	10 895 556	4 276 571	628 226	34 196 160	50 m
Iteration 3								
Allocate administration	3196 →	$\frac{3}{28} = 342$	$\frac{2}{28} = 228$	$\frac{3}{28} = 342$	$\frac{2.5}{28} = 285$	$\frac{0.5}{28} = 57$	$\frac{17}{28} = 1\,940$	
Allocate housekeeping	$\frac{30}{796} = 24$ ←	634 →	$\frac{8}{796} = 6$	$\frac{158}{796} = 126$	$\frac{30}{796} = 24$	$\frac{8}{796} = 6$	$\frac{562}{796} = 448$	
Allocate laundry	$\frac{0}{1500} = 0$	$\frac{80}{1500} = 12$	234	$\frac{120}{1500} = 19$	$\frac{25}{1500} = 4$	$\frac{75}{1500} = 12$	$\frac{1200}{1500} = 187$	

Table 4.6 (Continued)

	Administration	Housekeeping	Laundry	Other	Laboratory	NICU	Other	
New totals	24	12	0	10 896 043	4 276 884	628 301	34 198 735	50 m
Final direct allocations	24 →			$\frac{3}{23} = 3$	$\frac{2.5}{23} = 3$	$\frac{0.5}{23} = 1$	$\frac{17}{23} = 18$	
		12 →		$\frac{158}{758} = 3$	$\frac{30}{758} = 0$	$\frac{8}{758} = 0$	$\frac{562}{758} = 9$	
Final totals	0	0	0	10 896 049	4 276 887	628 302	34 198 762	50 m
Units					÷8 000 000	÷5 000		
Cost/unit					$0.53/WMU	$125.66/patient-day		

NICU, neonatal intensive care unit; WMU, workload measurement unit.

*Allocation denominator = sum of all departments except the one being allocated.

Table 4.7 Method 5—simultaneous allocation (reciprocal method)*

Administration $C_1 = 2\,000\,000 + \dfrac{2}{30}C_1 + \dfrac{30}{800}C_2$

Housekeeping $C_2 = 1\,500\,000 + \dfrac{3}{30}C_1 + \dfrac{4}{800}C_2 + \dfrac{80}{1500}C_3$

Laundry $\quad\quad C_3 = 1\,300\,000 + \dfrac{2}{30}C_1 + \dfrac{8}{800}C_2$

Laboratory $\quad C_4 = 4\,000\,000 + \dfrac{2.5}{30}C_1 + \dfrac{30}{800}C_2 + \dfrac{25}{1500}C_3$

NICU $\quad\quad\quad C_5 = 500\,000 + \dfrac{0.5}{30}C_1 + \dfrac{8}{800}C_2 + \dfrac{75}{1500}C_3$

$\dfrac{28}{30}C_1 - \dfrac{30}{800}C_2 = 2\,000\,000$

$-\dfrac{3}{30}C_1 + \dfrac{796}{800}C_2 - \dfrac{80}{1500}C_3 = 1\,500\,000$

$-\dfrac{2}{30}C_1 - \dfrac{8}{800}C_2 + C_3 = 1\,300\,000$

$-\dfrac{2.5}{30}C_1 - \dfrac{30}{800}C_2 - \dfrac{25}{1500}C_3 + C_4 = 4\,000\,000$

$-\dfrac{0.5}{30}C_1 - \dfrac{8}{800}C_2 - \dfrac{75}{1500}C_3 + C_5 = 500\,000$

The solution of this set of equation is

$C_1 = 2\,215\,531$
$C_2 = 1\,808\,772$
$C_3 = 1\,465\,790$
$C_4 = 4\,276\,886$
$C_5 = 628\,303$

Therefore, the cost/unit of output is

Laboratory $4\,276\,886/8\,000\,000 = \$0.53$/WMU

NICU: $628\,303/5\,000 = \$125.66$/patient-day

*Allocation denominator = sum of all departments.
WMU, workload meaurement unit; NICU, neonatal intensive care unit.

Table 4.8 Method 6—patient-day allocation of overhead

This is the simple method described earlier. It may be useful in some cases.

Laboratory costs would be charged without overhead: $0.50/WMU.

NICU costs would be the direct costs of $500 000 plus a share of all relevant other departments (2.0 m + 1.5 m + 1.3 m = 4.8 m) in proportion to patient-days (5 000/500 000 where the denominator is total annual hospital patient-days).

Thus,
NICU cost = $500 000 + $4 800 000 (5 000/500 000) = $548 000.
NICU cost/patient-day = $548 000/5 000 = $110/patient-day.

WMU, workload measurement unit; NICU, neonatal intensive care unit.

That is, as a result of treatment, the patient, or a family member currently providing informal care, may be able to return to work or be more productive at work. Also, in the case of life-saving therapy, extension of life may also imply extension of the patient's working life.

As was indicated earlier, the relevance of productivity changes depends on the viewpoint for the analysis. For example, if an evaluation is being undertaken from a government budget perspective, there may be interest in estimating the financial flows relating to employment (for example, the impact on tax receipts and sickness benefit payments). (We called these *transfer payments* earlier.) However, when a societal viewpoint is being adopted, the inclusion of productivity changes, either as costs or consequences, is contentious. The issue might arise as follows. Suppose one were evaluating two programmes in the field of mental health. One programme requires institutionalization of the patient for a given period; the other, being a community-based programme using community psychiatric nurses in association with out-patient hospital visits, means that patients can remain in their own homes. (For simplicity, let us assume that the programmes turn out to be equivalent in their medical effectiveness, as assessed by some agreed measure of clinical symptomatology; furthermore, let us assume that a survey of patients shows them to be indifferent to the treatment modes, providing they are cured.)

Suppose it turns out that the community care programme has higher costs to the health care system, but that the number of workdays lost by the cohort of patients on the community regimen is lower, as many more of them can remain at work. Would it be right to deduct these production gains from the higher health care costs of the community care programme? If so, how would the production gains be valued?

One might take the view that the production gains should be included in the analysis, since in principle there is no difference between these resource savings and any of the other labour inputs included in the health care cost estimates. Many analysts would follow this approach. The productivity changes would be estimated by using the extra earnings of patients on the community care regimen, gross of taxes and benefits (that is, gross earnings before deductions, plus employer-paid benefits). The logic here is that the gross wage reflects the value of the production at the margin.

Whilst the approach followed above is quite defensible, it gives rise to a number of wider considerations that should be noted. First, the approach assumes that the community loses production if the institutional-based programme removes patients from employment. However, it may be that, given a pool of unemployed labour, the jobs vacated by patients admitted to institutional care would be filled by other members of the community. If this were the case there may be few overall production gains from adopting the community care programme. Second, it may be that, at some later stage, the cost-effectiveness estimates obtained in this study are compared with those obtained in other fields of health care, say a community care programme for people with learning difficulties or for the elderly. Because the patients benefiting from these programmes are unlikely to be in employment, there is less potential for production gains. This would make the community care programme for mental illness patients seem relatively inexpensive in terms of net cost, particularly if it were for workers earning high incomes, such as business executives, psychiatrists, or, dare we say, economists! Thus, in making a choice on the basis of net cost-effectiveness estimates, decision-makers may be tacitly accepting priorities different from their stated ones—if these are for the care of the elderly or people with learning difficulties.

There are at least four concerns about the inclusion of productivity changes in evaluations undertaken from the societal perspective. The first concern is related to the *estimation* of changes in productivity. As mentioned above, these are typically estimates using the gross earnings (including employment overheads and benefits) of those in employment. (In the literature, this is known as the *human capital* approach.) Also, some studies impute an equivalent value for those not in paid employment (for example, homemakers) by one of a number of methods. These include the use of average wages, the cost of replacing the role fulfilled by the individual, or the opportunity cost of the production they could have contributed were they not at home.

However, it is frequently argued that these valuations overestimate the true cost to society if individuals were to be taken out of the workforce, either through illness or to receive health care. For example, for short-term absences, losses in production could be compensated for by the worker on their return to work, or by colleagues. Also, for many categories of worker the value of the productivity lost at the margin is likely to be lower than the average wage, on the grounds that all jobs contain tasks that are more or less important, and it is the less important ones that are usually forgone as a result of a short period of absence. Finally, for long-term absences the employer is likely to hire a replacement worker. Therefore, the amount of productivity lost depends on the time and cost of organizing the replacement, and the resulting adjustments in the economy more generally. That is, if the President gets sick, sooner or later one person will be removed from the ranks of the unemployed!

We should note that many of these points arose in the context of the valuation of health care costs above. Namely, it was argued that costs or savings at the margin may not be reflected by average costs, and that there are frequently costs or inefficiencies associated with changes in resource allocation. For example, the closure of a large mental illness institution cannot take place overnight and there may be times, during the closure process, where wards are underoccupied.

In the context of productivity losses, Koopmanschap *et al.*(1995) have proposed that these should be estimated by the *friction cost method*. The basic idea is that the amount of production lost due to disease depends on the time-span organizations need to restore the initial production level. This friction period is likely to differ by location, industry, firm, and category of worker. For example, it may only take half a day to train a replacement hamburger server at McDonalds, but at least 2 days to train a replacement health economist!

The challenge is therefore to estimate the relevant friction periods and some calculations have been made for the Netherlands (Koopmanschap *et al.* 1995; Koopmanschap and Rutten 1996). These give estimates of lost production much lower than those obtained from traditional methods, such as the human capital approach (see Table 4.9). Also, Goeree *et al.* (1999) compared the human capital and friction cost approaches in estimating the productivity costs due to premature mortality from schizophrenia in Canada. The estimates using the human capital approach were 69 times higher than those obtained using the friction cost approach.

Table 4.9 Human capital versus friction costs: Netherlands (1988, billions of gilders)

Cost category	Human capital	Friction costs
Absence from work	23.8	9.2
Disability	49.1	0.15
Mortality	8.0	0.15
Total	89.9	9.5
Percentage of net national income	18%	2.1%

From Koopmanschap et al. (1995).

In a sample of 40 studies, Pritchard and Sculpher (2000) found that the vast majority (26 out of 40) had estimated productivity costs using the human capital method, whereas only seven had used the friction cost method. However, irrespective of the chosen approach, questionnaires have been developed to estimate productivity changes more precisely (for example, Reilly et al. 1993; van Roijen et al. 1996).

The second concern relates to *double-counting*, especially in relation to productivity gains. If the value of improved health estimated in a given study already includes the value of the increased productivity that would result, then it would not be appropriate to include an additional estimate of the value of this item. This is most likely to be a problem in the case of the two forms of evaluation yet to be discussed, cost–utility and cost–benefit analysis. Here health state scenarios are presented to individuals for valuation, either in utility or monetary terms. Unless specifically told to ignore the impact that return to work would have on their income, respondents may factor this into their response.

This was a concern of the Public Health Service Panel on Cost-effectiveness in Health and Medicine (Gold et al. 1996). The panel's recommendation that the impact of productivity gains was best captured in the denominator of the cost-effectiveness ratio gave rise to a lively debate (Brouwer et al. 1997a; Weinstein et al. 1997). In the final exchange in the debate, Brouwer et al. (1997b) argued that, even if individuals did consider income when assessing the value to them of improved health, individual income may only have a weak link with production change, particularly in settings where individuals have protection against loss of income (for example, through sickness benefit payments) or where they experience reduced productivity whilst remaining at work. Therefore the best approach would be to estimate the value of improved health whilst asking individuals to ignore income effects and then to estimate productivity changes separately, for inclusion in the numerator of the cost-effectiveness ratio. This is consistent with the view we expressed in Section 2.4, in our discussion of the 'building blocks' for economic evaluation. See Currie et al. (2002) and Sculpher (2001) for more discussion of the double-counting issue and the estimation of productivity changes.

The third concern relates to the issue of *objectives and perspective* in the use of economic evaluation. For example, Gerard and Mooney (1993) argue that when the measure of benefit in an economic evaluation is health specific (for example, life-years gained, or quality-adjusted life-years gained), the opportunity cost of scarce health care resources is defined in terms only of health forgone. It then follows that the opportunity cost of interest in the context of cost-effectiveness analysis or cost–utility analysis is determined by the best alternative use of small increases to total health care budgets and not opportunity costs elsewhere in the economy. It would thus be confusing to include productivity changes, or indeed other non-health care costs such as patients' time, volunteer time, and costs falling on other agencies.

We take the view that, whilst the benefit measure in the denominator of many economic evaluations in health care is indeed often health specific, it is not helpful for economic analysis to reinforce artificial budgetary boundaries by limiting consideration to health care costs only. One way forward would be to present health care and non-health care costs and benefits separately in the analysis, so that the opportunity cost on the health care budget is clearly identified. This would be consistent with Gerard and Mooney's position and the notion, introduced in Chapter 2, that analyses can be undertaken from different viewpoints, including the societal viewpoint. In short, we believe that economic evaluations in health care should, where feasible, consider the societal viewpoint, although on occasions analytical difficulties will preclude the full measurement and valuation of all costs and consequences in monetary terms.

The fourth concern is the one hinted at in the discussion of the mental health programmes above; namely that the inclusion of productivity changes in an evaluation raises *equity* considerations. This takes us back to the different perspectives on the role of economic evaluation in health care, as represented by the three fictitious analysts in Chapter 2. As mentioned in the discussion of non-health care costs in future years (above), the extent to which productivity changes are included in the analysis may depend on the view one takes about equity. Olsen and Richardson (1999) argue that the value of productivity effects may be included to the extent that it results in increased resources being made available for health care.

Other ways the problem might be alleviated are by

(1) expressing productivity changes as the number of days of work or normal activity lost or gained, rather than the dollar amount;

(2) using a general wage rate to value productivity changes, rather than the actual wages of individuals affected by the health programme being evaluated.

Given the controversy surrounding the inclusion and estimation of productivity changes, we would suggest the following.

1 Report productivity changes separately so that the decision-maker can make a decision on whether or not to include them.

2 Report the quantities (in days of work, or normal activity lost or gained) separately from the prices (for example, earnings) used to value the quantities. (This mirrors the recommendation made earlier for costing.)

3 Consider whether earnings adequately reflect the value of lost production at the margin and whether an approach based on the adjustments necessary to restore productivity (for example, the friction approach) would be more valid.

4 Pay attention to the equity implications of the inclusion of productivity changes, and, where equity concerns are important, continue to conduct the base case analysis using the actual estimates of the impact of the programme; but also consider a sensitivity analysis to explore the impact of using more equitable estimates, for example, a general wage rate rather than age-, gender-, or disease-specific rates.

5 Consider whether the inclusion of productivity changes represents double counting. (As indicated above, this is particularly pertinent when undertaking a cost–utility or cost–benefit analysis, but less likely when the effectiveness measure does not incorporate any *valuation* of the health consequences.)

6 Take account of any official guidelines for conducting economic evaluation existing in the jurisdiction concerned. (These guidelines are discussed in Chapter 10.)

For a more theoretical discussion of some of the issues surrounding the inclusion and measurement of productivity changes in economic evaluation, see Olsen (1994), Posnett and Jan (1996), and Sculpher (2001).

4.5. **Exercise: costing alternative radiotherapy treatments**

Task

A clinical trial is being carried out comparing two forms of radiotherapy for patients with head and neck cancer and carcinoma of the bronchus. Patients receiving *conventional therapy* are treated once per day, 5 days per week, for about 6 weeks. They would normally travel on a daily basis to a hospital-based radiotherapy centre to receive care. Patients receiving *continuous hyperfractionated accelerated radiotherapy* (*CHART*) are treated three times on each of 12 consecutive days, including the weekend. Because of the intensity and frequency of treatment, patients would normally stay in hospital during therapy, either in a regular hospital ward or in a hostel owned by the hospital.

The different treatment regimens obviously give rise to different costs. However, in addition, there may be differences in the period following treatment for the following reasons:

(1) the higher intensity of the CHART regimen might give rise to more side-effects, and hence a greater need for community care after hospital discharge;

(2) the CHART regimen might give better tumour control, thereby slowing down the progression of the disease;

(3) CHART might reduce the extent of late radiation changes, and a lower incidence of necrosis may also reduce the need for salvage surgery.

The clinical trial will provide an opportunity to gather data on the use of resources by patients in the two treatment groups. You are asked to

(1) *identify* which categories of resource you feel it would be important to assess;

(2) indicate how you might *measure* the use of these resources in physical units;

(3) say how you might *value* the resource consumption in money terms.

1. Identification of resource categories

Resource use can be considered under the broad headings outlined in Chapters 2 and 3.

Health care resource use

Hospital resources	• Radiotherapy, bed days, out-patient attendances, overheads
Community care resources	• General practitioner (family physician) visits, nurse visits (types of nurse will vary by country or setting), ambulance or hospital car

Patient and family resource use

	• Patients' time, time of relatives, out-of-pocket expenses for transport (e.g. car, train, or taxi)

Resource use in other sectors

	• Social worker visits, home help (homemaker) visits

2. Measurement of resource use

The fact that a clinical trial is taking place greatly increases the opportunity for accurate data collection as case report forms are completed for patients enrolled in the trial. Normally these record data on clinical events, but they can be modified to include resource use, such as number and type of investigations, date of hospital admission and discharge. Also, the fact that patients are enrolled in a trial provides the opportunity to interview them about resource use in community care, time taken to travel to hospital, and personal expenditure. They can also be given diary cards to record expenditure or time spent by relatives in home nursing.

In the absence of a trial the two major sources of data on resource use are routine statistics kept at the hospital or by other agencies, and patients' case notes (charts). The quality of these records varies by agency and data are usually more comprehensive at the main place (clinic) where the patient is being treated. In addition, there are no routine records for patient and family resource use.

Turning to the specific resource items identified above, we might expect to record quantities used as follows:

Item	Possible measurements
(a) Hospital care	
Radiotherapy	• The number of treatment sessions could be recorded, possibly differentiating by length of session and time of day (e.g. normal working hours, after hours, weekends)
Bed days	• The number of bed days could be recorded, differentiating by type of hospital ward
Out-patient attendances	• The number of attendances could be recorded
Overheads	• These would probably be related to the number of bed days or other suitable resource item (see valuation below)
(b) Community care	
General practitioner visits	• The number could be ascertained, either by asking patients, or by consulting the general practitioners.

	It may make sense to differentiate between home visits and visits to the practitioner's office
Nurse visits	• The number could be recorded as for general practitioner visits above. The purpose of the nurse visit and type of nurse (e.g. general nurse, specialist cancer nurse) would be recorded
Ambulance and hospital car	• The number and length of trips could be recorded. Length of trip could be ascertained from the patient's place of residence

(c) Patient and family resources

Patients' time	• The time taken in seeking and receiving care could be estimated by asking the patient. Time off work could be estimated separately
Relatives' time	• Relatives could spend time in home nursing and in accompanying patients to hospital. It could be estimated as for patients' time above
Out-of-pocket expenses	• Some may be estimated directly in money terms (e.g. bus fares). Others may be estimated by asking patients (e.g. distance travelled in private car)

(d) Resources in other sectors

Social worker and home help visits	• These would be estimated in a similar way to nurse visits above.

3. Valuation of resource items

It is extremely difficult to give general advice on this because it is so dependent on the availability of local financial data. In some settings, like the USA, there may be data on hospital billings or charges. In other settings, detailed costing studies would be necessary. As mentioned elsewhere in this chapter, when using charge data it is important to

(1) investigate the relationship between charges and costs;

(2) record physical quantities as well as charges, so as to facilitate generalization of study results to other settings.

The general strategies for costing, ranging from the use of average costs (or *per diems*) to micro-costing, were outlined in Box 4.6. The skill in costing is to match the level of precision (and effort) to the importance (in quantitative terms) of the cost item. Turning to the specific resource items measured above, we might expect to value them as follows.

(a) Hospital care

Radiotherapy treatment sessions

In some settings there may be charge data, or average cost figures, for radiotherapy sessions. However, even if these exist, which is unlikely in many locations, they may not differentiate by type of session (for example, normal hours, out-of-hours, or weekend). This distinction is critical to understanding the relative costs of conventional radiotherapy and CHART. Therefore, it is likely that micro-costing would be required.

In micro-costing the approach would be to derive the cost of a treatment session from its component parts, namely consultant (medical) time, radiographer time, medical physics time, consumables, equipment, buildings, and departmental overheads. Some survey work may be required, plus data from the hospital finance department on staff salaries, overtime allowances, and equipment prices. Costing of equipment and buildings will require assumptions to be made about useful life and resale value. It would be necessary to express these costs first as *equivalent annual costs* (see the methods outlined on pp. 74–5) and then to apportion them to individual treatment sessions. Judgements would also need to be made about which components of hospital overheads (for example, cleaning, building maintenance, or administration) are most appropriately allocated to departments and the allocation basis (for example, square metres, cubic metres, number of staff, and so on). Some elements of overhead may be better allocated on the basis of in-patient days or number of patients.

Bed days
It may be possible to use the average daily costs (or *per diems*) for different types of wards, including hostel wards. However, these may be considered too imprecise, in which case micro-costing might be undertaken. This would derive a daily cost for a particular category of ward by considering nurse staffing levels, medical (consultant) input, and overheads.

Because hostel wards may not feature in the standard hospital accounts, micro-costing may be required for these, for example, they may be slightly off site or rely partly on staffing by volunteers. An opportunity cost for volunteer time may have to be inputed. In costing hospital beds it may be decided to make an allowance for the fact that there is usually less than 100% occupancy.

Out-patient attendances
There may be an average cost or charge available for an out-patient visit, although this may not differentiate between oncology and other clinical specialties. Depending on the quantitative importance of this item, micro-costing may be undertaken.

Overheads
As mentioned above, these could be allocated to the radiotherapy treatments, to out-patient attendances, or to hospital bed days, depending on the overhead item.

(b) Community care
General practitioner visits
There may be data available on physician fees for various types of visit (e.g. general assessment, home visit, etc.). Alternatively, there may be nationally available data on the average costs of various general practitioner services. Failing this, micro-costing may be required. This would calculate the cost of practitioners' time (per minute or per hour) and add the cost of travel for home visits. Drug costs would also need to be considered.

Nurse visits
The agencies providing the nurses may have data on the average cost of a visit. This may even distinguish between various types of visit. Failing this, micro-costing would have to be employed, taking into account nursing salaries, length of visits, travel time, and nurses time spent in general administration. There may also be some consumables to be accounted for in the cost of nurse visits.

Ambulance and hospital car

Estimates may be available for the average cost per mile travelled. This could be combined with data on the distances involved to generate total costs.

(c) Patient and family resources

Patients' time

If the time was taken from worktime, the gross salary (including employment benefits) could be used. Different assumptions could be made about the opportunity cost of leisure time.

Relatives' time

In general the valuation of this raises the same issues as the valuation of patients' time. The valuation of time spent in informal nursing care is complicated because the relative may also be able to carry out other tasks at the same time.

Out-of-pocket expenses

In general, the financial expenditures made (for example, bus fares) would suffice. However, for some items, such as use of one's private car, the expenditures (say) on fuel would underestimate the true cost. Here, motoring organizations can often provide data on the cost (per mile or kilometre) of running a car.

Finally, a few rare events, such as hospital admission for particular types of surgery, may be handled separately. Depending on how quantitatively important they seem, case-mix group costs or disease-specific *per diems* may suffice. Alternatively, micro-costing may be undertaken.

Final comment

This exercise was based on an actual costing study, undertaken in the UK. If you want to see how it was tackled in practice, see Coyle and Drummond (1997).

4.6. **Concluding remarks**

Cost analysis is a central feature of all economic evaluations, but it has received relatively little attention from analysts to date. Two recent reviews of the literature (Graves *et al.* 2002; Halliday and Darba 2003) have commented on the inadequacies of current practice. Deficiencies exist in the specification of the study perspective, the estimation of both quantities and prices, and even the identification of the year(s) to which costs apply. Therefore, users of economic evaluations would be wise to subject the costing methods to a fair degree of scrutiny. In particular they should be suspicious of any study that does not clearly state separately the sources and methods of estimating the quantities and prices used in the calculation of costs.

References

Adam, T., Evan, D. B., and Koopmanschap, M. A. (2003). Cost-effectiveness analysis: can we reduce the variability in costing methods? *International Journal of Technology Assessment in Health Care*, **19**, 407–20.

Black, A. J., Roubin, G. S., Sutor, C., Moe, N., Jarboe, J. M., Douglas, J. S., and King, S. B. (1988). Comparative costs of percutaneous transluminal coronary angioplasty and coronary bypass grafting in mutivessel coronary artery disease *American Journal of Cardiology*, **62**, 809–11.

Boyle, M. H., Torrance, G. W., Horwood, S. P., and Sinclair, J. C. (1982). *A cost analysis of providing neonatal intensive care to 500–1499-gram birth-weight infants*, Research Report No. 51, Programme for Quantitative Studies in Economics and Population. McMaster University, Hamilton, Ontario.

Brouwer, W., Koopmanschap, M., and Rutten, F. (1997*a*). Productivity costs measurement through quality of life? A response to the recommendation of the Washington Panel. *Health Economics*, **6**, 253–9.

Brouwer, W., Koopmanschap, M., and Rutten, F. (1997*b*). Productivity costs in cost-effectiveness analysis: numerator or denominator: a further discussion. *Health Economics*, **6**, 511–14.

Brouwer, W., Rutten, F., and Koopmanschap, M. (2001). Costing in economic evaluations. In: *Economic evaluation in health care: merging theory and practice* (ed. M. Drummond and A. McGuire), pp. 68–93. Oxford University Press, Oxford.

Bush, J. W. (1973). Discussion. In: *Health status indexes* (ed. R. L. Berg), p. 203. Hospital Research and Educational Trust, Chicago, Illinois.

Clements, R. M. (1974). *The Canadian hospital accounting manual supplement.* Livingston, Toronto.

Cohen, D. J., Breall, J. A., Kalon, K. L. H., *et al.* (1993). Economics of elective coronary revascularization: comparison of costs and charges for conventional angioplasty, directional atherectomy, stenting and bypass surgery. *Journal of the American College of Cardiology*, **22**, 1052–9.

Coyle, D. and Drummond, M. F. (1997). *Costs of conventional radical radiotherapy versus continuous hyperfractionated accelerated radiotherapy (CHART) in the treatment of patients with head and neck cancer and carcinoma of the bronchus.* Centre for Health Economics, University of York, York *(mimeo).*

Currie G. G., Donaldson, C., O'Brien, B. J., Stoddart, G. L., Torrance, G. W., and Drummond, M. F. (2002). Willingness-to-pay for what? A note on alternative definitions of health care program benefits for contingent valuation studies. *Medical Decision Making*, **22**, 493–7.

Daly, E., Roche, M., Barlow, D., Gray, A., McPherson, K., and Vessey, M. (1992). HRT: an analysis of benefits, risks and costs. *British Medical Bulletin*, **48**, 368–400.

Drummond, M. F., McGuire, A. L., and Fletcher, A. (1993). *Economic evaluation of drug therapy for hypercholesterolaemia in the United Kingdom*, Discussion Paper 104. Centre for Health Economics University of York, York.

Finkler, S. A. (1982). The distinction between costs and charges. *Annals of Internal Medicine*, **96(1)**, 102–9.

Gerard, K. and Mooney, G. H. (1993). QALY league tables: handle with care. *Health Economics*, **2**, 59–64.

Goeree, R., O'Brien, B. J., Blackhouse, G., Agro, K., and Goering, P. (1999). The valuation of productivity costs due to premature mortality: a comparison of the human-capital and friction-cost methods for schizophrenia. *Canadian Journal of Psychiatry*, **44**, 455–63.

Gold, M. R., Siegel, J. E., Russell, L. B., and Weinstein, M. C. (ed.) (1996). *Cost-effectiveness in health and medicine.* Oxford University Press, New York.

Graves, N., Walker, D., Raine, R., Hutchings, A., and Roberts, J. A. (2002). Cost data for individual patients included in clinical studies: no amount of statistical analysis can compensate for inadequate costing methods. *Health Economics*, **11**, 735–9.

Halliday, R. G. and Darba, J. (2003). Cost data assessment in multinational economic evaluations: some theory and review of published studies. *Applied Health Economics and Health Policy*, **2**, 149–55.

Henderson, R. A., Pocock, S. J., Sharp, S. J., Nanchahal, K., Sculpher, M. J., *et al.* (1998). Long-term results of RITA-1 trial: clinical and cost comparisons of coronary angioplasty and coronary-artery bypass grafting. *Lancet*, **352**, 1419–25.

Horngren, C. T. (1994). *Cost accounting: a managerial emphasis* (5th edn). Prentice Hall, Englewood Cliffs, New Jersey.

Hull, R., Hirsh, J., Sackett, D. L., and Stoddart, G. L. (1982). Cost-effectiveness of primary and secondary prevention of fatal pulmonary embolism in high-risk surgical patients. *Canadian Medical Association Journal*, **127**, 990–5.

Johannesson, M., Meltzer, D., and O'Conor, R. M. (1997). Incorporating future costs in medical cost-effectiveness analysis: implications for the cost-effectiveness of the treatment of hypertension. *Medical Decision Making*, **17**, 382–9.

Kaplan, R. S. (1973). Variable and self-service costs in reciprocal allocation models. *Accounting Review*, **XLVIII**, 738–48.

Koopmanschap, M. A. and Rutten, F. F. H. (1996). Indirect costs: the consequence of production loss or increased costs of production. *Medical Care*, **34 (suppl.)**, DS59–68.

Koopmanschap, M. A., Rutten F. F. H., van Ineveld, B. M., and van Roijen, L. (1995). The friction cost method for measuring indirect costs of disease. *Journal of Health Economics*, **14**, 171–89.

Krahn, M. and Gafni, A. (1993). Discounting in the economic evaluation of health care interventions. *Medical Care*, **31**, 403–18.

Levin, H. M. (1975). Cost-effectiveness analysis in evaluation research. In: *Handbook of evaluation research, Vol.* 2 (ed. M. Guttentag and E. L. Struening), pp. 89–122. Sage, London.

Lowson, K. V., Drummond, M. F., and Bishop, J. M. (1981). Costing new services: long-term domiciliary oxygen therapy. *Lancet*, **i**, 1146–9.

Meltzer, D. (1997). Accounting for future costs in medical cost-effectiveness analysis. *Journal of Health Economics*. **16**, 33–64.

Neuhauser, D. and Lewicki, A. M. (1975). What do we gain from the sixth stool guaiac? *New England Journal of Medicine*, **293**, 226–8.

Nigrovic, L. E. and Chiang, V. W. (2000). Cost analysis of enteroviral polymeras chain reaction in infants with fever and cerebrospinal fluid pleocytosis. *Archives of Pediatrics and Adolescent Medicine*, **154**, 817–21.

Olsen. J. A. (1994). Production gains: should they count in health care evaluations? *Scottish Journal of Political Economy*, **41**, 69–84.

Olsen, J. A. and Richardson, J. (1999). Production gains for health care: what should be included in cost-effectiveness analysis? *Social Science and Medicine*, **49**, 17–26.

Posnett, J. and Jan, S. (1996). Indirect cost in economic evaluation: the opportunity cost of unpaid inputs. Health Economics, **5**, 13–23.

Pritchard, C. and Sculpher, M. (2000). *Productivity costs: principles and practice in economic evaluation.* Office of Health Economics, London.

Ramsey, R. H. (1994). Activity-based costing for hospitals. *Hospital and Health Services Administration*, **39**, 385–96.

Reilly, M. C., Zbrozek, A. S., and Dukes, E. M. (1993). The validity and reproducibility of a Work Productivity and Activity Impairment Instrument. *PharmacoEconomics*, **4**, 353–65.

Richardson, A. W. and Gafni, A. (1983). Treatment of capital costs in evaluating health care programmes. *Cost and Management*, **Nov–Dec**, 26–30.

Schulman, K., Burke, J., Drummond, *et al.* (1998). Resource costing for multinational neurologic trials. *Health Economics*, **7**, 629–38.

Schulman, K. A., Glick, H. A., Rubin, H., and Eisenberg, J. M. (1991). Cost-effectiveness of HA-lA monoclonal antibody for gram-negative sepsis. *Journal of the American Medical Association*, **266**, 3466–71.

Sculpher, M. J., (2001). The role and estimation of productivity costs in economic evaluation. In: *Economic evaluation in health care: merging theory with practice* (ed. M. F. Drummond and A. McGuire), pp. 94–112. Oxford University Press, Oxford.

Sculpher, M. J., Seed, P., Henderson, R. A., Buxton, M. J., Pocock, S. J., and Parker, J. (1993). Health service costs of coronary angioplasty and coronary artery bypass surgery: the randomized intervention treatment of angina (RITA) trial. *Lancet*, **244**, 927–30.

Sherry, K. M., McNamara, J., Brown, J. S., and Drummond, M. F. (1996). An economic evaluation of propofol/fentanyl compared with midazolam/fentanyl on recovery of the ICU following cardiac surgery. *Anaesthesia*, **51**, 312–17.

Taira, D. A., Seto, T. B., Siegrist, R., Cosprove, R., Berezin, R., and Cohen, D. J. (2003). Comparison of analytic approaches for the economic evaluation of new technologies alongside multicenter clinical trials. *American Heart Journal*, **145**, 452–8.

van Roijen, L., Essink-Bot, M. L., Koopmanschap, M. A., Bonsel, G., and Rutten, F. F. H. (1996). Labor and health status in economic evaluation of health care. *International Journal of Technology Assessment in Health Care*, **12**, 405–15.

Weinstein, M. C. and Manning, W. G. (1997). Theoretical issues in cost-effectiveness analysis (editorial). *Journal of Health Economics*, **16**, 121–8.

Weinstein, M. C., Seigel, J. E., Garber, A. M., *et al.* (1997). Productivity costs, time costs and health-related quality of life: a response to the Erasmus Group. *Health Economics*, **6**, 505–10.

Weisbrod, B. A., Test, M. A., and Stein, L. I. (1980). Alternative to mental hospital treatment. II Economic benefit–cost analysis. *Archives of General Psychiatry*, **37**, 400–5.

Zupancic, J. A. F., Richardson, D. K., O'Brien, B. J., Eichenwald, E. C., and Weinstein, M. C. (2003). Cost-effectiveness analysis of predischarge monitoring for apnea of prematurity. *Pediatrics*, **111**, 146–52.

Annex 4.1. **Tutorial on methods of measuring and valuing capital costs**

We are indebted to Morris Barer of the University of British Columbia for producing these examples, which should clarify the treatment of capital costs.

As a first note, we need to distinguish two classes of 'capital'—land and equipment. This is an important consideration, because in costing exercises we assume land does not depreciate, while of course capital equipment does. You can think of there being a continuum along which materials and supplies 'depreciate' or are used up instantaneously and so are costed fully in the year of use; capital equipment depreciates more slowly and may be handled in a variety of ways; land does not depreciate at all.

As a second note, recall that capital equipment costs have three components—depreciation, opportunity cost, and actual operating costs. We will ignore the last of these here.

First, consider equipment, and let us use an example of a machine costing $200 000 that, at the end of 5 years, has a resale value of $20 000. Assume straight-line depreciation and a discount rate of 4%. There are, then, four approaches to costing.

1 One can assume all costs accrue at time 0. This amounts to treating the equipment as one would less durable materials and supplies.

Time	0	1	2	3	4	5
Depreciation	200 000	0	0	0	0	(20 000)
Undepreciated balance at beginning of period	0	0	0	0	0	
Opportunity cost	0	0	0	0	0	
Depreciation + opportunity cost	200 000	0	0	0	0	(20 000)
Present value (PV)	200 000	0	0	0	0	(16 439)
Net present value (NPV) of equipment cost = $183 561						

Alternatively, but equivalently, one can treat the machine as instantaneously depreciating, except for the $20 000 resale value, which then is maintained through the 5 years.

Time	0	1	2	3	4	5
Depreciation	180 000	—	—	—	—	—
Undepreciated balance at beginning of period		20 000	20 000	20 000	20 000	20 000
Opportunity cost		800	800	800	800	800
Depreciation + opportunity cost		800	800	800	800	800
PV	180 000	769	740	711	684	658
NPV of equipment cost = $183 562						

2 One can compute depreciation and opportunity costs separately. They are related in that the opportunity cost of equipment refers to the use of the resources embodied in the equipment, in their next best use—this is 'approximated' by calculating the return on the funds implicit in the undepreciated value of the equipment at each point in time. Hence, the higher the rate of depreciation, the lower the opportunity cost, all else equal. Again, one has the choice of building the $20 000 resale in at the end, or just depreciating less of the machine. It works out the same.

Time	1	2	3	4	5
Depreciation	36 000	36 000	36 000	36 000	36 000
Undepreciated balance at beginning of period	200 000	164 000	128 000	92 000	56 000
Opportunity cost	8 000	6 560	5 120	3 680	2 240
Depreciation + opportunity cost	44 000	42 560	41 120	39 680	38 240
PV	42 308	39 349	36 556	33 919	31 430
NPV of equipment cost = $183 562					

Time	1	2	3	4	5
Depreciation	40 000	40 000	40 000	40 000	20 000
Undepreciated balance at beginning of period	200 000	160 000	120 000	80 000	40 000
Opportunity cost	8 000	6 400	4 800	3 200	1 600
Depreciation + opportunity cost	48 000	46 400	44 800	43 200	21 600
PV	46 154	42 899	39 827	36 928	17 754
NPV of equipment cost = $183 562					

3 One can compute an equivalent annual cost. This may be useful in a situation where other operating costs are the same each year, making necessary the comparison of only a single year of cost data for each alternative in the economic evaluation:

$$NPV = E \cdot AF_{5,4\%} \text{ (where } AF_{5,4\%} \text{ is the annuity factor for 5 years at an}$$
interest rate of 4%; see Table 2 in Annex 4.2)

$$183\ 562 = E \cdot 4.4518 \rightarrow E = \$41\ 233.$$

In other words, an *equal* stream of costs amounting to $41 233 in *each* of the 5 years of the programme has a present value equivalent to any of the *unequal* cost streams in (1) or (2) above. Note, therefore, that the equivalent annual cost embodies both depreciation and opportunity cost.

4 One can use equivalent or actual rental costs, if available or estimable. Note that because the renter will need to recover not only depreciation of the rental equipment but also a rate of return at least as good as that from the next best use of the resource, one can take rental cost to embody both depreciation and opportunity cost.

Second, the treatment of *land* is quite different because of the lack of depreciation.

A land purchase of $200 000 at time 0 would generate the following cost time stream.

Time	1	2	3	4	5
Depreciation	—	—	—	—	—
Undepreciated balance at beginning of period	200 000	200 000	200 000	200 000	200 000
Opportunity cost	8 000	8 000	8 000	8 000	8 000
Depreciation + opportunity cost	8 000	8 000	8 000	8 000	8 000
PV	7 692	7 396	7 112	6 838	6 575
NPV = $35 613					

Converted to an equivalent annual cost
$$NPV = E \cdot AF_{5,4\%}$$
$$\$35\ 613 = E \cdot 4.4518$$
It comes as no particular surprise that $E = \$8000$!

Annex 4.2. Discount tables

Discount Table 1

Present value of $1

N	1%	2%	3%	4%	5%	6%	7%	8%	9%	10%	11%	12%	13%	14%	15%
1	0.9901	0.9804	0.9709	0.9615	0.9524	0.9434	0.9346	0.9259	0.9174	0.9091	0.9009	0.8929	0.8850	0.8772	0.8696
2	0.9803	0.9612	0.9426	0.9246	0.9070	0.8900	0.8734	0.8573	0.8417	0.8264	0.8116	0.7972	0.7831	0.7695	0.7561
3	0.9706	0.9423	0.9151	0.8890	0.8638	0.8396	0.8163	0.7938	0.7722	0.7513	0.7312	0.7118	0.6931	0.6750	0.6575
4	0.9610	0.9238	0.8885	0.8548	0.8227	0.7921	0.7629	0.7350	0.7084	0.6830	0.6587	0.6355	0.6133	0.5921	0.5718
5	0.9515	0.9057	0.8626	0.8219	0.7835	0.7473	0.7130	0.6806	0.6499	0.6209	0.5935	0.5674	0.5428	0.5194	0.4972
6	0.9420	0.8880	0.8375	0.7903	0.7462	0.7050	0.6663	0.6302	0.5963	0.5645	0.5346	0.5066	0.4803	0.4556	0.4323
7	0.9327	0.8706	0.8131	0.7599	0.7107	0.6651	0.6227	0.5835	0.5470	0.5132	0.4817	0.4523	0.4251	0.3996	0.3759
8	0.9235	0.8535	0.7894	0.7307	0.6768	0.6274	0.5820	0.5403	0.5019	0.4665	0.4339	0.4039	0.3762	0.3506	0.3269
9	0.9143	0.8368	0.7664	0.7026	0.6446	0.5919	0.5439	0.5002	0.4604	0.4241	0.3909	0.3606	0.3329	0.3075	0.2843
10	0.9053	0.8203	0.7441	0.6756	0.6139	0.5584	0.5083	0.4632	0.4224	0.3855	0.3522	0.3220	0.2946	0.2697	0.2472
11	0.8963	0.8043	0.7224	0.6496	0.5847	0.5268	0.4751	0.4289	0.3875	0.3505	0.3173	0.2875	0.2607	0.2366	0.2149
12	0.8874	0.7885	0.7014	0.6246	0.5568	0.4970	0.4440	0.3971	0.3555	0.3186	0.2858	0.2567	0.2307	0.2076	0.1869
13	0.8787	0.7730	0.6810	0.6006	0.5303	0.4688	0.4150	0.3677	0.3262	0.2897	0.2575	0.2292	0.2042	0.1821	0.1625
14	0.8700	0.7579	0.6611	0.5775	0.5051	0.4423	0.3878	0.3405	0.2992	0.2633	0.2320	0.2046	0.1807	0.1597	0.1413

15	0.8613	0.7430	0.6419	0.5553	0.4810	0.4173	0.3624	0.3152	0.2745	0.2394	0.2090	0.1827	0.1599	0.1401	0.1229
16	0.8528	0.7284	0.6232	0.5339	0.4581	0.3936	0.3387	0.2919	0.2519	0.2176	0.1883	0.1631	0.1415	0.1229	0.1069
17	0.8444	0.7142	0.6050	0.5134	0.4363	0.3714	0.3166	0.2703	0.2311	0.1978	0.1696	0.1456	0.1252	0.1078	0.0929
18	0.8360	0.7002	0.5874	0.4936	0.4155	0.3503	0.2959	0.2502	0.2120	0.1799	0.1528	0.1300	0.1108	0.0946	0.0808
19	0.8277	0.6864	0.5703	0.4746	0.3957	0.3305	0.2765	0.2317	0.1945	0.1635	0.1377	0.1161	0.0981	0.0829	0.0703
20	0.8195	0.6730	0.5537	0.4564	0.3769	0.3118	0.2584	0.2145	0.1784	0.1486	0.1240	0.1037	0.0868	0.0728	0.0611
21	0.8114	0.6598	0.5375	0.4388	0.3589	0.2942	0.2415	0.1987	0.1637	0.1351	0.1117	0.0926	0.0768	0.0638	0.0531
22	0.8034	0.6468	0.5219	0.4220	0.3418	0.2775	0.2257	0.1839	0.1502	0.1228	0.1007	0.0826	0.0680	0.0560	0.0462
23	0.7954	0.6342	0.5067	0.4057	0.3256	0.2618	0.2109	0.1703	0.1378	0.1117	0.0907	0.0738	0.0601	0.0491	0.0402
24	0.7876	0.6217	0.4919	0.3901	0.3101	0.2470	0.1971	0.1577	0.1264	0.1015	0.0817	0.0659	0.0532	0.0431	0.0349
25	0.7798	0.6095	0.4776	0.3751	0.2953	0.2330	0.1842	0.1460	0.1160	0.0923	0.0736	0.0588	0.0471	0.0378	0.0304
26	0.7720	0.5976	0.4637	0.3607	0.2812	0.2198	0.1722	0.1352	0.1064	0.0839	0.0663	0.0525	0.0417	0.0331	0.0264
27	0.7644	0.5859	0.4502	0.3468	0.2678	0.2074	0.1609	0.1252	0.0976	0.0763	0.0597	0.0469	0.0369	0.0291	0.0230
28	0.7568	0.5744	0.4371	0.3335	0.2551	0.1956	0.1504	0.1159	0.0895	0.0693	0.0538	0.0419	0.0326	0.0255	0.0200
29	0.7493	0.5631	0.4243	0.3207	0.2429	0.1846	0.1406	0.1073	0.0822	0.0630	0.0485	0.0374	0.0289	0.0224	0.0174
30	0.7419	0.5521	0.4120	0.3083	0.2314	0.1741	0.1314	0.0994	0.0754	0.0573	0.0437	0.0334	0.0256	0.0196	0.0151
35	0.7059	0.5000	0.3554	0.2534	0.1813	0.1301	0.0937	0.0676	0.0490	0.0356	0.0259	0.0189	0.0139	0.0102	0.0075
40	0.6717	0.4529	0.3066	0.2083	0.1420	0.0972	0.0668	0.0460	0.0318	0.0221	0.0154	0.0107	0.0075	0.0053	0.0037
45	0.6391	0.4102	0.2644	0.1712	0.1113	0.0727	0.0476	0.0313	0.0207	0.0137	0.0091	0.0061	0.0041	0.0027	0.0019
50	0.6080	0.3715	0.2281	0.1407	0.0872	0.0543	0.0339	0.0213	0.0134	0.0085	0.0054	0.0035	0.0022	0.0014	0.0009

Discount Table 2

Present value of annuity of $1 in arrears

N	1%	2%	3%	4%	5%	6%	7%	8%	9%	10%	11%	12%	13%	14%	15%
1	0.9901	0.9804	0.9709	0.9615	0.9524	0.9434	0.9346	0.9259	0.9174	0.9091	0.9009	0.8929	0.8850	0.8772	0.8696
2	1.9704	1.9416	1.9135	1.8861	1.8594	1.8334	1.8080	1.7833	1.7591	1.7335	1.7125	1.6901	1.6681	1.6467	1.6257
3	2.9410	2.8839	2.8286	2.7751	2.7232	2.6730	2.6243	2.5771	2.5313	2.4869	2.4437	2.4018	2.3612	2.3216	2.2832
4	3.9020	3.8077	3.7171	3.6299	3.5460	3.4651	3.3872	3.3121	3.2397	3.1699	3.1024	3.0373	2.9745	2.9137	2.8550
5	4.8534	4.7135	4.5797	4.4518	4.3295	4.2124	4.1002	3.9927	3.8897	3.7908	3.6959	3.6048	3.5172	3.4331	3.3522
6	5.7955	5.6014	5.4172	5.2421	5.0757	4.9173	4.7665	4.6229	4.4859	4.3553	4.2305	4.1114	3.9975	3.8887	3.7845
7	6.7282	6.4720	6.2303	6.0021	5.7864	5.5824	5.3893	5.2064	5.0330	4.8684	4.7122	4.5638	4.4226	4.2883	4.1604
8	7.6517	7.3255	7.0197	6.7327	6.4632	6.2098	5.9713	5.7466	5.5348	5.3349	5.1461	4.9676	4.7988	4.6389	4.4873
9	8.5660	8.1622	7.7861	7.4353	7.1078	6.8017	6.5152	6.2469	5.9952	5.7590	5.5370	5.3282	5.1317	4.9464	4.7716
10	9.4713	8.9826	8.5302	8.1109	7.7217	7.3601	7.0236	6.7101	6.4177	6.1446	5.8892	5.6502	5.4262	5.2161	5.0188
11	10.3676	9.7868	9.2526	8.7605	8.3064	7.8869	7.4987	7.1390	6.8052	6.4951	6.2065	5.9377	5.6869	5.4527	5.2337
12	11.2551	10.5753	9.9540	9.3851	8.8633	8.3838	7.9427	7.5361	7.1607	6.8137	6.4924	6.1944	5.9176	5.6603	5.4206
13	12.1337	11.3484	10.6350	9.9856	9.3936	8.8527	8.3577	7.9038	7.4869	7.1034	6.7499	6.4235	6.1218	5.8424	5.5831
14	13.0037	12.1062	11.2961	10.5631	9.8986	9.2950	8.7455	8.2442	7.7862	7.3667	6.9819	6.6282	6.3025	6.0021	5.7245
15	13.8651	12.8493	11.9379	11.1184	10.3797	9.7122	9.1079	8.5595	8.0607	7.6061	7.1909	6.8109	6.4624	6.1422	5.8474

16	14.7179	13.5777	12.5611	11.6523	10.8378	10.1059	9.4466	8.8514	8.3126	7.8237	7.3792	6.9740	6.6039	6.2651	5.9542
17	15.5623	14.2919	13.1661	12.1657	11.2741	10.4773	9.7632	9.1216	8.5436	8.0216	7.5488	7.1196	6.7291	6.3729	6.0472
18	16.3983	14.9920	13.7535	12.6593	11.6896	10.8276	10.0591	9.3719	8.7556	8.2014	7.7016	7.2497	6.8399	6.4674	6.1280
19	17.2260	15.6785	14.3238	13.1339	12.0853	11.1581	10.3356	9.6036	8.9501	8.3649	7.8393	7.3658	6.9380	6.5504	6.1982
20	18.0456	16.3514	14.8775	13.5903	12.4622	11.4699	10.5940	9.8181	9.1285	8.5135	7.9633	7.4694	7.0248	6.6231	6.2593
21	18.8570	17.0112	15.4150	14.0292	12.8212	11.7641	10.8355	10.0168	9.2922	8.6487	8.0751	7.5620	7.1016	6.6870	6.3125
22	19.6604	17.6580	15.9369	14.4511	13.1630	12.0416	11.0612	10.2007	9.4424	8.7715	8.1757	7.6446	7.1695	6.7429	6.3587
23	20.4558	18.2922	16.4436	14.8565	13.4886	12.3034	11.2722	10.3711	9.5802	8.8832	8.2664	7.7184	7.2297	6.7921	6.3988
24	21.2434	18.9139	16.9355	15.2470	13.7986	12.5504	11.4693	10.5288	9.7066	8.9847	8.3481	7.7843	7.2829	6.8351	6.4338
25	22.0232	19.5235	17.4131	15.6221	14.0939	12.7834	11.6536	10.6748	9.8226	9.0770	8.4217	7.8431	7.3300	6.8729	6.4641
26	22.7952	20.1210	17.8768	15.9828	14.3752	13.0032	11.8258	10.8100	9.9290	9.1609	8.4881	7.8957	7.3717	6.9061	6.4906
27	23.5596	20.7069	18.3270	16.3296	14.6430	13.2105	11.9867	10.9352	10.0266	9.2372	8.5478	7.9426	7.4086	6.9352	6.5135
28	24.3164	21.2813	18.7641	16.6631	14.8981	13.4062	12.1371	11.0511	10.1161	9.3066	8.6016	7.9844	7.4412	6.9607	6.5335
29	25.0658	21.8444	19.1885	16.9837	15.1411	13.5907	12.2777	11.1584	10.1983	9.3696	8.6501	8.0218	7.4701	6.9830	6.5509
30	25.8077	22.3965	19.6004	17.2920	15.3725	13.7648	12.4090	11.2578	10.2737	9.4269	8.6938	8.0552	7.4957	7.0027	6.5660
35	29.4086	24.9986	21.4872	18.6646	16.3742	14.4982	12.9477	11.6546	10.5668	9.6442	8.8552	8.1755	7.5856	7.0700	6.6166
40	32.8347	27.3555	23.1148	19.7928	17.1591	15.0463	13.3317	11.9246	10.7574	9.7791	8.9511	8.2438	7.6344	7.1050	6.6418
45	36.0945	29.4902	24.5187	20.7200	17.7741	15.4558	13.6055	12.1084	10.8812	9.8628	9.0079	8.2825	7.6690	7.1232	6.6543
50	39.1961	31.4236	25.7298	21.4822	18.2559	15.7619	13.8007	12.2335	10.9617	9.9148	9.0417	8.3045	7.6752	7.1327	6.6605

Chapter 5

Cost-effectiveness analysis

5.1. **Some basics**

Cost-effectiveness analysis (CEA) is one form of full economic evaluation where both the costs and consequences of health programmes or treatments are examined. Therefore, all the points discussed in Chapter 4 on cost analysis apply here also. This chapter introduces some additional issues that need to be confronted when undertaking a CEA; in addition to the general introduction, it contains a study design exercise in Section 5.2, followed by a critical appraisal exercise in Section 5.3. Then, in Section 5.4, the use of quality of life scales in CEA is discussed. In Section 5.5, the interpretation of incremental cost-effectiveness ratios is discussed, and, finally, in Section 5.6, the relationship between the cost-effectiveness ratio and net benefit is explained. As before, the chapter progresses by attempting to answer some of the questions that analysts might need to consider when undertaking a CEA.

5.1.1. **When should cost-effectiveness analysis be used?**

It was mentioned in Chapter 2 that CEA is of most use in situations where a decision-maker, operating with a given budget, is considering a limited range of options within a given field. For example, a person with responsibility for organizing cancer screening programmes might be interested in maximizing the number of cases detected. Therefore it would be relevant to know the incremental cost per case detected from a range of alternative screening programmes.

However, even this limited application of CEA relies on the chosen outcome, 'cases detected', being an appropriate measure of achievement for the desired objective. Presumably the objective of introducing screening programmes is to prevent premature morbidity and mortality. Therefore, 'cases detected' may not be a reliable outcome measure if the consequences, for morbidity and mortality, vary in relation to the type of cancer detected and its stage of development.

Thus, 'life-years saved' might be a better outcome measure to use in a CEA of cancer screening programmes, although even this would not allow consideration of the morbidity consequences (that is, gains health-related quality of life) resulting from introducing screening. Where there are multiple objectives of treatments or programmes, one approach would be to present an array of the differential achievements, along each dimension, for the various alternatives. These data can then be presented to the decision-makers, so that they can make their own trade-off between effects. We called this form of evaluation a *cost-consequences analysis* in Chapter 2.

Table 5.1 Examples of effectiveness measures used in cost-effectiveness analyses

Study reference	Clinical field	Effectiveness measure
Logan *et al.*(1981)	Treatment of hypertension	mm Hg blood pressure reduction
Schulman *et al.*(1990)	Treatment of hypercholesterolaemia	Percentage serum cholesterol reduction
Hull *et al.*(1981)	Diagnosis of DVT	Cases of DVT detected
Sculpher and Buxton (1993)	Asthma	Episode-free days
Mark *et al.*(1995)	Thrombolysis	Years of life gained

DVT, deep-vein thrombosis.

However, the main problem with this approach is that the trade-offs are not made explicit, so it is not possible to judge the basis on which they are being made. For this reason, cost–utility analysis (CUA) (discussed in Chapter 6) is now becoming more popular, because it is recognized that most health treatments and programmes impact upon both length and quality of life. The outcome measures used in CUA, such as the quality-adjusted life-year (QALY), do incorporate explicit weightings of the various components of outcome.

Table 5.1 gives examples of effectiveness measures used in CEAs in the published literature. Some are final, health-related measures of outcome, such as 'life-years gained' or 'episode-free days'. Others are expressed as intermediate outcomes, such as 'percentage cholesterol reduction' or 'cases detected'. Intermediate outputs are admissible, although care must be taken to establish a link between these and a final health output, or to show that the intermediate outputs themselves have some value. For example, correct diagnosis of cases and the consequent confirmation of true negatives can provide reassurance both to the patient and to the doctor, and therefore may have a value in its own right quite apart from the health effects resulting from subsequent treatment. In general though, one should choose an effectiveness measure relating to a final output. (This is discussed further below and in Chapter 9.) However, the most important issue to consider is whether the measure is relevant, given the objectives of the decision-maker concerned. As more jurisdictions request economic evaluations as part of the formal decision-making process for health technologies, measures that relate to broader objectives, such as maximizing health gain, are becoming the most relevant.

5.1.2. How are the effectiveness data to be obtained?

Although primarily a clinical issue, the availability of good quality data on the effectiveness of the programmes or treatments being assessed is crucial to the cost-effectiveness analyst. (In fact CEAs are more often criticized for the quality of the effectiveness evidence on which they are based, rather than for the subsequent economics.)

A major source of effectiveness data is the existing medical literature. Use of such data in economic evaluations raises three issues: quality, relevance, and comprehensiveness.

Table 5.2 The relationship between levels of evidence and grades of recommendation

Level of evidence		Grade of recommendation
Level I	Large randomized trials with clear-cut results (and low risk of error)	Grade A
Level II	Small randomized trials with uncertain results (and moderate to high risk of error)	Grade B
Level III	Non-randomized, contemporaneous controls	Grade C
Level IV	Non-randomized, historical controls	Grade D
Level V	No controls, case series only	Grade E

A full discussion of appraisal of the *quality* of medical evidence is beyond the scope of this book and the reader should consult (for example) the users' guides to the medical literature produced by the Department of Clinical Epidemiology and Biostatistics, McMaster University. (They are collected together in the book by Guyatt and Rennie (2002).) These papers set out a checklist of questions to ask of any published study of diagnostic or therapeutic interventions. Although there are a number of important methodological features of a well-designed study to assess effectiveness, probably the most important aspect is the random allocation of patients to treatment groups.

In general, economists support the quality criteria laid down by clinical epidemiologists for clinicians seeking evidence to support clinical recommendations. One example is the relationship between levels of evidence and grades of recommendation proposed by Cook *et al.* (1992) (see Table 5.2). However, whilst they recognize that estimates of treatment effect are usually best obtained from randomized studies, economists are also aware that the complete dataset for an economic evaluation may have to be drawn from a wider set of study designs. For example, an estimate of the probability of occurrence of a rare side-effect, or the resources used in treating it, may have to be obtained from an (uncontrolled) observational study (Drummond 1998). Indeed, it is rare for the data on clinical outcomes used in economic evaluations to be drawn solely from clinical trials.

In judging the *relevance* of results published in the literature, one would have to consider how close one's own situation is to those where the published clinical studies were conducted. Important factors to consider are the patient case-load, the expertise of medical and other staff, and the existence of backup facilities.

Potentially, the criteria laid down to judge quality of evidence may conflict with those for judging relevance. This is because many randomized controlled trials are undertaken under atypical conditions. For example, the patients enrolled in the trial may be highly selective, the patient and doctor may be blind to the treatment assignment, a comparison may be made with placebo rather than another active agent, the trial protocol may require additional tests or procedures to be performed, and patients may be closely monitored to ensure compliance with therapy. These conditions usually make sense when the objective is to assess the therapy's ability to do more good than harm. (We called this *efficacy* in Chapter 2.) However, assessments made under these conditions may not tell us much about the therapy's performance in actual clinical use. (We called this *effectiveness* in Chapter 2.)

Ideally, economic evaluations should incorporate clinical data on effectiveness (rather than efficacy) but these may not be available, at least from controlled trials. This is particularly true in the case of pharmaceuticals, where the bulk of the clinical research before the medicine's launch concentrates on establishing efficacy and safety for licensing purposes. Economic analysts are consequently often in a dilemma. Do they argue for additional randomized controlled trials, with more naturalistic designs, to accommodate economic evaluation, or alternatively do they adjust or supplement the data from controlled trials in an economic model? (Buxton *et al.* 1997). (These issues are discussed further in Chapters 8 and 9.)

Undertaking economic analysis alongside clinical trials raises a number of practical and methodological challenges, which have been widely discussed (Drummond and Davies 1991; Adams *et al.* 1992; Coyle *et al.* 1998; Glick *et al.* 2001). These challenges relate both to the suitability of particular trials as vehicles for economic analysis and the additional burdens in data capture. (We discuss this further in Chapter 8.)

The question of whether any adjustments should be made to published clinical data to increase its relevance for economic evaluation is much more complicated. For example, should adjustments be made for the possibility that clinical practices or conventions differ from those in the trial setting, or vary from place to place? (The study by Palmer *et al.* (2004), discussed in Chapters 9 and 10, tackles these issues.) Also, should adjustments be made for the possibility that the trial protocol itself affects costs or benefits? For example, should data from trials of ulcer medications, where patients are endoscoped every month, be adjusted for the fact that many ulcers would not come to the notice of the patient or clinician in regular practice? (See Hillman and Bloom (1989), O'Brien *et al.* (1995), and Box 5.1.)

The third criterion for judging the effectiveness evidence in economic evaluations is that of *comprehensiveness*. That is, are the clinical data used in the economic evaluation representative of the medical literature as a whole? This issue was highlighted by Freemantle and Maynard (1994), who argued that the selective use of clinical data in an economic evaluation of antidepressants resulted in a more favourable cost-effectiveness assessment than would have been the case if all the available data were used. This point was demonstrated more generally by Coyle and Lee (2002), who showed that the clinical evidence base used in a range of economic studies had a big impact on results.

This issue is handled in the clinical literature through the conduct of systematic reviews of effectiveness. Those who undertake systematic reviews have a series of methodological principles covering issues such as the description of the literature search techniques, inclusion/exclusion criteria for individual studies, choice of (clinical) endpoints, records of individual study characteristics (for example, patient characteristics), details about the therapy (for example, drug dose), tests of statistical homogeneity, statistical pooling procedures, and sensitivity analysis (L'Abbe *et al.* 1987; Detsky 1995; Khan *et al.* 2001).

One of the earliest economic evaluations using clinical data from a systematic review was that by Mugford (1989), who used data from a review of 58 controlled

Box 5.1 **Adjustments to trial-based data in a study of ulcer therapy**

O'Brien *et al.* (1995) wanted to assess the cost-effectiveness of *Helicobacter Pylori* eradication relative to alternative pharmacologic strategies in the long-term management of persons with confirmed duodenal ulcer. A key factor in the calculation was the probability of ulcer recurrence (at 6 months and 12 months) under the various regimens.

Given the large number of randomized trials, they obtained the probabilities by undertaking a meta-analysis (systematic overview). However, in most ulcer trials the rates of recurrence are estimated by endoscopic examination. This is problematic for the economic analysis as this seeks to estimate costs and consequences *as they would occur in normal clinical practice*. In normal practice patients would not be endoscoped unless they had bothersome symptoms and consulted their physicians.

Therefore, it is likely that some of the ulcers detected by endoscopy would be asymptomatic, or silent. In order to account for this O'Brien *et al.* reviewed the trials that reported symptomatic and asymptomatic recurrence separately and estimated that about 75% of recurrences determined by endoscopy are symptomatic. The *adjusted* rates of ulcer recurrence were used in their cost-effectiveness model. Because the adjustment was made for all regimens, it did not change the ranking of programmes (in cost-effectiveness) in this study, but it does affect the *absolute value* of *H. Pylori* eradication or maintenance therapy for ulcer.

Ulcer recurrences per 1000 patients

Strategy	Total	Symptomatic	Expected 1 year cost per patient ($)
1. Heal and wait; treat duodenal ulcer recurrence with			
(a) ranitidine	108	81	329
(b) omeprazole	108	81	341
2. Heal and *H. Pylori* eradication immediately with			
(a) omeprazole and amoxicillin	20	15	272
(b) triple therapy	20	15	253

Adapted from O'Brien *et al.* 1995.

trials to estimate the cost-effectiveness of giving prophylactic antibiotics routinely to reduce the incidence of wound infection after caesarean section. In another study, Jefferson and Demicheli (1994) undertook a systematic review of both the epidemiological and economic variables pertaining to vaccination against hepatitis B.

Nowadays, many more economic evaluations use data from a review of clinical trials and a well-conducted synthesis of available data is a central element of studies incorporating decision analytic modelling. (The methodology of these studies is discussed in more detail in Chapter 9.)

As more economic evaluations are undertaken using data from systematic reviews, it will be interesting to see whether economists have a different perspective on issues such as inclusion/exclusion criteria and the reliability or relevance of particular clinical endpoints. Saint *et al.* (1999) discuss some of the issues arising from the use of meta-analysis in CEA. In general they are supportive of its use, but argue that the homogeneity and quality of the primary studies needs to be considered when interpreting the overall estimate of treatment effect.

The choice of approach for integrating clinical and resource use data in economic evaluations is one of the main methodological issues facing economic analysts. It is discussed further in Chapters 8 and 9. Also, issues of generalizing and interpreting economic data from one location to another are discussed further in Chapter 10. Although raised here first in the context of CEA, these issues apply equally to all four forms of full economic evaluation.

Finally, in situations where no good clinical evidence exists, the cost-effectiveness analyst may proceed by making assumptions about the clinical evidence and then undertaking a sensitivity analysis of the economic results to different assumptions. The underlying logic is that if the final result is not sensitive to the estimate used for a given variable, then it is not worth much effort to obtain a more accurate estimate.) It may be that in some cases a CEA based on existing medical evidence, with an appropriate sensitivity analysis, can obviate the need for a costly and time-consuming data collection. This might be the case in extreme situations where a very small improvement in effectiveness (much smaller than that expected to be observed) would make the new programme or treatment cost-effective, or where even high effectiveness of the new programme (much higher than that observed before in similar programmes) would not make the new programme cost-effective (Sculpher *et al.* 1997). In more recent studies these issues are explored more formally, through the use of *probabilistic sensitivity analysis* and *value of information analysis*. This is discussed further in Chapters 9 and 10.

5.1.3. **How does one link intermediate and final outcomes?**

We mentioned earlier that although intermediate outcomes may themselves have some value (or clinical meaning), the economic analyst should ideally choose an effectiveness measure relating to a final outcome. Establishing the link between intermediate and final outcomes is not straightforward. Many of the issues are discussed in Gold *et al.* (1996) and later in Chapter 9. However, in many cases the available clinical literature may report only intermediate endpoints. This is often true of the literature on prevention, mainly because studies to estimate an improvement in final endpoints are costly and time consuming to conduct. Here, apart from conducting the CEA using the intermediate endpoint, the only option for the economic analyst is to establish a link with a final outcome. For example, Oster and Epstein (1987) used an epidemiological model, based on the risk equations from the Framingham Heart Study, to link reduction in total serum cholesterol with coronary heart disease risk and survival. The success of this approach depends on the extent to which the link between intermediate and final outcome has been established.

In some cases, where the size of the relative risk (for example, of death) comparing individuals with and without the risk factor is large, it may be possible to establish the link through observational or case–control studies. An example here is the link between smoking and lung cancer. However, in many situations it might be necessary to establish the link through studies of stronger methodology, such as intervention studies with random assignment of subjects to treatment groups. For example, the Framingham Heart Study shows that individuals who have lived their lives with cholesterol levels towards the lower end of the distribution have a lower incidence of coronary heart disease. This is different from saying that lowering serum cholesterol by drug therapy actually increases survival. Accordingly, until the publication of large, long-term, intervention studies measuring final endpoints (for example, the Scandinavian Simvastatin Survival Study Group (1994) and Shepherd *et al.* (1995)), there was scepticism in some quarters over whether lowering cholesterol by drugs did indeed increase overall survival. Therefore, economic evaluations based on models have, in such circumstances, been viewed with suspicion.

We give more examples of the use of modelling in economic evaluation in Chapter 9. However, when undertaking a CEA using effectiveness data relating to an intermediate endpoint the economic analyst should either (1) make a case for the intermediate endpoint having value or clinical relevance in its own right, (2) be confident that the link between intermediate and final outcomes has been adequately established by previous research, or (3) ensure that any uncertainty surrounding the link is adequately characterized in the economic study.

5.1.4. Should effects occurring in the future be discounted?

In Chapter 4, the logic and procedures for discounting costs to present values were outlined. Because CEA also considers effects, should these be discounted too? This issue has aroused controversy, although it should be pointed out that in many CEAs it does not arise because the effects occur in a short period of time. (Capital costs may have to be converted to an annual amount using the annuitization procedure outlined in Chapter 4, however.) Nevertheless, the discounting of effects does have major practical consequences for the economic evaluation of preventive programmes. It is often argued that these are penalized by discounting.

The reasons often given for not discounting effects are as follows.

1 Unlike resources, it is difficult to conceive of individuals investing in health or trading flows of healthy years through time.

2 Discounting years of life gained in the future gives less weight to future generations in favour of the present one. Whereas this may make sense in the context of resources, where one would expect future generations to be wealthier, it might not make sense in the context of health. (On the other hand, it might, if one expects future generations to have better therapeutic technologies available.)

3 Empirical evidence suggests that individuals discount health at a different rate from monetary benefits (see Cairns (1992), Parsonage and Neuburger (1992), Gold *et al.* (1996), and Viscusi (1995) for a fuller discussion of these issues).

However, there are several arguments in favour of discounting effects as well as costs.

1 It can be shown, by the use of simple numerical examples, that leaving effects undiscounted while discounting costs, or discounting costs and effects at different rates, can lead to inconsistencies in reasoning. For a simple numerical example see Weinstein and Stason (1977); for a theoretical treatment see Keeler and Cretin (1983).

2 Leaving effects undiscounted leads to quite impossible conclusions. For example, a health programme giving rise to $1 of health benefits each and every year stretching into the future would be worthwhile whatever the size of the initial capital sum.

3 Contrary to the argument set out above, one *can* conceive of investments in health and the trading of health through time (Grossman 1972). Although it is not possible to give up a year now in return for a year at the end of one's life, individuals can trade reductions in health status or other goods and services now, in return for healthy time in the future (and *vice versa*). If this were not the case, people would not abstain from pleasurable but potentially unhealthy (in the long term) pursuits.

4 Whereas one of the arguments for not discounting effects is to avoid the problem of giving less weight to future generations, it may lead one to defer decisions *whenever* they are considered, this generation or next! This is because, with discounting of costs, the present value of a stream of expenditure starting next year is always lower than the present value of the same stream starting today. Therefore, it will be better to build the hospital next year; until we get to next year, when it will then be better to build the hospital the year after that!

5 Treating health care projects differently from those in other sectors of the economy may lead to inconsistencies in the overall allocation of resources. That is, health care projects would get an inside track.

Much has been written about the discount rate for health effects in recent years. van Hout (1998) demonstrated that the 'inconsistency' arguments of Weinstein and Stason (1977) and Keeler and Cretin (1983) only hold under certain circumstances. The crucial assumption underlying the reasoning of Weinstein and Stason is that 'life years are valued the same in relation to dollars in the present as in future'. However, it is not clear that growth rates of health and wealth, and the marginal utilities with respect to each, will be constant over time.

The crucial assumption underlying the reasoning of Keeler and Cretin is that programmes are stopped after 1 year, or that the budget being allocated is intended for one cohort of individuals at a time. However, as Cohen (2003) points out, health care budgets are multiyear budgets that are roughly constant from year to year.

Gravelle and Smith (2001) argue that, when health effects can be valued in monetary terms, as in cost–benefit analysis, they should be discounted at the same rate as costs. If health effects are measured in quantities (for example, life-years or QALYs) as in CEA or CUA, and the value of health effects is increasing over time, discounting the volume of health effects at a lower rate than costs would be a valid method of taking account of the increase in the future value of health effects.

In reviewing all the arguments that have appeared in the literature over the past 25 years, Lazaro (2002) concludes that the heart of the debate is polarized. Those who defend the uniform discount rate (for both costs and effects), believe that health can be exchanged for money at a rate that remains constant over time. Those who argue for a differential discount rate feel that this requirement cannot be accepted.

Lazaro proposes more empirical research on the relationship between individual time preferences for money and individual time preferences for health. Much of the existing empirical work is summarized by Cairns (2001), who highlights the complexities of this type of research. One recent empirical investigation of the consistency proposition found that respondents were inconsistent in their preferences over present and future costs and health effects, and whether they discounted costs and effects at the same rate (Brouwer and van Exel 2004).

Despite these concerns, the balance of opinion is probably still in favour of discounting both costs and effects at the same rate (Viscusi 1995; Gold *et al.* 1996). Smith and Gravelle (2001) reviewed existing practice in discounting and found only one jurisdiction, the UK, where the official guidance was to discount health effects by a lower rate than costs (6% per annum for costs, 1.5% per annum for effects). Even this guidance has recently changed, with the current recommendation that both costs and effects should be discounted at the rate of 3.5% (National Institute for Clinical Excellence 2004). Also, whilst acknowledging the debates in the literature, the World Health Organization guide to CEA recommends a discount rate of 3% per annum for both costs and effects in the base case, with a sensitivity analysis using 0% for effects and 6% for costs (Tan-Torres Edejer *et al.* 2003).

Bearing all this in mind, what should the analyst do? First, as mentioned in Chapter 4, it is important to take account of any official guidance on discounting in the jurisdiction concerned. In the absence of this, the base case analysis should probably use a discount rate of 3–5% for both costs and effects. In addition, a sensitivity analysis should be carried out, to illustrate the impact of using a lower rate of discount for effects. As argued by Severens and Milne (2004), in the absence of a clear theoretical or empirical argument for an optimal discount rate for discounting health outcomes, it is important that consistent principles of discounting are established both nationally and internationally.

5.2. **Exercise: designing a cost-effectiveness study**

Imagine that you have been consulted on the following issue. Try to apply the knowledge you have gained so far.

5.2.1. **Description of situation**

Occasionally patients die from pulmonary embolism (that is, clots in the blood vessels leading to the lung) following general surgery. Although death is relatively rare, the incidence is higher in patients over the age of 40 years who have undergone surgery lasting at least 30 minutes under general anaesthetic. Existing studies suggest that about eight in 1000 patients will die.

The current approach is to treat post-operatively as and when venous thrombo-embolism becomes clinically apparent. The clinical signs might include (for pulmonary embolism) pleuritic chest pain, shortness of breath or coughing up blood, or (for deep-vein thrombosis (DVT), a related condition) pain and tenderness in the thigh or calf. Once the signs occur, the diagnosis is confirmed by lung scanning (for pulmonary embolism) or by venography (for DVT). The treatment for both types of venous thromboembolism is the same—full-dose anticoagulant therapy consisting of heparin given intravenously for 7–10 days, followed by out-patient treatment with sodium warfarin for 12 weeks. Anticoagulant therapy prolongs hospital stay following surgery and some patients will have major bleeding complications.

Recently there has been an interest in prophylaxis. The options include the following.

1. Primary prophylaxis

(a) *Subcutaneous administration of heparin in low doses.* In this approach all patients would be given heparin subcutaneously for 2 hours pre-operatively and then every 8 hours for 7 days post-operatively. If clinically suspected DVT or pulmonary embolism were to develop, venography or lung scanning would be performed. If this confirmed the diagnosis, full-dose anticoagulant therapy (with heparin) would be given. The low dose prophylaxis is not associated with significant bleeding.

(b) *Intravenous administration of dextran.* In this approach all patients would be given dextran intravenously for 4 days, post-operatively. If clinically suspected DVT or pulmonary embolism develops, venography or lung scanning would be performed. If this confirms the diagnosis, full-dose anticoagulant therapy would be given, as in (a). Dextran prophylaxis carries slight risks of complications but these can be reduced to less than 2% by careful administration.

(c) *Intermittent pneumatic compression of legs.* In this approach, an inflatable cuff is strapped to the patient's leg, enabling gentle pressure to be applied to the calf in a regular cycle. The procedure typically begins during the operation and is continued until the patient is considered no longer at risk, for example, when the patient is ambulant. The cuff is worn continuously but is removed once per nursing shift. The modern devices that provide intermittent pneumatic compression are free of clinically significant side-effects; in particular, there is no risk of bleeding. As in (b), if clinically suspected DVT or pulmonary embolism developed, venography or lung scanning would be performed. If this confirmed the diagnosis, full-dose anticoagulant therapy (with heparin) would be given.

2. Secondary prevention

The approach here would be to perform leg scanning using iodine-125-labelled fibrinogen daily for 3 days following surgery and then on alternate days for up to 5 days, or up to the time of discharge if the patient was not ambulant. Leg scanning is free of complications.

If a positive scan was obtained, venography would be performed to confirm that diagnosis. Also, lung scanning would be performed on patients showing clinical signs of pulmonary embolism. If the diagnosis was confirmed, patients would undergo full-dose anticoagulant therapy, as in the case of primary prophylaxis above.

5.2.2. Tasks

(A) Set out the five alternatives in a clear form, showing the sequence of diagnostic and therapeutic actions arising under each. (You may find that a diagrammatic representation helps.)

(B) Consider the following methodological issues, important in designing the cost-effectiveness study.

1 What should be the viewpoint for the study? (In particular, whose costs should be considered?)

2 What broad categories of cost should be considered for each alternative?

3 What would you choose as the main measure of effectiveness of the alternatives?

4 Are there any other attributes of the alternatives that should also be considered in addition to the main effectiveness measure?

5 What kind of medical evidence will be required for the cost-effectiveness study?

6 What are likely to be the main uncertain factors for which a sensitivity analysis might be required?

Do not turn to Task (C) until Task (B) has been completed.

(C) Assume that the following data have been made available. Use them to calculate the cost-effectiveness of the alternatives. Also, indicate the major points you would make in a discussion of the cost-effectiveness results.

Costs ($)

1 *Prophylactic procedures (per patient)*

Intermittent pneumatic compression of the legs	33
Leg scanning with iodine-125-labelled fibrinogen	85
Intravenous administration of dextran	103
Subcutaneous administration of heparin in low doses	20

2 *Diagnostic procedures (per patient)*

Venography	88
Lung scanning	117

3 *Full-dose anticoagulant therapy (per patient)*

Hospitalization costs (for 7 extra days at $290 per day)	2030
Intravenous heparin therapy	30
Laboratory tests	104
Warfarin therapy	10
Physician fees	35
Total	2209

Outcomes (obtained from controlled clinical trials and given for a cohort of 1000 patients receiving each regimen)

1 *Current (no programme) approach*

Number of patients with clinically suspected DVT	40
Number of patients with clinically suspected pulmonary embolism	30
Number of positive venograms	19
Number of positive lung scans	14
Deaths	8

2 *Subcutaneous administration of heparin*

Number of patients with suspected DVT	10
Number of patients with suspected pulmonary embolism	10
Number of positive venograms	4
Number of positive lung scans	4
Deaths	1

3 *Intravenous administration of dextran*

Number of patients with suspected DVT	20
Number of patients with suspected pulmonary embolism	10
Number of positive venograms	9
Number of positive lung scans	4
Deaths	1

4 *Intermittent pneumatic compression of legs*

Outcomes as for subcutaneous administration of heparin, except that number of deaths not known. However, it is known that the approach is effective in preventing DVT.

5 *Leg scanning*

Number of positive scans	135
Number of patients with suspected pulmonary embolism	15
Number of positive venograms	107
Number of positive lung scans	7

Deaths (not known, although it is thought that leg scanning is effective in preventing fatal pulmonary embolism).

5.2.3. **Solutions**

1. Description of the alternatives

An algorithm of the clinical alternatives is given in Fig. 5.1. This diagrammatic representation is useful in getting a feel for those clinical options involving not just one action, but a sequence of interrelated actions. In this example, the number of objective tests performed (that is, venography and lung scanning) depends on the number of patients developing clinically suspected DVT or pulmonary embolism under each approach. The number of patients receiving full-dose anticoagulant therapy will then depend on the results of the diagnostic tests.

The option involving leg scanning is somewhat different from the others in that it employs a further objective diagnostic test in order to identify possible cases at an early stage. It can be seen from the figure that the cost of this strategy for 1000 patients will be crucially dependent on the number of positive leg scans and the number of these that are subsequently ruled out (as cases of DVT) by venography (the gold standard test for DVT).

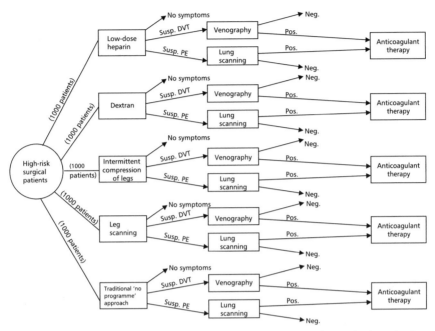

Fig. 5.1 Algorithm of clinical alternatives. Susp., suspected; DVT, deep-vein thrombosis; PE, pulmonary embolism; Pos., positive, Neg., negative.

A slightly more advanced method of setting out complex sequences of clinical alternatives is the *decision tree*. This approach has gained considerable popularity as a vehicle for undertaking economic evaluations and is described in Fineberg (1980) and Weinstein and Fineberg (1980). A decision tree flows from left to right beginning with an initial clinical choice or decision (indicated by a box) on a defined category of patient (or cohort of patients). As a result of the decision made there will be outcomes of given prior probabilities, depicted in the decision tree at a chance node (indicated by a circle). The sum of prior probabilities at each chance node (for example, $P_1 + P_2 + P_3$) is equal to unity. Our example is redrawn in decision tree format in Fig. 5.2. (Decision trees are the cornerstone of decision analytic modelling; this approach to economic evaluation is discussed in more detail in Chapter 9.)

2. Methodological issues in study design

(a) *Viewpoint for the study*. One viewpoint from which to undertake the analysis would be that of the third-party payer. Therefore, it would be most relevant to compare the health care costs of the alternative regimens (including physician charges). Then the issue would be one of whether alternative (or broader) viewpoints would change the kind of results that merely a health care cost comparison would give. See the example below.

From the patient's viewpoint,

- is length of hospital stay the same?
- is recovery time the same?

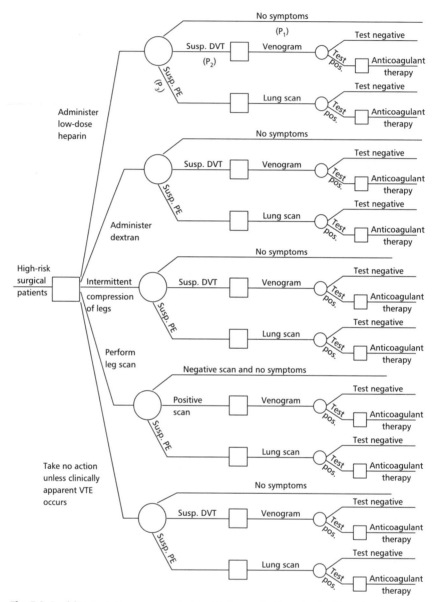

Fig. 5.2 Decision tree. Susp., suspected; DVT, deep-vein thrombosis; PE, pulmonary embolism; Pos., positive; VTE, venous thromboembolism.

- are health outcomes the same; death, complications?
- will expenditure be the same under all options, for example, out-patient visits?

From the society's viewpoint,

- are there any spillover costs or savings to other public or private sector agencies?

In this case, apart from the patient's interest in outcome there does not seem to be much conflict between the third-party payer (for example, Ministry of Health) and other viewpoints.

(b) *Categories of cost to be considered.* Obviously these depend on viewpoint, but one would definitely want to consider

- hospital hotel costs
- prophylaxis costs (for the three preventive measures)
- treatment costs (that is, full-dose anticoagulant therapy).

The main issues are

- do we consider costs common to all the alternatives as well as the differences? (This affects mainly the costing of hospital in-patient stay.)
- how accurate are the hospital *per diem* costs?

(c) *Measure of effectiveness and other attributes of the regimens.* The most obvious choice for the main measure of effectiveness would be deaths averted or life-years gained. Life-years gained would be preferable but would require some assumptions to be made about the likely life expectancy of patients undergoing this type of surgery. Other relevant attributes of the regimens include

- unpleasantness of the diagnostic approaches, particularly venography
- complications (for example, bleeding) either from the prophylaxis or, more importantly, from the full-dose anticoagulant therapy
- prolongation of hospital stay by anticoagulant therapy.

An alternative approach would be to use an intermediate effectiveness measure, such as cases of venous thromboembolism averted. Although less generic than life-years gained, one might argue that a case of venous thromboembolism is a clinically and economically relevant event in its own right. Certainly it is a surrogate for the other relevant attributes mentioned above. An advantage of choosing this endpoint is that it would be much easier to design and execute a clinical study to determine any difference between the alternative strategies. As deaths are rare for all options, a study powered to detect a difference in deaths would be very large.

Perhaps the cost-effectiveness study should use both endpoints, with cases of venous thromboembolism being estimated directly from a clinical trial and the number of deaths and life-years gained being obtained by extrapolation, using assumptions and the existing literature.

(d) *Source of medical evidence.* Ideally one would like evidence on the outcomes for each alternative, generated by controlled clinical trials. The variables that would be important to estimate include

- the number of patients developing clinically suspected pulmonary embolism or DVT
- the number of positive venograms or lung scans (for those patients tested) and hence the number of patients receiving full-dose anticoagulant therapy
- the number of complications from therapy
- the number of deaths from pulmonary embolism.

As mentioned above, it would be much easier to design a controlled clinical trial to detect a difference in cases of venous thromboembolism, rather than a difference in deaths.

(e) *Factors requiring a sensitivity analysis.* This will depend on which of the medical parameters can be established by randomized controlled trials—either in conjunction with this study or drawn from other sources.

Obviously, cost-effectiveness of the regimens would be highly sensitive to the number of deaths resulting from the no programme approach, the number of deaths averted by prophylaxis, and the sensitivity and specificity of the leg scanning, venography, and lung scanning procedures. Also, as primary prophylaxis involves giving everyone the low-dose therapy, the cost-effectiveness results would be highly sensitive to the cost of this. Finally, hospitalization costs are a large part of the total cost. Therefore, it would be important to explore the sensitivity of results to variations in these costs and it would be worthwhile varying both the daily rate and the prolongation of hospital stay assumed.

3. Calculations of cost-effectiveness of the alternatives

The data on the flow of patients under each regimen are added to the algorithm of clinical alternatives in Fig. 5.3. Of particular note is the fact that leg scanning identifies a large number of cases of possible DVT, few of which are ruled out by venography.

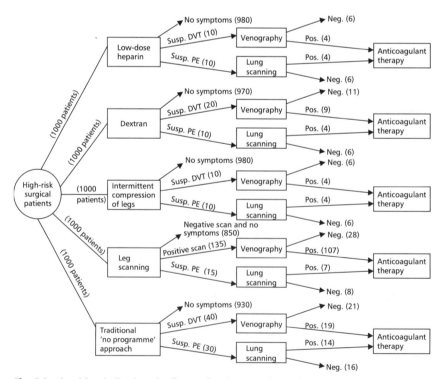

Fig. 5.3 Algorithm indicating the flows of patients under regimen.

Table 5.3 Alternative strategies for prevention of fatal pulmonary embolism in high-risk surgical patients

Strategy	Data		Incremental comparison		
	Cost/1000 ($)	Deaths/1000	Cost	Lives saved	C/E ratio (cost/per life saved)
No programme	80 000	8			
Intravenous dextran	135 000	1	55 000	7	7900
Low-dose subcutaneous heparin	40 000	1	−40 000	7	<0
Intermittent pneumatic compression of legs	53 000	?	−27 000	?	?
Leg scanning with ^{125}I-fibrinogen	350 000	?	270 000	?	?

This means that many more patients are given full anticoagulant therapy under this approach with consequent high costs.

The number treated is much greater than the cases of suspected DVT under the no programme approach. This signifies that leg scanning is detecting a number of cases that would otherwise not become clinically apparent.

These data can then be combined with the cost data to give the total cost (per 1000 patients) for the five options. This cost is shown in Table 5.3, along with the effects, in terms of deaths. Table 5.3 also shows the incremental analysis in terms of costs and lives saved. It can be seen that the most cost-effective option is subcutaneous administration of heparin, which has the lowest costs yet saves seven lives. That is, it is dominant over the no programme approach.

The following points might be raised in a discussion of the results.

1 How sensitive is this result to the assumptions made about the cost of prophylaxis and the cost of hospitalization?

2 Is the effectiveness of intermittent pneumatic compression worth evaluating through a randomized controlled trial? (This approach is almost as inexpensive as subcutaneous administration of heparin, yet does not carry any risk of bleeding or wound complications due to prophylaxis.)

The same data are presented in decision tree form in Fig. 5.4. Rather than presenting flows of patients, the decision tree includes the probabilities of events occurring at each chance node. For example, if low-dose heparin is given to 1000 patients, 980 will have no symptoms, 10 will develop suspected DVT, and 10 will develop suspected pulmonary embolism. On the tree these translate to probabilities of 0.980, 0.010, and 0.010 respectively.

5.2.4. A published study

The situation upon which this exercise is based was, in fact, real. A group of Canadian researchers designed and undertook a cost-effectiveness study to address the issue

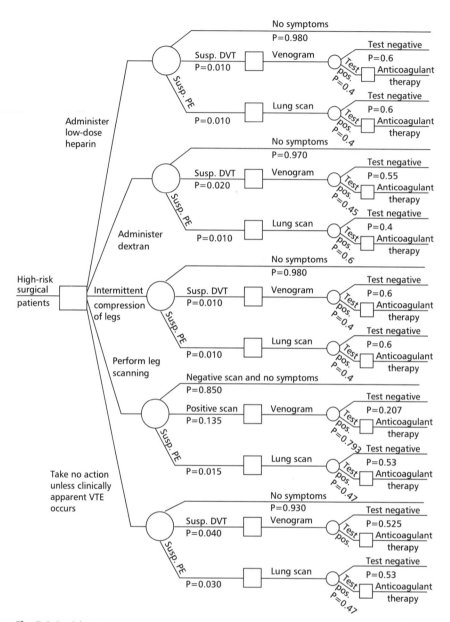

Fig. 5.4 Decision tree.

concerned and this was published in the *Canadian Medical Association Journal* (Hull *et al.* 1982). The paper is assessed in Section 5.3 using the 10 questions set out in Chapter 3. It is suggested that you locate the article and consider the comments below in the light of your own attempt at the problem and the solution given in Section 5.2.3.

5.3. **Critical appraisal of a published article**

Reference: Hull, R. D., Hirsh, J., Sackett, D. L., and Stoddart, G. L. (1982). Cost-effectiveness of primary and secondary prevention of fatal pulmonary embolism in high-risk surgical patients. *Canadian Medical Association Journal*, **127**, 990–5.

1. Was a well-defined question posed in answerable form?

   _X_ YES ___NO ___CAN'T TELL

The authors considered both the dollar costs and the effects (deaths due to pulmonary embolism averted) of several strategies for preventing fatal pulmonary embolism in high-risk general surgical patients. The five alternatives compared are stated on p. 990, column 2, of the article: (1) primary prevention with subcutaneous administration of heparin; (2) primary prevention with intravenous administration of dextran; (3) primary prevention with intermittent pneumatic compression of the legs; (4) secondary prevention with iodine 125-labelled fibrinogen leg scanning; and (5) treatment of clinically apparent thromboembolism. The viewpoint for the analysis could have been more explicitly stated. From p. 991, paragraph 2, column 1, it appears that the analytical viewpoint is that of the third-party paying agency responsible for reimbursement of hospital and medical costs in the province of Ontario.

2. Was a comprehensive description of the competing alternatives given?

   _X_ YES ____NO ____CAN'T TELL

The competing alternatives are reasonably well described. Details on the administration of heparin (p. 991, column 1), dextran (p. 992, column 1), and leg scanning (p. 992, column 1), are provided in subsections of the article, which describe the initial strategy and its subsequent investigations. (Unfortunately, the layout of the article headings might confuse a reader, because it appears that this information is being provided under a section entitled 'Costs of the strategies'.) Intermittent pneumatic compression of the legs (p. 992, column1) and treatment of clinically apparent thromboembolism, called traditional (no programme) approach (p. 992, column 2), are dealt with similarly though in less detail; however, the authors have provided references for all clinical protocols used. The list of competing alternatives appears complete and, as the authors have stated, option (5) is, in essence, the *do-nothing* alternative. In complex comparisons such as this, it is useful to visualize the comparison in terms of a flow chart of patients or in a decision tree form. It might have been helpful for readers if the authors had done so in this case. An example of such a chart, showing the clinical options and the distribution of patients among the various pathways, was presented earlier in Fig. 5.3. The chart is based on the authors' use of an illustrative cohort of 1000 patients in each alternative.

3. Was there evidence that the programmes' effectiveness had been established?

   _X_ YES _____NO ____CAN'T TELL

The authors have addressed the clinical evidence directly (p. 992, column 2). Most of the evidence is drawn from well-referenced randomized controlled trials, some from the authors' own setting. It is noted that evidence on the effectiveness of leg scanning and intermittent compression was inferred from knowledge of venous thrombosis and its relationship to fatal pulmonary embolism, because no randomized control trials with fatal pulmonary embolism as an endpoint exist for these two alternatives. This lack of evidence is taken into account in subsequent analyses. However, it would make the analyses problematic only if either leg scanning or intermittent compression were likely to be *more effective* prophylactic strategies than heparin.

4. Were all important and relevant costs and consequences for each alternative identified?

　X　YES ＿＿＿NO ＿＿＿＿CAN'T TELL

This may be a debatable assessment because the identification of consequences appears to be handled more clearly than that of costs. Deaths due to pulmonary embolism averted are clearly indicated as the effect of interest. Clinical complications of the alternative strategies also are identified, especially the risk of bleeding with heparin and the risk of anaphylactoid reaction and fluid overload with dextran (p. 993, column 2). Whilst detailed discussion of potential clinical complications is not provided, the authors have referenced their view that more explicit consideration of such complications would not change the basic results of the analysis.

With respect to the range of costs identified, the cost of each strategy is defined as the direct cost of the prophylactic procedure plus the diagnostic and treatment costs of non-fatal venous thromboembolism (p. 991, column 1). Although further detail is provided in Tables I and II of the article, the description of individual cost components could perhaps be clearer and more comprehensive. For example, it is not possible to ascertain whether capital costs are considered.

Other categories of costs and consequences, such as out-of-pocket costs, indirect costs, and indirect benefits to patients, are excluded from the analysis because it has not been performed from a societal viewpoint. However, these would only be of significance if they were higher for primary prophylaxis (especially heparin) than for the traditional approach of waiting to treat clinically apparent venous thromboembolism.

5. Were costs and consequences measured accurately in appropriate physical units?

　X　YES ＿＿＿＿NO ＿＿＿＿CAN'T TELL

The measurement of deaths due to pulmonary embolism averted is straightforward. With respect to costs, the ideal presentation would give both the quantities of all resources used and the unit costs of each resource, prior to multiplying the two and summing across all resources or cost items in order to derive the total cost for any alternative. The authors have attempted to summarize the quantities of resources used in a textual description (p. 991–2) and in Tables I and II. Whilst this could perhaps be more thorough, it may be unreasonable to expect journal editors to be interested in a more detailed presentation! The authors have dealt with the issue of shared costs (especially overheads) by separating items used differentially by patients with venous thromboembolism from other hospital cost items, and by measuring the former separately while implicitly accepting average *per diem* measurements (and values) for the latter. Whilst more sophisticated methods exist for handling this problem, there does not appear to be a compelling case for their use in this instance.

6. Were costs and consequences valued credibly?

___YES ___NO _X_ CAN'T TELL

Because the analysis deals (appropriately for the specific clinical focus) with effects measured in natural units, the progression to valuation of these effects in terms of their dollar benefit or utility is not applicable. The reporting of the valuation of costs is handled less adequately than readers might expect, however.

The only statement that deals directly with the issue suggests that costs are derived from the third party and operating costs incurred in a university teaching hospital in Ontario (p. 991, column1). This leaves readers to make at least two assumptions, both of which may be warranted, but which should have been made explicit. They are that (1) the unit costs of specific items were based upon market values as represented by entries on hospital budgets, reimbursement schedules for specific procedures, or prevailing market prices for the prophylactic agents, and (2) no significant imputations or adjustments to these values were required for any reason. While possible variations in these values are handled partially in the following sensitivity analysis, more explicit reporting of the valuation procedures would seem appropriate.

7. Were costs and consequences adjusted for differential timing?

____YES _X_ NO _____CAN'T TELL

Costs and consequences are not discounted to present values. However, discounting to present values is inappropriate in the context of this study, because all costs and effects relevant to the analysis, as framed by the comparison statement and viewpoint, occur in the present. That is, the analysis is conducted at one point in time, and the analytic horizon, from the beginning of the interventions to their resolution in outcomes of interest, is well inside 1 year.

8. Was an incremental analysis of costs and consequences of alternatives performed?

_X_ YES ____NO _____CAN'T TELL

The presentation of the results provided at the bottom of p. 992 and top of p. 993 does this implicitly. However, the explicit presentation of the incremental analysis could be significantly improved. The increment in effectiveness associated with primary and secondary prophylaxis strategies is the number of deaths due to pulmonary embolism averted. This is found in the text. The increment in cost associated with primary and secondary prophylaxis is the difference in the total cost per 1000 patients between each alternative and the traditional (no programme) approach. Incremental cost is rather tersely reported in the text at the top of p. 993: the traditional approach costs twice as much as subcutaneous heparin prophylaxis and about half as much as intravenous dextran prophylaxis. The incremental analysis probably warrants a separate table, space permitting. An example of such a table was given earlier (Table 5.3). The use of a hypothetical cohort of 1000 patients managed by each of the clinical strategies facilitates considerably the presentation of the results.

9. Was allowance made for uncertainty in the estimates of costs and consequences?

_X_ YES ____NO _____CAN'T TELL

Sensitivity analysis is performed on several variables, as reported in Tables III and IV, p. 993. No specific justification is provided for the ranges of variables employed.

The quite wide variation in cost values does, however, seem to deflect some of the criticism made above, because the study result is relatively robust. Of particular note is the joint possibility that the costs of prophylaxis have been underestimated and hospitalization costs overestimated in the initial analysis, because this would bias the analysis against the traditional (no programme) approach. Sensitivity analysis on these assumptions simultaneously (Table IV, last column), rather than one-at-a-time as is typically done, showed that heparin became only slightly more costly than the traditional approach, while still saving seven lives. At the time this study was undertaken, one-way sensitivity analysis was the most common approach, with a few studies (such as this) including a multiway analysis. If the study were undertaken today, probabilistic sensitivity analysis might be employed. (See Chapter 9 for more details.)

10. Did the presentation and discussion of study results include all issues of concern to users?

　　　 YES _X_ NO ____ CAN'T TELL

The analysis does not explicitly provide cost-effectiveness ratios for the alternatives; rather, it discusses directly the large incremental effectiveness of heparin and the likely cost saving that would accompany its use. The results are not compared with those of other investigators because this is the initial CEA of these methods. Based on the limited task of this analysis and the nature of the recommended strategy of subcutaneous heparin prophylaxis, further issues of generalizability, ethics, distributional considerations such as equity, and implementation would not appear problematic and are, therefore, not addressed in any detail by the authors.

5.4. Use of quality of life scales in economic evaluation

In recent years there has been increasing interest in assessing the health consequences of interventions in terms of their impact on quality of life. Indeed, for some conditions, such as arthritis, impact on quality of life might be the primary measure of the effectiveness of therapy. In other conditions, such as cancer, one might be interested in the quality of life during any increased survival from therapy, because many therapies are known to have toxic side-effects.

Because improvement in health-related quality of life is one of the main *economic* benefits of treatment, it clearly needs to be incorporated in economic evaluation. In CEA the relative costs of treatments are compared with their relative consequences, measured in natural units. Therefore, the question arises as to whether health-related quality of life scales can be used in the denominator of CEAs, either alone or alongside other measures of the success of therapy, such as life-years gained (O'Brien 1994).

5.4.1. Types of health-related quality of life scales

The different types of quality of life scale have been reviewed by Guyatt *et al.* (1993). There are three main types:

(1) specific measures (for example, disease specific, age specific, and so on);

(2) general health profiles;

(3) preference-based measures.

Preference-based (or utility) measures are extensively used in CUA and will therefore be discussed in Chapter 6. Our interest here is in the potential and problems of using specific measures or general health profiles in economic evaluation. These descriptive measures often do not generate a single index measure, which limits their usefulness to economic analysts.

Specific measures, as the name implies, focus on health outcomes specific to an individual disease, medical condition, or patient population. They usually concentrate on the dimensions (or domains) of quality of life that are most relevant to the disease in question. For example, a disease-specific measure in arthritis is likely to include assessments of pain and mobility.

The main advantages of such measures are (1) that, being focused, they are more likely to be responsive to changes in the patients condition and (2) that they are likely to be seen as most relevant to patients and physicians and therefore more accepted (for inclusion in a study). Their main disadvantage, from the economist's viewpoint, is that they do not give comprehensive measures of quality of life and therefore cannot be used to compare the cost-effectiveness of programmes in different disease areas. Also, on occasions their focus may be too narrow even to capture fully the relevant dimensions of quality of life in a given disease area. For example, in a comparison of two drugs (say) for arthritis, a specific scale focusing on physical functioning and pain may miss some of the impacts on quality of life caused by side-effects of the medications (for example, rashes).

General health profiles, on the other hand, *are* comprehensive measures of health-related quality of life. Typically, they include consideration of physical functioning, ability for self-care, psychological status, level of pain or distress, and amount of social integration. Therefore, in principle they can be applied across different patient populations and in different disease areas.

There are now several well-known general health profiles, the most widespread being the Short Form (SF) 36, the Nottingham Health Profile, and the Sickness Impact Profile (Brazier 1993). The main advantage of using these scales is that they have been widely applied and have established reliability and validity. However, in some situations they may exhibit a lower responsiveness to change than disease-specific measures. See the paper by Dowie (2002) and the responses in the same issue of *Health Economics* for a lively debate on the merits and demerits of specific and general quality of life measures.

General health profiles are useful in an economic evaluation as supplementary information, but there are several disadvantages from the economist's viewpoint to their use as an outcome measure. First, except for the Sickness Impact Profile, the instruments do not produce a single quality of life score, but rather produce a profile of scores across the different domains of the instrument. (Indeed, some of the developers of general health profiles would regard such aggregation as counter-productive.) This means it is not possible to compare directly an improvement in one dimension with another, or to compare across different programmes that produce outcomes of different types. Second, because the scoring for the instruments is not, in general, based on preferences of individuals for the various possible outcomes, it is not clear that higher scores are necessarily associated with outcomes that are more preferred.

Third, because the scores for these instruments are not calibrated on to a scale where dead = 0 and healthy = 1, they cannot be used to combine quality of life with quantity of life, as, for example, in the QALY calculation.

A preference-weighted version of the SF-36, the SF-6D, has recently been developed (Brazier *et al.* 2002). In principle, this offers the potential to calculate health state preference values (utilities) from general quality of life data collected using the SF-36. This is discussed in more detail in Chapter 6.

5.4.2. Problems and potential of using quality of life scales

Economic evaluations using either specific measures or general health profiles are best regarded as sophisticated examples of cost-effectiveness or cost-consequences analyses. Therefore, they suffer from the limitation, mentioned in Chapter 2, of telling us nothing about the *value* of the health consequences produced, and are most suited to answering more restrictive questions, such as 'Is treatment A or treatment B better for a given category of patients?' Even then, some judgements are likely to be required on the part of the decision-maker, unless one treatment is superior to the other on all dimensions of quality of life.

When using specific or health profile measures in an economic evaluation the economic analyst should consider the following issues.

1 Is the measure recognized as being clinically relevant in the disease area concerned?
2 Has the measure been validated for use in this disease or on a similar patient population?
3 Is there a widely agreed interpretation of what would constitute a quantitatively important change in the dimension(s) of health-related quality of life being measured?

Finally, whilst specific and health-profile measures may have limited use as effectiveness measures in CEA, the information produced may be indirectly relevant to CUA (discussed in Chapter 6). That is, it may be possible to convert the descriptive quality of life information to a utility or preference-based measure, either by

(1) mapping health states from a specific or health profile measure on to an established preference-weighted classification (Chancellor *et al.* 1997); or
(2) using the quality of life information gained from the scales to construct scenarios for health state preference valuation.

This potential has been explored by Brazier and Dixon (1995). They concluded that, whilst potential exists, much more research is required. Therefore, in the short term specific or health profile measures are likely to be used alongside the preference-based measures discussed in Chapter 6.

5.5. Interpreting incremental cost-effectiveness ratios

In Chapter 3 we pointed out that the appropriate comparison between two health care programmes or interventions was in terms of the *incremental* cost-effectiveness ratio (see Fig. 3.2). We also discussed the notion of *dominance*, where one programme could be said to dominate another if its effectiveness were higher and its costs lower.

In this section we discuss the same concepts, but in the context of a more complicated situation, where there are three competing programmes, each of which can be delivered with varying degrees of intensity. For example, suppose we are comparing three treatment programmes for three different groups of 1000 patients each. All three programmes are for life-threatening conditions (for example, different types of cancer, end-stage renal disease, or myocardial infarction), so a simple effectiveness measure, such as life-years saved, can be used for purposes of comparison. Also, more intensive programmes of treatment are more effective in each case, but at increased cost. How would we decide on an efficient allocation of resources among the three programmes if saving life-years was our objective?

Tables 5.4 and 5.5, adapted from the paper by Karlsson and Johannesson (1996), give the data on costs, effects, and incremental cost-effectiveness ratios for the three programmes. In essence there are 11 alternatives (A–M) to be considered, with the additional alternative (O) of doing nothing. (For simplicity this is assumed to have zero costs and zero effects, although often this is *not* the case.) Also, the various alternatives within each programme are assumed to be *mutually exclusive*, in that if a patient receives one of

Table 5.4 Cost per patient (C) and effectiveness per patient (E) for the available alternatives in each of three treatment strategies. (There are 1000 patients to be treated in each group.)

Treatment strategy I			Treatment strategy II			Treatment strategy III		
Alternative	C	E	Alternative	C	E	Alternative	C	E
A	100	10	F	200	12	K	100	5
B	200	14	G	400	16	L	200	8
C	300	16	H	550	18	M	300	12
D	400	19						
E	500	20						

From Karlsson and Johannesson (1996).

Table 5.5 Incremental cost (ΔC), incremental effectiveness (ΔE), and incremental cost-effectiveness ratio ($\Delta C/\Delta E$) per patient for the different treatment alternatives shown in Table 5.4 (there are 1000 patients in each patient group)

Treatment strategy I				Treatment strategy II				Treatment strategy III			
Alternative	ΔC	ΔE	ΔC/ΔE	Alternative	ΔC	ΔE	ΔC/ΔE	Alternative	ΔC	ΔE	ΔC/ΔE
A	100	10	10	F	200	12	17	K	100	5	20
B	100	4	25	G	200	4	50	L	100	3	33
C	100	2	50	H	150	2	75	M	100	4	25
D	100	3	33								
E	100	1	100								

From Karlsson and Johannesson (1996).

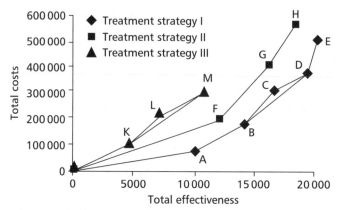

Fig. 5.5 Total costs and effectiveness of alternative treatment options (A–M) for the three treatment strategies (each has 1000 patients) (from Karlsson and Johannesson, 1996).

the treatments in the programme, they will not receive the others. Additionally, the treatment used in one patient group is assumed to be *independent* of the treatments used in other groups. That is, the costs and health effects of a treatment in one patient group are not affected by the treatment alternative chosen in any other patient group.

In Table 5.5 the incremental cost-effectiveness ratios are calculated for each successive alternative, from the least costly to the most. The same data are presented in Fig. 5.5. Here the incremental cost-effectiveness ratios are given by the slope of the line joining any two points (alternatives). (This is a development of the idea first presented in Fig. 3.2.)

The figure enables us to explore another notion of dominance, called *extended dominance* (Weinstein 1990). This is where the incremental cost-effectiveness ratio for a given treatment alternative is higher than that of the next, more effective, alternative. There are two cases of extended dominance in Fig. 5.5: alternatives C and L. For example, if all 1000 patients were given alternative C, this would cost 300 000 and 16 000 life-years would be gained. However, if 500 patients were given alternative B and 500 alternative D, the total cost would still be 300 000 but 16 500 life-years would be gained in total.

Graphically, we can see that points B and D can be connected with a line of lower slope (that is, lower cost-effectiveness ratio), in essence missing out point C. This is the same as saying that alternative C should be excluded from consideration as it is dominated. The same applies to alternative L. However, it should be noted that this analysis requires two simplifying assumptions: (1) that the treatments are perfectly divisible; and (2) that there are constant returns to scale. In other words, it has to be possible to deliver alternatives B and D to smaller numbers of patients without any reduction in cost-effectiveness. In real life this may not be possible and more complicated approaches are needed (see below).

Finally, this example can be used to determine how a fixed budget could be spent, if the objective is to maximize the number of life-years gained. With the budget as the decision-making constraint, the choice of treatments depends on the size of the budget. In order to maximize the life-years gained for a given budget, we order all the treatments in terms of their incremental cost-effectiveness ratios, starting with the do-nothing

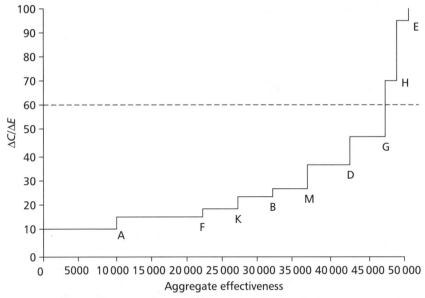

Fig. 5.6 The marginal cost of producing effectiveness (hypothetical treatments A–M) (from Karlsson and Johannesson, 1996).

or status quo option. We then begin by implementing the treatment with the lowest incremental ratio and then add independent treatments or replace mutually exclusive treatments until the budget is exhausted.

Figure 5.6 shows the alternatives that would be adopted, given increased sizes of budget. The steps in the curve indicate the increases in the incremental cost of producing life-years ($\Delta C/\Delta E$) as successive alternatives are added, beginning with A, which has an incremental ratio (over doing nothing) of 10.

Each budgetary limit defines a shadow price of life-years gained. For example, if the budget enabled us to adopt alternatives of successively higher incremental cost-effectiveness ratio up to and including G, the implied shadow price would be 50. That is, the implication of setting a budget of this size is that we are not willing to pay more than 50 for a unit of effectiveness. The alternative approach would be to state what we are willing to pay for a unit of effectiveness and to see what size of budget this implies.

The application of the logic implied by this hypothetical example raises a number of issues. Birch and Gafni (1993) argue that the two simplifying assumptions, perfect divisibility of programmes and constant returns to scale, are unlikely to apply in practice and that therefore the decision rules will not apply. Johannesson and Weinstein (1993) argue that the methods of dealing with indivisibility of programmes, through integer programming or dynamic programming, are well known and that, in any case, the simple rules give good approximations. In another paper, Stinnett and Paltiel (1996) demonstrate that a general programming framework can accommodate much more complex information regarding returns to scale, partial and complete indivisibility and programme interdependence. They also present methods for incorporating ethical constraints into the recourse allocation process, including explicit identification of the cost of equity.

However, the application of mathematical programming models in health care is still in its infancy. In a recent paper, Earnshaw and Dennett (2003) review a range of applications, ranging from radiotherapy treatment planning to the allocation of funds for HIV prevention. They argue that one of the main advantages of these methods is the simultaneous consideration of multiple constraints and a built-in sensitivity analysis.

One restriction is that the usefulness of models of this type is limited by the need for information about the costs and effects of all candidate programmes. For a decision-maker with a large budget covering many fields of health care this is clearly difficult, and probably impossible. However, Stinnett and Paltiel (1996) argue that even in these situations, the use of informed but imperfect estimates is preferable to the alternatives of either making uninformed decisions or relying on assumptions that lack face validity.

Nevertheless, decision-makers wishing to optimize the allocation of resources across a large budget require a reliable method for narrowing down the number of choices. One such approach is programme budgeting/marginal analysis (PBMA). The main features of PBMA involve identifying the range of available options (including current options and new proposals), the resources they would consume, and their likely effectiveness. By doing this, PBMA helps focus on those choices at the margin where shifts in the allocation of resources can generate more benefits in total. One finding of PBMA exercises is that decision-makers would at least like a systematic approach to priority setting, where all claims on resources are treated equally and judged at one time against agreed criteria (Mitton and Donaldson 2001 and 2003).

5.6. **From cost-effectiveness ratios to net benefits**

The incremental cost-effectiveness ratio remains the most popular method of presenting the results of CEA and CUA. However, as was mentioned in Chapters 1 and 2, it does have drawbacks. For example, the ratio gives no idea of the size or scale of the treatments or programmes being considered. Also, in Chapter 8, we will discover that testing for statistical differences between ratios gives rise to some additional complications. This has led some to propose *net benefit* as an alternative summary measure of the value for money of health-care programmes (Phelps and Mushlin 1991; Stinnett and Mullahy 1998).

In the discussion of the cost-effectiveness plane in Chapter 3, it was explained that the slope of the line joining the point determined by the incremental costs and effects of a programme and the origin (representing existing care) is the incremental cost-effectiveness ratio. Therefore, consider the cost-effectiveness plane, as drawn in Fig. 5.7, where point A represents a treatment or programme. The incremental ratio, compared to existing care (O), is OA. In addition, suppose that the dotted line, passing through the origin, represents our 'acceptable' cost-effectiveness ratio. That is, our maximum (or 'threshold') willingness-to-pay for a unit of effect (for example, a life-year or a QALY). The fact that this line passes through the origin, into the south-west quadrant on the cost-effectiveness plane, illustrates another problem with ratios. Namely, the same ratio is obtained when dividing a reduction in costs by a

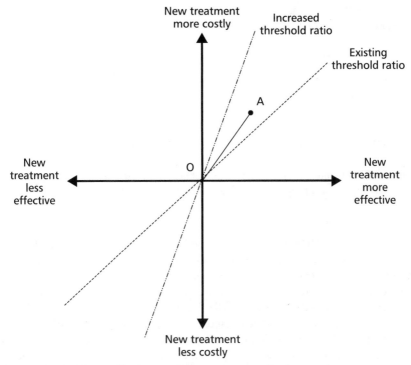

Fig. 5.7 Threshold cost-effectiveness ratios on the cost-effectiveness plane.

reduction in effects, whereas this has a different interpretation from the same ratio in the north-east quadrant.

It can be seen that the incremental ratio for programme A falls outside the acceptable range and the programme might therefore be deemed 'not cost-effective'. In fact the area to the right of the dotted line is our region of cost-effectiveness. It can also be seen that the region of cost-effectiveness is determined by our threshold willingness-to-pay. If our willingness-to-pay were zero—that is, our only interest is in saving costs—then the dotted line would be horizontal, passing through the origin. On the other hand, if our threshold willingness-to-pay is represented by the dashed line, then programme A would be deemed cost-effective.

The net benefit approach employs a simple re-arrangement of the cost-effectiveness decision rule in order to overcome the problems with cost-effectiveness ratios. If our threshold ratio is R_T, a programme is deemed cost-effective if

$$\Delta C / \Delta E < R_T$$

This expression can be re-arranged, showing that the programme is cost-effective if

$$R_T \Delta E - \Delta C > 0$$

$R_T \Delta E - \Delta C$ is called the *net monetary benefit* (*NMB*) of the programme. It is the increase in effectiveness (ΔE), multiplied by the amount the decision-maker is willing to pay per unit of increased effectiveness (R_T), less the increase in cost (ΔC). Thus, using the NMB approach, a programme is deemed cost-effective if

$$\text{NMB} = R_T \Delta E - \Delta C > 0$$

Of course, if R_T were actually known, or had been estimated from individuals' willingness-to-pay, this net benefit expression would be equivalent to the calculation performed in a cost-benefit analysis. For NMB to be positive, $R_T \Delta E$ has to be greater than ΔC.

Whilst the NMB expression is probably most familiar to economists, and is the one most often referred to as '*net benefit*' in the literature, it is also possible to re-arrange the inequality in another way to define the *net health benefit* (*NHB*). In this case, using the NHB approach, a programme is deemed cost-effective if

$$\text{NHB} = \Delta E - (\Delta C / R_T) > 0$$

That is, for the NHB to be positive, the health gain (ΔE) has to be greater than that from investing the same resources in an alternative, marginally cost-effective programme, having the cost-effectiveness ratio R_T.

When operating within the CEA paradigm, where the real value of R_T is not known, it is common to present the results of a study giving NMB or NHB as a function of R_T. In a plot of NMB as a function of the threshold ratio, NMB is zero when the incremental cost-effectiveness ratio for the health programme being studied is equal to the threshold ratio. Also, when R_T is zero, the intercept on the y axis represents the negative value of the incremental costs of programme A compared with existing care (see Fig. 5.8).

The discussion here has been conducted within a deterministic framework (that is, one where the incremental costs and benefits of a given programme are known with certainty). We will return to this issue in Chapter 8, when the concept of uncertainty around the estimates of cost-effectiveness ratios and net benefits is introduced.

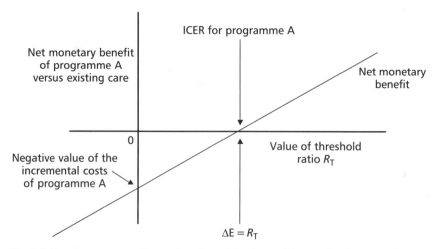

Fig. 5.8 Net monetary benefit as a function of the threshold cost-effectiveness ratio.

5.7. **Concluding remarks**

Cost-effectiveness analysis is a form of full economic evaluation where both costs and consequences are considered. Many of the issues raised in this chapter, such as the sources of clinical data, the discounting of health effects and the ways of combining clinical and resource data, are also pertinent to the other forms of economic evaluation discussed below.

Cost-effectiveness analysis has been very popular to date and is a very useful approach where there is a single unambiguous objective of therapy. However, many health care programmes have multiple objectives or outcomes and the issue of assigning preferences or values to these outcomes becomes central to the evaluation. This issue is tackled in Chapters 6 and 7.

References

Adams, M. E., McCall, N. T., Gray, D. T., *et al.* (1992). Economic analysis in randomized control trials. *Medical Care*, **30**, 231–43.

Birch, S. and Gafni, A. (1993). Changing the problem to fit the solution: Johannesson and Weinstein's (mis)application of economics to real world problems. *Journal of Health Economics*, **12**, 469–76.

Brazier, J. (1993). The SF-36 Health Survey Questionnaire—a tool for economists. *Health Economics*, **2**, 213–15.

Brazier, J. and Dixon, S. (1995). The use of condition specific outcome measures in economic appraisal. *Health Economics*, **4**, 255–64.

Brazier, J., Roberts, J., and Deverill, M. (2002). The estimation of a preference-based measure of health from the SF-36. *Journal of Health Economics*, **21**, 271–92.

Brouwer, W. B. F. and van Exel, N. J. A. (2004). Discounting in decision making: the consistency argument revisited empirically. *Health Policy*, **67**, 187–94.

Buxton, M. J., Drummond, M. F., van Hout, B. A., *et al.* (1997). Modelling in economic evaluation: an unavoidable fact of life? *Health Economics*, **6**, 217–27.

Cairns, J. (1992). Discounting and health effects for medical decisions. In: *Valuing health care: costs, benefits and effectiveness of pharmaceuticals and medical technologies* (ed. F. A. Sloan), pp. 123–45. Cambridge University Press, New York.

Cairns, J. (2001). Discounting in economic evaluation. In: *Economic evaluation in health care: merging theory with practice* (ed. M. F. Drummond and A. McGuire), pp. 236–255. Oxford University Press, Oxford.

Chancellor, J., Coyle, D., and Drummond, M. F. (1997). Constructing health state preference values from descriptive quality of life data: mission impossible? *Quality of Life Research*, **6**, 159–68.

Cohen, B. J. (2003). Discounting in cost-utility analysis of healthcare interventions: reassessing current practice. *PharmacoEconomics*, **21**, 75–87.

Cook, D. J., Guyatt, G. H., Laupacis, A., and Sackett, D. L. (1992). Rules of evidence and clinical recommendations on the use of antithrombitic agents. *Chest*, **102**, 305S–11S.

Coyle, D. and Lee, K. M. (2002). Evidence-based economic evaluation: how the use of different data sources can impact results. In: *Evidence-based health economics* (ed. C. Donaldson, M. Mugford, and L. Vale), pp. 55–66. BMJ Books, London.

Coyle, D., Davies, L. M., and Drummond, M. F. (1998). Trials and tribulations: emerging issues in designing economic evaluations alongside clinical trials. *International Journal of Technology Assessment in Health Care*, **14**, 135–44.

Detsky, A. S. (1995). Evidence of effectiveness: evaluating its quality. In: *Valuing health care.* (ed. F. A. Sloan), pp. 15–29. Cambridge University Press, New York.

Dowie, J. (2002). Decision validity should determine whether a generic or condition-specific HRQOL measure is used in health care decisions. *Health Economics*, **11**, 1–8 (see also the commentaries on pages 9–22).

Drummond, M. F. (1998). Experimental versus observational data in the economic evaluation of pharmaceuticals. *Medical Decision Making*, **18**, S12–S18.

Drummond, M. F. and Davies, L. M. (1991). Economic analysis alongside clinical trials: revisiting the methodological issues. *International Journal of Technology Assessment in Health Care*, **7**, 561–73.

Earnshaw, S. R. and Dennett, S. L. (2003). Integer/linear mathematical programming models: a tool for allocating healthcare resources. *PharmacoEconomics*, **21**, 839–51.

Fineberg, H. V. (1980). Decision trees: construction, uses, and limits. *Bulletin du Cancer*, **67**, 395–404.

Freemantle, N. and Maynard, A. (1994). Something rotten in the state of clinical and economic evaluations? *Health Economics*, **3**, 63–7.

Glick, H. A., Polsky, D. P., and Schulman, K. A. (2001). Trial-based economic evaluations: an overview of design and analysis. In: *Economic evaluation in health care: merging theory with practice* (ed. M. F. Drummond and A. McGuire), pp. 113–140. Oxford University Press, Oxford.

Gold, M. R., Siegel, J. E., Russell, L. B., and Weinstein, M. C. (ed.) (1996). *Cost-effectiveness in health and medicine.* Oxford University Press, New York.

Gravelle, H. and Smith, D. (2001). Discounting for health effects in cost-benefit and cost-effectiveness analysis. *Health Economics*, **10**, 587–99.

Grossman, M. (1972). *The demand for health: a theoretical and empirical investigation*, NBER Occasional Paper 119. National Bureau of Economic Research, New York.

Guyatt, G. and Rennie, D. (2002). *Users' guides to the medical literature: a manual for evidence-based clinical practice.* AMA. Press, Chicago.

Guyatt, G. H., Feeny, D. H., and Patrick, D. L. (1993). Measuring health-related quality of life. *Annals of Internal Medicine*, **118**, 622–9.

Hillman, A. L. and Bloom, B. S. (1989). Economic effects of prophylactic use of misoprostol to prevent gastric ulcer in patients taking nonsteroidal anti-inflammatory drugs. *Archives of Internal Medicine*, **149**, 2061–5.

Hull, R. D., Hirsh, J., Sackett, D. L., and Stoddart, G. L. (1981). Cost-effectiveness of clinical diagnosis, venography and non-invasive testing in patients with symptomatic deep-vein thrombosis. *New England Journal of Medicine*, **304**, 1561–7.

Hull, R. D., Hirsh, J., Sackett, D. L., and Stoddart, G. L. (1982). Cost-effectiveness of primary and secondary prevention of fatal pulmonary embolism in high-risk surgical patients. *Canadian Medical Association Journal*, **127**, 990–5.

Jefferson, T. and Demicheli, V. (1994). Is vaccination against Hepatitis B efficient? A review of world literature. *Health Economics*, **3**, 25–37.

Johannesson, M. and Weinstein, M. C. (1993). On the decision rules of cost-effectiveness analysis. *Journal of Health Economics*, **12**, 913–17.

Karlsson, G. and Johannesson, M. (1996). The decision rules of cost-effectiveness analysis. *PharmacoEconomics*, **9**, 113–20.

Keeler, E. and Cretin, S. (1983). Discounting of life savings and other non-momentary effects. *Management Science*, **29**, 300–6.

Khan, K. S., ter Riet, G., Glanville, J., Sowden, A. J., and Kleijnen, J. (ed.) (2001). *Undertaking systematic reviews of research on effectiveness*, CRD Report Number 4 (2nd edn). Centre for Reviews and Dissemination, University of York, York.

L'Abbe, K. A., Detsky, A. S., and O'Rourke, K. (1987). Meta-analysis in clinical research. *Annals of Internal Medicine*, **107**, 224–33.

Lazaro, A. (2002). Theoretical arguments for the discounting of health consequences: where do we go from here? *PharmacoEconomics*, **20**, 943–61.

Logan, A. G., Milne, B. J., Achber, C., Campbell, W. P., and Haynes, R. B. (1981). Cost-effectiveness of a worksite hypertension treatment programme. *Hypertension*, **3**, 211–18.

Mark, D. B., Hlatky, M. A., Califf, R. M., *et al.* (1995). Cost-effectiveness of thrombolytic therapy with tissue plasminogen activator as compared with streptokinase for acute myocardial infarction. *New England Journal of Medicine*, **332**, 1418–24.

Mitton, C. and Donaldson, C. (2001). Twenty-five years of programme budgeting and marginal analysis in the health sector, 1974–1999. *Journal of Health Service Research and Policy*, **6**, 239–48.

Mitton, C. and Donaldson, C. (2003). Setting priorities and allocating resources in health regions: lessons from a project evaluating program budgeting and marginal analysis (PBMA). *Health Policy*, **64**, 335–48.

Mugford, M. (1989). Reducing the incidence of infection after caesarian section: implications of prophylaxis with antibiotics for hospital resources. *British Medical Journal*, **299**, 10003–6.

National Institute for Clinical Excellence (2004). *Guide to the methods of technology appraisal*. National Institute for Clinical Excellence, London.

O'Brien, B. (1994). Measurement of health-related quality of life in the economic evaluation of medicines. *Drug Information Journal*, **28**, 45–53.

O'Brien, B., Goeree, R., Mohamed, A. H., and Hunt, R. (1995). Cost-effectiveness of *Helicobacter pylori* eradication for the long-term management of duodenal ulcer in Canada. *Archives of Internal Medicine*, **155**, 1958–64.

Oster, G. and Epstein, A. M. (1987). Cost-effectiveness of antihyperlipidemic therapy in the prevention of coronary heart disease: the case of cholestyramine. *Journal of the American Medical Association*, **258**, 2381–7.

Palmer, S., Sculpher, M., Philips, Z., *et al.* (in press). Management of non-ST-elevation acute coronary syndromes: how cost-effective are glycoprotein IIb/IIIa antagonists in the UK National Health Service? *International Journal of Cardiology*.

Parsonage, M. and Neuburger, H. (1992). Discounting and health benefits. *Health Economics*, **1**, 71–6.

Phelps, C. E. and Mushlin, A. (1991). On the (near) equivalence of cost-effectiveness and cost–benefit analyses. *International Journal of Technology Assessment in Health Care*, **7**, 12–21.

Saint, S., Veenstra, D. L., and Sullivan, S. D. (1999). The use of meta-analysis in cost-effectiveness analysis: issues and recommendations. *PharmacoEconomics*, **15**, 1–8.

Scandinavian Simvastatin Survival Study Group (1994). Randomised trial of cholesterol lowering in 4444 patients with coronary heart disease. *Lancet*, **344**, 1383–9.

Schulman, K. A., Kinosian, B., Jacobson, J. A., *et al.* (1990). Reducing high blood cholesterol level with drugs. *Journal of the American Medical Association*, **264**, 3025–33.

Sculpher, M. J. and Buxton, M. J. (1993). The episode-free day as a composite measure of effectiveness. *PharmacoEconomics*, **4**, 345–52.

Sculpher, M. J., Drummond, M. F., and Buxton, M. J. (1997). The iterative use of economic evaluation as part of the process of health technology assessment. *Journal of Health Services Research and Policy*, **2(1)**, 26–30.

Severens, J. L. and Milne, R. J. (2004). Discounting health outcomes in economic evaluation: the ongoing debate. *Value in Health*, **7**, 397–401.

Shepherd, J., Cobbe, S. M., Ford, I., *et al.* (1995). Prevention of coronary heart disease with pravastatin in men with hypercholesterolemia. *New England Journal of Medicine*, **333**, 1301–7.

Smith, D. and Gravelle, H. (2001). The practice of discounting economic evaluations of health care interventions. *International Journal of Technology Assessment in Health Care*, **17**, 236–43.

Stinnett, A. and Mullahy, J. (1998). Net health benefits: a new framework for the analysis of uncertainty in cost-effectiveness analysis. *Medical Decision Making*, **18**, S68–S80.

Skinnett, A. A. and Paltiel, A. D. (1996). Mathematical programming for the efficient allocation of health care resources. *Journal of Health Economics*, **15**, 641–53.

Tan-Torres Edejer, T., Baltussen, R., Adam, T., *et al.* (2003). *Making choices in health care: WHO guide to cost-effectiveness analysis.* World Health Organization, Geneva.

van Hout, B. A. (1998). Discounting costs and effects: reconsideration. *Health Economics*, **7**, 581–94.

Viscusi, W. K. (1995). Discounting health effects for medical decisions. In: *Valuing health care: costs, benefits and effectiveness of pharmaceuticals and medical technologies* (ed. F. A. Sloan), pp. 123–145. Cambridge University Press, New York.

Weinstein, M. C. (1990). Principles of cost-effective resource allocation in health care organizations. *International Journal of Technology Assessment in Health Care*, **6**, 93–105.

Weinstein, M. C. and Fineberg, H. V. (1980). *Clinical decision analysis.* Saunders, Philadelphia.

Weinstein, M. C. and Stason, W. B. (1977). Foundations of cost-effectiveness analysis for health and medical practices. *New England Journal of Medicine*, **296**, 716–21.

Chapter 6

Cost–utility analysis

6.1. Some basics

Cost–utility analysis (CUA) is a form of evaluation that focuses particular attention on the quality of the health outcome produced or forgone by health programmes or treatments. It has many similarities to cost-effectiveness analysis (CEA), and thus all the points discussed in Chapter 4 on cost analysis and many of those discussed in Chapter 5 on CEA also apply here. The first section of this chapter reviews some of the general issues the analyst would need to consider when undertaking a CUA. Later sections discuss particular issues in more detail.

6.1.1. How does cost–utility analysis differ from cost-effectiveness analysis?

In CEA, the incremental cost of a programme from a particular viewpoint is compared to the incremental health effects of the programme, where the health effects are measured in natural units related to the objective of the programme, for example, average blood pressure improvement in mm Hg, cases found, cases of disease averted, patients significantly improved, lives saved, or life-years gained. The results are usually expressed as a cost per unit of effect. In CUA, the incremental cost of a programme from a particular viewpoint is compared to the incremental health improvement attributable to the programme, where the health improvement is measured in quality-adjusted life-years (QALYs) gained, or possibly some variant, like disability-adjusted life-years (DALYs) gained. The results are expressed as a cost per QALY gained. Thus, there are many similarities between CEA and CUA. For example, the questions of whether or not to include productivity changes (Section 4.4) and whether or not to discount future effects (Section 5.1.4) still apply.

Cost-effectiveness analysis and CUA are similar, if not identical, on the cost side, but differ on the outcomes side. As described in Box 6.1, outcomes in CEA are single, programme specific, and unvalued. In contrast, outcomes in CUA may be single or multiple, are generic as opposed to programme specific, and incorporate the notion of value. Cost–utility analysis, because of its broad applicability, is more useful to decision-makers with a broad mandate than is CEA.

Both CEA and CUA require valid effectiveness data (from the literature, from your own study, or from expert judgement supplemented by sensitivity analysis), but in the case of CUA only final outcome effectiveness data will suffice (for example, lives saved, disability-days averted). Intermediate output data (for example, cases found,

Box 6.1 **Why was cost–utility analysis developed?**

In cost-effectiveness analysis the outcomes are measured in programme-specific units such as millimetres of blood pressure reduction, disability-days averted, cases cured, lives saved, and life-years gained. Typically the main outcome is designated as the primary effectiveness measure and used as the denominator in the cost/effectiveness ratio. There are four problems. First, because the measure of primary effectiveness may differ from programme to programme, cost-effectiveness analysis cannot be used to make comparisons across a broad set of interventions. Second, decision-makers with a limited budget must not only determine if a new programme is cost-effective but must also determine which programme to reduce to free up funds for the new programme. Cost-effectiveness analysis cannot typically address this issue of the opportunity cost of funding the new programme. Third, in any one programme there is often more than one outcome of interest. In fact, normally there is a large number of relevant outcomes; for example, outcomes of any specific intervention often include life extension, long-term quality of life changes, side-effects, both major and minor, from the intervention, as well as the short-term quality of life effects of the intervention itself. Fourth, some outcomes are more important, or more valued, than others.

Cost–utility analysis was developed to address these problems. It enables a broad range of relevant outcomes to be included by providing a method through which the various disparate outcomes can be combined into a single composite summary outcome. This, in turn, allows broad comparisons across widely differing programmes. And, finally, cost–utility analysis provides a method to attach values to the outcomes so the more important outcomes are weighted more heavily.

patients appropriately treated) are unsuitable, because they cannot directly be converted into an outcome measure like QALYs gained which is required for CUA. As an aside, intermediate outcomes may well be suitable for clinical decision analysis using a patient's utilities for the intermediate outcomes, but they are simply unsuitable for CUA where the outcomes must be expressed in an outcome measure like QALYs gained.

By converting the effectiveness data to a common unit of measure, like QALYs gained, CUA is able to incorporate simultaneously both the changes in the quantity of life (mortality) and the changes in the quality of life (morbidity). In the QALY approach, the quality adjustment is based on a set of values or weights called utilities, one for each possible health state, which reflect the relative desirability of the health state.

Because of the similarities between CUA and CEA some authors do not distinguish between the two, particularly in the USA. For example, Weinstein and Stason (1977) and Gold *et al.* (1996*b*) treat CUA as a particular case of CEA. Thus, be aware in reading the literature that CUA may appear under other labels.

Although technically CUA can be seen as simply a specific type of CEA, we have continued to use the separate label because we believe it is useful for several reasons. First, it clearly distinguishes between those studies that use a generic measure of outcome and thus are potentially comparable across studies (CUA), and those that use a measure of outcome specific to the programme under study (CEA). Second, it highlights the crucial role of consumer preferences (utilities) in valuing the outcomes. Third, because of the need to incorporate consumer preferences, there is much that is special about CUA. And, finally, we have continued with the CUA label to maintain consistency with the previous editions, and with much of the field of health economics, which has now adopted the distinction. (See Box 6.2. for a brief history of CUA.)

Box 6.2 **History of cost–utility analysis**

In the beginning the approach described in this chapter was not called cost–utility analysis. Because it relaxed the narrow restrictiveness of traditional cost-effectiveness analysis, it was first called generalized cost-effectiveness analysis (Torrance 1971). Later it was called utility maximization (Torrance *et al.* 1972) and the health status index model (Torrance 1976*b*). The health status index approach was also the initial label used for a similar development from the Bush group at San Diego (Fanshel and Bush 1970; Bush *et al.* 1972). The label 'cost–utility analysis' was first used by our group in 1981 (Sinclair *et al.* 1981) and by the Bush group in 1982 (Kaplan and Bush 1982). Since then the cost–utility label has stuck, except in the USA where many analysts still call it cost-effectiveness.

We adopted the CUA label to distinguish the approach from CEA. The distinguishing features of CUA are that multiple outcomes can be incorporated and the outcomes are not just counted but are valued according to their desirability. In addition, a distinguishing feature of CUA, as we practise it, is that the relative desirability of outcomes is measured using von Neumann-Morgenstern utility theory. Hence, the origin of the name cost-UTILITY analysis. Although we believe the name is useful, it has caused its own confusion. On the one hand, there are those who correctly point out that, from a theoretical point of view, CUA as conventionally practised, even using von NM utilities as the quality-adjustment weights, would maximize utility only under very restrictive assumptions (Weinstein and Fineberg 1980; Torrance and Feeny 1989; Mehrez and Gafni 1991; Garber and Phelps 1995) and so one might argue the label is misleading. On the other hand, there are many studies, including our own (Oldridge *et al.* 1993), that have used the CUA label regardless of how the quality-adjustment weights were determined (Kaplan and Bush 1982; Kaplan *et al.* 1988; Goel and Detsky 1989; Hall *et al.* 1992; Kennedy *et al.* 1995). Our view is that the CUA label is useful in describing a certain class of studies, and thus helps to communicate. However, use of the label does not guarantee that all studies have used a uniform methodology (Gerard 1992; Chapman *et al.* 2000), and readers need to assess for themselves how the study has been conducted.

6.1.2. **When should cost–utility analysis be used?**

The following are a number of situations where you might wish to use CUA.

1 When health-related quality of life is *the* important outcome. For example, in comparing alternative programmes for the treatment of arthritis, no programme is expected to have an impact on mortality, and the interest is focused on how well the different programmes improve the patient's physical function, social function, and psychological well-being.

2 When health-related quality of life is *an* important outcome. For example, in evaluating neonatal intensive care for very-low-birth-weight infants, not only is survival an important outcome, but also the quality of that survival is critical.

3 When the programme affects both morbidity and mortality and you wish to have a common unit of outcome that combines both effects. For example, treatments for many cancers improve longevity and improve long-term quality of life, but decrease quality of life during the treatment process itself.

4 When the programmes being compared have a wide range of different kinds of outcomes and you wish to have a common unit of output for comparison. For example, if you are a health planner who must compare several disparate programmes applying for funding, such as an expansion of neonatal intensive care, a programme to locate and treat hypertensives, and a programme to expand the rehabilitative services provided to post-myocardial infarction patients.

5 When you wish to compare a programme to others that have already been evaluated using CUA.

6 When you are dealing with a limited budget situation such that the decision-maker must determine which programmes or services to reduce or eliminate to free up funding for the new programme.

7 When your objective is to allocate limited resources optimally by considering all alternatives and using constrained optimization (for example, mathematical programming) to maximize the health gain achieved.

6.2. **Utilities**

The term 'utility' has been around for several centuries, has been used by a variety of disciplines, and has a number of related but different meanings (Cooper and Rappoport 1984; Miyamoto 1988; Sen 1991). Thus, it creates a significant potential for confusion and for people to talk past each other. In a broad way the term has always been synonymous with preference; the more preferable an outcome, the more utility associated with it. The differences in meaning arise when approaches are developed to define the concept more precisely and especially when attempts are made to measure it.

Measured preferences may be ordinal or cardinal. For ordinal preferences, outcomes simply need to be rank ordered, with ties allowed, from most preferred to least preferred. For cardinal preferences, a number must be attached to the outcome that in some sense represents the strength of preference for the outcome relative to the others. These numbers should be measured such that they fall on an interval scale, in two senses. First, in terms of measurement theory, the scale should be an interval scale as described later in Section 6.5.2; that is, a scale like temperature in °F, that has no natural zero and is unique under a positive linear transformation. Second, in terms of the individual's preferences, the scale must have the equal interval property in the sense that the interval from 0.2 to 0.3 has the same meaning to the individual as the interval from 0.8 to 0.9 (Bossert 1991).

6.2.1. **History of utility theories**

This is an optional section that readers may skip, if they wish, without loss of continuity.

In 1944, a mathematician, John von Neumann, and an economist, Oscar Morgenstern, first published their theory of rational decision-making under uncertainty, now called expected utility theory, or sometimes von Neumann–Morgenstern utility theory (von Neumann and Morgenstern 1944). Interestingly, they developed the theory, not for its own sake, but only because they needed it as a small part of a theory of games they were developing. History now remembers them only secondarily for their contributions to game theory, and primarily for their enormous contribution in developing a theory of decision-making that has dominated the field for over half a century.

Von Neumann and Morgenstern developed a normative model; that is, they prescribed how a rational individual 'ought' to make decisions when faced with uncertain outcomes. To do this they defined, in a set of fundamental axioms, what they meant by rational behaviour under uncertainty (see Box 6.3). The axioms are compelling, have withstood vigorous debate, and have remained the dominant normative definition of rational behaviour under uncertainty for over half a century. The axioms are certainly not without controversy, and to this day they are constantly under attack with many variations and alternatives being proposed (Allais 1991; Schoemaker 1991; Currim and Sarin 1992; Schoemaker 1992; Tversky and Kahneman 1992; Kleindorfer *et al.* 1993; Wakker *et al.* 1994; Fishburn and Wakker 1995; Cohen 1996; Nease 1996). However, no alternative has dislodged them from their position as the dominant normative paradigm. The axioms of von Neumann and Morgenstern provide the foundation for modern decision theory, which has been widely applied in business, government, health care, and many other fields for several decades. See, for example, the applications described in Chapter 9. Their work also represented a seminal contribution to the economic theory of behaviour under uncertainty.

It is doubly unfortunate, however, that von Neumann and Morgenstern called their new approach 'utility theory' and called the associated preference measures 'utilities'. First, in their usage, utility did not mean usefulness as it does in normal language. Second, in their usage utility meant neither what it had traditionally meant to economists and philosophers during the nineteenth century nor what it meant to modern economists. In developing consumer theory during the nineteenth century, economists assumed the existence of a cardinal utility function that represented the consumer's satisfaction for various bundles of commodities received with certainty. Nineteenth-century philosophers used this concept of utility as the foundation for

Box 6.3 **Axioms of von Neumann–Morgenstern utility theory**

The original axioms of von Neuman and Morgenstern have been refined and restated over the years by various authors. Bell and Farquhar (1986) present the axioms as follows.

1 *Preference exist and are transitive.* For any pair of risky prospects y and y' eithery y is preferred to y', y' is preferred to y or the individual is indifferent between y and y'. In addition, for any three risky prospects, y, y', and y'', if y is preferred to y', and y' is preferred to y'', then y is preferred to y''; similarly, if y is indifferent to y', and y' is indifferent to y'', then y is indifferent to y''.

2 *Independence.* An individual should be indifferent between a two-stage risky prospect and its probabilistically equivalent one-stage counterpart derived using the ordinary laws of probability. For example, consider two risky prospects y and y' where y is made up of outcome x_1 with probability p_1 and outcome x_2 with probability $(1 - p_1)$, indicated symbolically as $y = \{p_1, x_1, x_2\}$, and $y' = \{p_2, x_1, x_2\}$. This axiom implies that an individual would be indifferent between the two-stage risky prospect (p, y, y'), and its probabilistically equivalent one-stage counterpart $\{pp_1 + (1 - p)p_2, x_1, x_2\}$.

3 *Continuity of preferences.* If there are three outcomes such that x_1 is preferred to x_2, which is preferred to x_3, there is some probability p at which the individual is indifferent between outcome x_2 with certainty or receiving the risky prospect made up of outcome x_1 with probability p and outcome x_3 with probability $1 - p$.

utilitarian ethics in which utilities among individuals were compared and aggregated to decide on the socially optimal policy. Ultimately, this approach, particularly the comparison and aggregation of these individual utilities, was rejected.

At the turn of the century, the Italian economist, Vilfredo Pareto, discovered that ordinal utilities were sufficient to support consumer theory. More recently, Arrow and Debreu (1954) further refined the theory based on the concept of consumers' preference orderings, including risk. As a result, students of micro-economics have been taught that cardinal utility (under certainty) is unnecessary, probably immeasurable, and may not even exist. For a discussion of this history see Russell and Wilkinson (1979) or Allais (1991). For a discussion of the relationship of von Neumann–Morgenstern utilities within micro-economics see Hey (1979).

The key point here is that cardinal utilities under uncertainty, as defined by von Neumann and Morgenstern, are quite different from both the ordinal utilities underlying contemporary micro-economics and the cardinal utilities (under certainty) of nineteenth-century economists. To avoid these potential confusions, it is frequently recommended that users of modern utility theory under uncertainty refer to their measures as 'von Neumann–Morgenstern (NM) utilities'. Unfortunately, very few writers take this precaution. From this point in the book, unless otherwise specified, we use utility to mean NM utility.

Following the initial work by von Neumann and Morgenstern, the field has expanded rapidly and there is now a vast literature. Some representative books include those by Luce and Raiffa (1957), Raiffa (1968), Holloway (1979), and Keeney and Raiffa (1976, 1993).

It is important to appreciate that the von Neumann–Morgenstern axioms and utility theory are not intended as descriptions of how individuals actually make decisions in the face of uncertainty, but as a prescriptive or normative model of how they 'ought' to make such decisions if they wish to act rationally as defined by the basic axioms. Although there is some evidence that individuals in some circumstances do follow the model (Fischer 1979; Currim and Sarin 1992; Nease 1996), there is much more evidence that they do not (Loomes 1991; Luce 1992).

We should not be surprised that individual behaviour does not necessarily follow a normative model; normative models are not behavioural models. Normative models are used to define approaches that individuals should take to be consistent with underlying theories; behavioural models are used to describe actual behaviour as found in reality. As Howard (1988) points out, 'the whole idea of a normative model arises when we are not satisfied with our functioning . . . [In] view of the many easily demonstrated lapses in human decision-making that we can observe, who would want to rely on unaided judgement for a complex and important decision problem?'.

6.2.2. **Utility, value, and preference**

Many people use the terms 'utility', 'value', and 'preference' interchangeably, but in fact there are differences. Preference is the umbrella term that describes the overall concept; utilities and values are different types of preferences. What you get depends on how you do the measurements (see Table 6.1). There are two key aspects of the measurement process. One is the way in which the question is framed, specifically whether the outcomes in the question are certain or uncertain. The other is the way in

Table 6.1 Methods of measuring preferences

Response method	Question framing	
	Certainty (values)	**Uncertainty (utilities)**
Scaling	1 Rating scale Category scaling Visual analogue scale Ratio scale	2
Choice	3 Time trade-off Paired comparison Equivalence Person trade-off	4 Standard gamble

which the subject is asked to respond, specifically whether the subject is asked to perform a scaling task based on introspection or to make a choice.

Consider a subject being asked preference questions for health outcomes, where each outcome is a specific lifetime path for the subject. That is, each outcome describes a path from now to death consisting of one or more health states for specified time periods. This, in fact, is the most general case of measuring preferences for health outcomes, and all health state preference measurement uses, or should use, this format. Even measuring preferences for single temporary states, such as 1 week of hospitalization for an acute episode of some disease, cannot be done in isolation of what will follow. What will follow should always be described explicitly, else the subject will implicitly assume something and it will affect the measurement in unknown ways.

A question framed under certainty would ask the subject to compare two or more outcomes and to choose between them or to scale them. In thinking about each outcome, the subject is asked to assume that the outcome would occur with certainty. There are no unknowns and no probabilities in the way the various futures are described. A question framed under uncertainty would ask the subject to compare two alternatives, where at least one of the alternatives contained uncertainty; that is, it contained probabilities. The conventional standard gamble question, described in Section 6.3.2, is a common example. The difference between these two forms of questioning is that the certainty method does not capture the subject's risk attitude, while the uncertainty method does.

Risk attitude is a well-known concept in preference measurements and utility theory (Keeney and Raiffa 1976; Holloway 1979; Gafni and Torrance 1984). The intuitive notion is that if a person shies away from more risky alternatives in favour of less risky alternatives, they are risk averse. If they are indifferent, they are risk neutral, and if they prefer risky situations, they are risk seeking. Mathematically, the concept can only be operationalized when measuring preferences over outcomes that are themselves defined on an interval scale. Then, the definition is that if the subject prefers the expected value of an uncertain alternative to the uncertain alternative itself, the subject is risk averse; indifference between the two represents risk neutrality; and a preference for the gamble indicates a risk-seeking attitude.

For example, a subject who prefers $100 for sure to a 50/50 gamble of receiving $0 or $200 would be said to be risk averse with respect to money. On the other hand, if the subject was indifferent between the two, they would be risk neutral; and if the gamble was preferred, they would be risk-seeking. Similarly, a subject who rated three health outcomes, A, B, and C, on a visual analogue scale (VAS) as valued at 0.4, 0.6, and 0.8, who then preferred outcome B for sure to a 50/50 gamble of receiving outcome A or C, would be said to be risk averse with respect to value. As in the case for money, if the subject had been indifferent, they would have been classed as risk neutral; and if they had preferred the gamble, they would be called risk seeking. Risk attitude with respect to values is sometimes called relative risk attitude (Dyer and Sarin 1979, 1982; Torrance et al. 1995) to differentiate it from risk attitudes with respect to fundamental consequences like dollars or years of healthy life (YHL).

Note that the risk attitude really only pertains to a specific question. There is no requirement that a person have a consistent risk attitude over multiple questions.

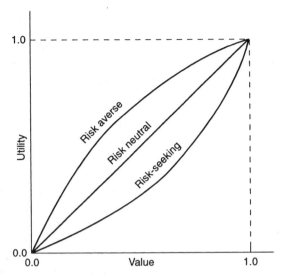

Fig. 6.1 The three generic types of relative risk attitude. From Torrance *et al.* (1995), Fig. 1.

For example, it is often found empirically that people are risk averse for large gains, risk seeking for small gains, and risk seeking for losses (Holloway 1979; Fischer *et al.* 1986). However, the existence of a consistent risk attitude that can be modelled mathematically is often assumed for practical convenience. For example, the three generic types of relative risk attitude are shown in Fig. 6.1. As the figure shows, a person whose relative risk attitude is consistently risk averse over the length of the scale will have utilities (preferences adjusted for risk) that exceed their values (riskless preferences). Empirically, this is the common finding.

The second dimension of Table 6.1 refers to the response method. A subject can be asked to determine a strength of preference by introspection and to indicate the result on a numerical scale. Alternatively, a subject can be asked to choose between two alternatives, thus revealing the preference indirectly. The first approach is primarily rooted in psychology and psychometric scaling, although it is also described in the field of decision science as a measurable value function (Dyer and Sarin 1979, 1982; Loomes 1995). The second method comes primarily from economics and decision sciences, and is a particular application of the revealed preference approach. (Revealed preference is a general approach in economics whereby the underlying preferences are revealed by the choices that individuals make.) The advantage of scaling is that it takes less respondent time. The advantage of the choice-based methods is that choosing, unlike scaling, is a natural human task at which we all have considerable experience, and furthermore it is observable and verifiable. Thus, many analysts, including ourselves, prefer the choice-based methods in designing studies.

Table 6.1 is divided into four cells. Cell 1 contains instruments that require the subject to think introspectively about outcomes presented with certainty and to provide a rating or a score. Rating scales (assign a number), category scales (assign a category), and VASs (mark a line) are all variations on the same theme. Ratio scaling, as used by Rosser and colleagues (Rosser and Kind 1978; Rosser and Watts 1978), also belongs in this category. In ratio scaling, subjects were asked to indicate how many times worse one outcome was compared to the next best outcome. The outcomes were defined with certainty and the task was one of introspection. There are no instruments that fall in cell 2 to our knowledge, although presumably one could ask subjects to rate their preferences for gamble alternatives. Cell 3 contains the time trade-off (TTO) approach (see Section 6.3.3), the paired comparison approach (Streiner and Norman 1989; Hadorn et al. 1992; Hadorn and Uebersax 1995), and the old equivalence approach (Patrick et al. 1973; Patrick and Erickson 1993), now renamed the person trade-off (PTO) approach (Nord et al. 1993; Nord 1995, 1996, 1999; Green 2001). Finally, cell 4 contains the well-known standard gamble in all its variations (Torrance 1986; Torrance and Feeny 1989; Furlong et al. 1990; O'Brien et al. 1994; Bennett and Torrance 1996; Torrance et al. 2002).

To summarize, all of the methods in Table 6.1 measure preferences. Those in cells 1 and 3 measure values; those in cell 4 measure utilities. Because the task is different in each cell, one should not be surprised that the resulting preference scores will differ. Indeed, the common finding is that, for states preferred to death, standard gamble scores are greater than TTO scores, which in turn are greater than visual analogue scores (Torrance 1976a; Wolfson et al. 1982; Read et al. 1984; Churchill et al. 1987; Bass et al. 1994; Stiggelbout et al. 1994; O'Leary et al. 1995; Rutten-van Molken et al. 1995; Bennett and Torrance 1996). However, one study produced the contrary finding of TTO scores exceeding standard gamble scores (Dolan et al. 1996a). The reason given for the differences between cells 3 and 4 is risk attitude, which is only captured in cell 4. The reason for the difference between cells 1 and 3 presumably lies in the difference between choosing and scaling.

Which method is best? As indicated earlier, other things being equal, we prefer choice-based methods over scaling methods. In practice, other things are not equal, notably the time required to use the different approaches, and we typically use a mixture of scaling and choice questions (see Section 6.4.5). In choosing between values and utilities we can get some help from the underlying theories. Von Neumann–Morgenstern utility theory indicates that utilities are appropriate for problems that involve uncertainty *or* certainty or both; note that outcomes with certainty can be included as a degenerate probability distribution (that is, a probability distribution with a single outcome that has a probability of 1.0). On the other hand, again based on the underlying theory, values are *only* appropriate for problems that involve certainty; thus, values are much more restricted in their applicability. Another way to think of it is that only utilities capture the individual's risk attitude and this is essential for problems that contain uncertainty. Hence we, and others (Mehrez and Gafni 1991; Gold et al. 1996b), argue that because future health outcomes are clearly uncertain in the real world, the preferences measured under uncertainty (utilities) are the more appropriate. It should be noted, however, that these theoretical arguments are technically only valid at the individual level. Von Neumann–Morgenstern utility theory only covers individual decision-making, and once we aggregate the utilities across the respondents and use the results to inform societal decision-making, the theory no longer directly applies. On the other hand, the theory would apply if we assume that society is a single individual with utilities equal to the mean utilities of the community. Finally, cells 3 and 4 are similar with respect to time and complexity of the methods. So, on balance, we recommend utilities rather than values.

As a final caveat, users of economic evaluation studies and preference-scored health status classification systems should be aware that all of these methods are in use. Users should check carefully to determine what method was used in studies or pre-scored instruments of interest to them, and to ensure that the method suits their purpose.

6.3. Measuring preferences

The various methods for measuring preferences are summarized briefly in this section, and a simulated interview of the three main instruments is provided in Annex 6.1. Further descriptions of most of the methods are available in the literature. A detailed technical manual describing how to build and use standard gamble boards, TTO boards, and feeling thermometers (VASs) is available (Furlong *et al.* 1990). A video demonstrating an interview using these instruments can also be obtained (O'Brien *et al.* 1994). The book by Spilker (1996) contains descriptions of the standard gamble, the TTO, and VASs in Chapters 12 and 27. The book by Gold *et al.* (1996*b*) contains a brief summary of a variety of measurement approaches in Chapter 6. Journal articles covering the three main techniques are also available (Torrance 1986, Torrance *et al.* 2002).

The three most widely used techniques to measure directly the preferences of individuals for health outcomes are the rating scale and its variants, the standard gamble, and the TTO. These three are summarized below.

6.3.1. Rating scale, category scaling, and visual analogue scale

The simplest approach to measuring preferences is to ask subjects first to rank health outcomes from most preferred to least preferred, and second, to place the outcomes on a scale such that the intervals or spacing between placements correspond to the differences in preference as perceived by the subject. That is, outcomes that are almost equally desirable would be placed close together while outcomes that are very different in desirability would be placed far apart. The subject should be instructed to concentrate on these intervals and comparisons of one interval to another, rather than on the scores themselves. The purpose is to encourage the subject to produce an interval scale of preferences. Note that because ratios of scale values are meaningless in an interval scale it is inappropriate for subjects to make comparisons like 'outcome A is twice as desirable as outcome B and so I will place it twice as high on the scale'. The correct comparisons are ones like, 'the difference in desirability between outcomes A and B is twice as great as the difference between C and D, hence I will make the interval between A and B twice as large'.

There are a number of variations on the rating scale approach. The scale can have numbers (for example, 0–100), categories (for example, 0–10), or just consist of a

10 cm line on a page. The different variations often have different names. Rating scale usually refers to a scale of numbers, often 0–100. Category rating or category scaling is the variation that consists of a small number of categories, often 10 or 11, that the subject is to assume to be equally spaced. Visual analogue scaling consists of a line on a page, often 10 cm in length, with clearly defined endpoints and with or without other marks along the line. Sometimes several techniques are combined. For example, many of the studies from McMaster University use a 'feeling thermometer' which is a combination of VAS and a 0–100 rating scale (Furlong *et al.* 1990; Bennett and Torrance 1996; Feeny *et al.* 1996).

Preferences for chronic states can be measured on a rating scale. The chronic states are described to the subject as irreversible; that is, they are to be considered permanent from age of onset until death. The subject must be provided with the age of onset and the age of death, and these should be the same for all states that are measured together relative to each other in one batch. States with different ages of onset and/or ages of death can be handled by using multiple batches. Two additional chronic states are added to each batch as reference states for the scale—healthy (from age of onset to age of death) and death (at age of onset).

The subject is asked to select the best health state of the batch, which presumably would be 'normal healthy life' and the worst state, which may or may not be 'death at age of onset' and to place these at the ends of the scale. They are then asked to locate the other states on the rating scale relative to each other such that the distances between the locations are proportional to their preference differences. The rating scale is measured between 0 at one end and 1 at the other end. If death is judged to be the worst state and placed at 0 on the rating scale, the preference value for each of the other states is simply the scale value of its placement. If death is not judged to be the worst state but is placed at some intermediate point on the scale, say d, the preference values for the other states are given by the formula $(x - d)/(1 - d)$, where x is the scale placement of the health state.

Note that if the respondent places the best and/or the worst state near, but not at, the ends of the scale, the formula above must be modified. A simple way to handle this situation is to linearly rescale the interval between the worst and best states on to 0–1, and then to proceed with the formulae as shown above. This approach, for example, is needed when using the VAS included in the EuroQoL Group's EQ-5D instrument, assuming the researcher wants the scores on the conventional dead–healthy 0–1 scale. The approach is needed because the VAS in the EQ-5D has ends labelled 'best imaginable health state' and 'worst imaginable health state', which encourages respondents to place actual states not at the ends (one can always imagine something better or worse). Another feature of the VAS in the EQ-5D instrument is the fact that the health states are typically of 1-day duration which makes it difficult to place death on the same scale, and thus difficult to get a rating on the conventional dead–healthy 0–1 scale.

Preferences for temporary health states can also be measured on a rating scale. Temporary states are described to the subject as lasting for a specified duration of time at the end of which the person returns to normal health. As with chronic states, temporary states of the same duration and same age of onset should be batched together for measurement. Each batch should have one additional state, 'healthy', added to it. The subject is then asked to place the best state (healthy) at one end of the scale and the worst temporary state at the other end. The remaining temporary states are located on the scale such that the distances between the locations are proportional to the subject's preference differences.

If the programmes being evaluated involve only morbidity and not mortality and if there is no need to compare the findings to programmes that do involve mortality, the procedure described above for temporary health states is sufficient. However, if this is not the case, the interval preference values for the temporary states must be transformed on to the standard 0–1 health preference scale. This can be done by redefining the worst temporary health state as a chronic state of the same duration, and measuring its preference value by the technique described for chronic states. The values for the other temporary health states can then be transformed on to the standard 0–1 dead–healthy scale by a positive linear transformation (just like converting °F to °C).

Scores from a rating scale give the investigator a firm indication of the ordinal rankings of the health outcomes, and some information on the intensity of those preferences. However, rating scales are subject to measurement biases, and the empirical findings are that when compared to preferences measured by the standard gamble or the TTO, the rating scale scores are not an interval scale of preferences (Torrance 1976a; Torrance et al. 1982, 1996a; Bleichrodt and Johannesson 1997; Robinson et al. 2001; Torrance et al. 2001a). Notable biases that seem to be at work are the end-of-scale bias in which subjects tend to shy away from using the ends of the scale, and the context bias in which subjects tend to space out the outcomes over the scale regardless of how good or bad the states are (Bleichrodt and Johannesson 1997; Torrance et al. 2001a). Empirical findings indicate that rating scale scores can be converted to standard gamble or TTO scores by using a power curve conversion (Torrance 1976a; Torrance et al. 1982, 1996a, 2001a). Thus, one approach is to use the rating scale method, which is quick and efficient, and to convert the resulting scores to utilities by a suitable power curve conversion. A second approach, which is not mutually exclusive, is to use the rating scale task primarily as a warm up for subjects, to familiarize them with the descriptions of the outcomes, and to have them begin to think hard about their preferences prior to measuring the important preferences by some other technique.

6.3.2. Standard gamble

The standard gamble is the classical method of measuring cardinal preferences. It is based directly on the fundamental axioms of utility theory, first presented by von Neumann and Morgenstern (1944) (see Box 6.3). In fact, the standard gamble method is a direct application of the third axiom in Box 6.3. The method has been used extensively in the field of decision analysis, and good descriptions of the methods are available in books in this field; for example, see Holloway (1979).

The method can be used to measure preferences for chronic states but the method varies somewhat depending upon whether or not the chronic state is preferred to death or considered worse than death. For chronic states preferred to death the method is displayed in Fig. 6.2. The subject is offered two alternatives. Alternative 1 is a treatment with two possible outcomes: either the patient is returned to perfect health and lives for an additional t years (probability P), or the patient dies immediately (probability $1 - P$). Alternative 2 has the certain outcome of chronic state i for life (t years). Probability P is varied until the respondent is indifferent between the two alternatives, at which point the required preference score for state i for time t is simply P; that is, $h_i = P$. Here, h_i is measured on a utility scale where perfect health for t years is 1.0 and immediate death is 0.0.

Because most subjects cannot readily relate to probabilities, the standard gamble is often supplemented with the use of visual aids, particularly a probability wheel (Torrance 1976a; Furlong et $al.$ 1990). This is an adjustable disk with two sectors, each of different colour, and constructed so that the relative size of the two sectors can be readily changed. The alternatives are displayed to the subject on cards, and the two outcomes of the gamble alternative are colour-keyed to the two sectors of the probability wheel. The subject is told that the chance of each outcome is proportional to the similarly coloured area of the disk.

Preferences for temporary health states can be measured relative to each other using the standard gamble method as shown in Fig. 6.3. Here intermediate states i

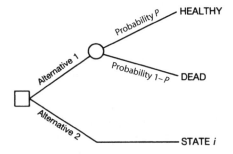

Fig. 6.2 Standard gamble for a chronic health state preferred to death.

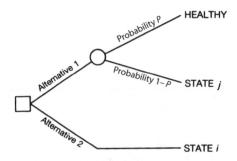

Fig. 6.3 Standard gamble for a temporary health state.

are measured relative to the best state (healthy) and the worst state (temporary state j). Note that all states must last for the same duration, say t, followed by a common state, usually healthy. In this format the formula for the utility of state i for time t is $h_i = P + (1 - P)h_j$, where i is the state being measured and j is the worst state. Here h_i is measured on a utility scale where perfect health for duration t is 1.0. If death is not a consideration in the use of the utilities, h_j can be set equal to zero and the h_i values determined from the formula, which then reduces to $h_i = P$. However, if it is desired to relate these values to the 0–1 dead–healthy scale, the worst of the temporary states (state j) must be redefined as a short duration chronic state for time t followed by death and measured on the 0–1 scale by the technique described above for chronic states. This gives the value for h_j for time t which can then, in turn, be used in the above formula to find the value for h_i for time t.

Variations on this method are also possible. For example, in Figure 6.3 state j can be the state considered next best compared to state i, rather than being the worst state. This does not change the formula $h_i = P + (1 - P)h_j$ but it does mean that the h values for the states have to be solved in sequence, starting with the worst state. This variation is used in the simulated interview in Section 6.8 of this chapter.

The traditional method of obtaining standard gamble measurements is through individual one-on-one face-to-face interviews with the subjects, complete with carefully scripted interviews and helpful visual aids (Furlong *et al.* 1990). Other, more efficient techniques are, however, being developed. These include interactive computer approaches (Lenert 2001), paper-based approaches (Ross *et al.* 2003), and group interviews with paper-based response (Gorber 2003).

6.3.3. **Time trade-off**

The TTO method was developed specifically for use in health care by Torrance *et al.* (1972). It was originally developed as a simple, easy-to-administer instrument that gave comparable scores to the standard gamble (Torrance 1976*a*). Subsequently, its theoretical properties have been explored (Mehrez and Gafni 1990; Bleichrodt 2002), and further empirical work indicates that TTO scores require adjustment before they can be used as NM utilities (Martin *et al.* 2000).

The application of the TTO technique to a chronic state considered better than death is shown in Fig. 6.4. The subject is offered two alternatives:

(1) state i for time t (life expectancy of an individual with the chronic condition) followed by death;

(2) healthy for time $x < t$ followed by death.

Time x is varied until the respondent is indifferent between the two alternatives, at which point the required preference score for state i is given, $h_i = x/t$.

Preferences for temporary health states can be measured relative to each other using the TTO method as shown in Fig. 6.5. As with the rating scale and the standard gamble, intermediate states i are measured relative to the best state (healthy) and the

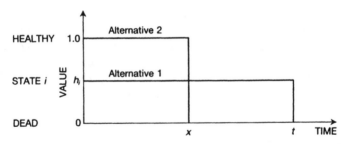

Fig. 6.4 Time trade-off for a chronic health state preferred to death.

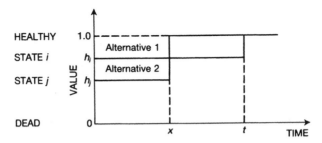

Fig. 6.5 Time trade-off for a temporary health state.

worst state (temporary state *j*). The subject is offered two alternatives:

(1) temporary state *i* for time *t* (the time duration specified for the temporary states), followed by healthy;

(2) temporary state *j* for $x < t$, followed by healthy.

Time *x* is varied until the respondent is indifferent between the two alternatives, at which point the required preference score for state *i* is $h_i = 1 - (1 - h_j)x/t$. If we set $h_j = 0$, this reduces to $h_i = 1 - x/t$. Figure 6.5 shows the basic format, but other variations are possible. State *j* need not be the worst state as long as it is any state worse than *i*. In using variations, however, care must be taken to ensure that all preference values can be calculated. In one systematic variation that has been used (Torrance *et al.* 1972; Torrance 1976a; Sackett and Torrance 1978), state *j* is always the next worse state to state *i*. This variation is used in the simulated interview in this section. Although the formula is still the same, $h_i = 1 - (1 - h_j)x/t$, the states must now be solved in sequence from worst to best.

Finally, as with the rating scale and the standard gamble, if the preference scores for the temporary states are to be transformed to the 0–1 dead–healthy scale, the worst of the temporary states must be redefined as a short duration chronic state and measured by the method for chronic states described above.

The methods described above represent the conventional approach to TTO as developed by Torrance and colleagues. Variations have been suggested by others. Buckingham *et al.* (1996) experimented with three approaches to trading off time: conventional TTO where the respondent trades against unwanted premature death, annual TTO where the trade is against unwanted convalescence, and daily TTO with a trade against unwanted sleep. Based on ease of use and relationship to independent variables they recommended daily TTO. However, one potential problem with this recommendation is that if the TTO scores are used for calculating QALYs, they are in fact being used to represent trade-offs between living states and death, and it would seem that scores based on trades against death would be more appropriate for the task.

Cook *et al.* (1994) investigated the second stage of using TTO for temporary states (Cook *et al.* 1994). This is the stage where the worst temporary state is redefined as a short-term chronic state followed by death and measured using the method for chronic states. They were concerned that the imminence of death in such a scenario would inappropriately distort the result. Accordingly, in an application where the short duration was 12 weeks, they chose to present the state at two longer durations, 12 months and 12 years, in part to determine if the duration would affect the results. To their surprise there was no effect of duration on the TTO score. Although this is only one study, it is encouraging that TTO scores measured at one duration also apply to a different duration.

6.3.4. Other methods

In the early work of Rosser and colleagues a 'ratio scaling' method was used to measure health state preferences (Rosser and Kind 1978). The method took advantage of the fact that the disability scale could be considered a ratio scale with perfect health representing a natural zero of no disability. Then each successively more undesirable disability was compared to the next better one, and the subject was asked how many times worse it was. The result was computed into a ratio scale of disability (x) and converted to an interval scale of preference (y) through the conversion $y = 1 - x$. This was the source of the scores for the original Rosser Index (Rosser and Kind 1978; Rosser and Watts 1978). Interestingly, the scores were very different from those obtained from the traditional instruments (Buxton and Ashby 1988). To our knowledge, the ratio scaling method has never been used since.

In the early work of the San Diego group that developed the Quality of Well-Being scale, an 'equivalence' preference measurement technique was used in which respondents were asked to state how many patients in the designated state of health should have their lives extended by 1 year in order to be equivalent to extending the lives of 100 healthy patients by 1 year (Patrick *et al.* 1973; Patrick and Erickson 1993). They reported that the technique gave similar values to their main technique, category scaling. Accordingly, there has been little further interest in the approach until recently. Now the approach has been revived under a new name, person trade-off (Nord *et al.* 1993; Nord 1995, 1996, 1999; Green 2001). Nord reports that PTO results do not match the results from traditional techniques like rating scale, standard gamble, and TTO and that the differences can be quite large. Moreover, Nord argues that the PTO scores are more appropriate for use in resource allocation, because they are based directly on the trade-offs that society considers appropriate.

On the other hand, the traditional scores are based directly on the trade-offs that each person considers appropriate for themselves, while the PTO scores are based on trade-offs considered appropriate for others in general. The issue of which approach is best for resource allocation is currently unresolved, and may in the end be unresolvable other than by fiat. Further research and debate no doubt will enlighten the situation, but ultimately the choice between the two approaches hinges less on analytical correctness than it does on normative values. See further discussion of this topic in Chapter 10.

Disease-specific utility measurement refers to a relatively new approach to attempt to combine the advantages of utility instruments, as described in this section, with the advantages of disease-specific instruments, specifically disease-specific health-related quality of life instruments. The utility instruments have the advantage of providing scores that are generalizable across all diseases and conditions, and are appropriate for calculating QALYs and for use in CUA. Disease-specific instruments, on the other hand, have the advantage of being more focused on the disease or condition under study and thus being more sensitive and responsive. The general approach that has been used has been to measure the utility in two stages. In the first stage, utility is measured on a scale focused on the disease. The lower anchor of the scale is the disease in its most serious form. In the second stage, the utilities from the first stage are placed into the larger context of the traditional health utility scale in which dead is 0.0 and healthy is 1.0. The intent is that the disease-specific utilities from the first stage will be of primary interest to patients and clinicians specializing in this disease, and will be all that is required for resource allocation decision-making within the disease. The utilities from the second stage, on the other hand, will be of primary interest to decision-makers with broader responsibilities, and will be suitable for the calculation of QALYs and for traditional CUAs. Moreover, it is expected that the measurement noise will be less with this approach because the first stage focuses the subject's attention more closely on the disease and does not introduce the possibility of death. This approach has been used in osteoarthritis of the knee (Bennett *et al.* 1997), in unipolar depression (Bennett *et al.* 2000), and in erectile dysfunction (Torrance *et al.* 2004). In the latter two cases the system also included a new disease-specific health status classification system focused on health-related quality of life. This is completed by the patient as the first step of the instrument and provides traditional health-related quality of life data complementary to the utility data provided by stages 1 and 2.

6.4. **Multi-attribute health status classification systems with preference scores**

Measuring preferences for health outcomes, as described in the previous section, is a very time consuming and complex task. An alternative that is very attractive and widely used is to bypass the measurement task by using one of the pre-scored multi-attribute health status classification systems that exist. The four most widely used systems will be described here in some detail: Quality of Well-Being (QWB), Health Utilities Index (HUI), EQ-5D from the EuroQoL Group, and Short Form

6D (SF-6D). Other systems include the 15D (Sintonen 2001) and the Assessment of Quality of Life (AQoL) (Hawthorne *et al.* 2001).

In this section we first describe the applicable theory, multi-attribute utility theory, and then the four main systems.

6.4.1. Multi-attribute utility theory

Traditional von Neumann–Morgenstern utility theory was extended to cover multi-attribute outcomes by Keeney and Raiffa (1976). To accommodate the extension they had to add one additional assumption to the three axioms of utility theory. This assumption is that the utility independence among the attributes can be represented by at least first-order utility independence, and perhaps by stronger utility independence (mutual utility independence, additive independence). This is best explained by example. Consider the Health Utilities Index Mark 2 (HUI2) which is a multi-attribute health status classification system consisting of the following six core attributes: sensation, mobility, emotion, cognition, self-care, pain. Each attribute in turn consists of four or five levels of specified impairment from no impairment to full impairment. See Section 6.4.5 for a full description of the system.

First-order utility independence implies that there is no interaction (synergism or antagonism) between preferences among levels on any one attribute and the fixed levels for the other attributes. An example would be the case where level 3 mobility has a utility of 0.6 on the mobility subscale, regardless of the health status levels on the other attributes. The mobility subscale is the single attribute utility function for mobility, scaled such that the best level of mobility is 1.0 and the worst level of mobility is zero. Note that the overall weight for mobility could change on the basis of health status on the other attributes, and thus the overall effect of changes in mobility could change without violating first-order utility independence. For example, a change from level 1 mobility to level 3 mobility could reduce overall utility by 0.2 if that were the only health status deficit, but by less than 0.2 if the individual already had other major health status deficits. All that is required for first-order utility independence is that the relative scaling *within* the mobility subscale stays constant.

Mutual utility independence is a stronger assumption. It requires that there be no interaction between preferences for levels on *some* attributes and the fixed levels for other attributes. This characteristic must hold for all possible subsets of attributes. An example of mutual utility independence would be the case where level 2 on sensation coupled with level 3 on mobility has a utility of 0.7 on the sensation–mobility subscale, regardless of the health status levels on the other attributes. The sensation–mobility subscale is the subscale for these two attributes combined, such that the worst level on sensation coupled with the worst level of mobility is zero and the best level on sensation coupled with the best level on mobility is 1. Note that the weight of this subscale for sensation and mobility could change given different health status on other attributes, so that the overall impact of changes within sensation and mobility could differ without violating mutual utility independence. For example, a change from level 1 on sensation and level 1 on mobility to level 2 on sensation and level 3 on mobility could reduce overall utility by 0.25 if those were the only deficits, but by less than 0.25 if the individual already had other major deficits. What is required for mutual utility independence is that the relative scaling *within* the sensation–mobility subscale stays constant.

Additive utility independence implies that there is no interaction for preferences among attributes at all. That is, the overall preference depends only on the individual levels of the attributes and not on the manner in which the levels of the different attributes are combined. An example of additive independence would be the case where a change from level 1 mobility to level 3 mobility would reduce the overall utility by 0.2 regardless of the levels on the other attributes.

The three independence assumptions lead to three different multi-attribute functions. The simplest assumption, first-order utility independence, leads to the most complex mathematical function, the multilinear function. The second possible assumption, mutual utility independence, leads to the multiplicative function. The strongest assumption (most difficult to fulfil), additive independence, leads to the simplest function, the additive function. See Box 6.4 for the three multi-attribute utility functions.

6.4.2. Quality of Well-Being

The QWB scale (Kaplan and Anderson 1988, 1996) classifies patients according to four attributes: mobility, physical activity, social activity, and symptom–problem complex. If the patient has multiple symptoms or problems, the one the patient finds to be most undesirable is used. The scoring function is based on category scaling measurements previously taken on a random sample of the general public in San Diego, California. The scores are values, not utilities. Respondents were asked to rate a single day in the various states on a scale anchored by death and perfect health. The resulting scoring function is on the 0.0 (death) to 1.0 (full health) preference scale. The original QWB questionnaire required a trained interviewer and was time consuming to use, taking about 15 minutes for a patient to be classified. Subsequently, a self-administered version, the QWB-SA, has been developed and tested (Andresen *et al.* 1998). It too, however, is relatively time consuming, taking a mean time of 14 minutes for completion (Andresen *et al.* 1998).

The QWB system and scoring function is shown in Tables 6.2 and 6.3.

6.4.3. EQ-5D

The EuroQoL Group, a consortium of investigators in western Europe, initially developed a system with six attributes: mobility, self-care, main activity, social relationships, pain, and mood (EuroQoL Group 1990). Subsequently it was revised to include five attributes: mobility, self-care, usual activity, pain/discomfort, and anxiety/depression (Essink-bot *et al.* 1993; Brooks 1996; Kind 1996). Each attribute has three levels: no problem, some problems, and major problems, thus defining 243 possible health states, to which has been added 'unconscious' and 'dead' for a total of 245 in all. Preferences for the scoring function were measured with the TTO technique on a random sample of approximately 3000 members of the adult population of the UK (Dolan *et al.* 1995, 1996b). The scoring function was developed using econometric modelling as opposed to multi-attribute utility theory. The scores fall on the 0.0 (dead) to 1.0 (perfect health) value scale.

Box 6.4 **Types of multi-attribute utility functions**

Additive

$$u(x) = \sum_{j=1}^{n} k_j u_j(x_j)$$

where $\sum_{j=1}^{n} k_j = 1$.

Multiplicative

$$u(x) = (1/k)\left[\prod_{j=1}^{n} (1 + kk_j u_j(x_j)) - 1\right]$$

where $(1 + k) = \prod_{j=1}^{n}(1 + kk_j)$.

Multilinear

$$\begin{aligned}
u(x) = {} & k_1 u_1(x_1) + k_2 u_2(x_2) + \cdots \\
& + k_{12} u_1(x_1) u_2(x_2) + k_{13} u_1(x_1) u_3(x_3) + \cdots \\
& + k_{123} u_1(x_1) u_2(x_2) u_3(x_3) + \cdots \\
& + \cdots
\end{aligned}$$

where the sum of all ks equals 1.

Hybrid

Various hybrid models are possible, based on hierarchically nested subsets of attributes.

Notation: $u_j(x_j)$ is the single attribute utility function for attribute j.

$u(x)$ is the utility for health state x, represented by an n-element vector.

k and k_j are model parameters.

Σ is the summation sign.

Π is the multiplication sign.

The multiplicative model contains the additive model as a special case. In fitting the multiplicative model, if the measured k_j sum to 1, then $k = 0$ and the additive model holds.

The full system and the original scoring function are shown below in Tables 6.4 and 6.5 (Dolan *et al.* 1995). A second scoring function has also been published (Dolan and Roberts 2002) with the recommendation that one be used as primary and one as secondary to determine what difference, if any, it makes. Further details on the EQ-5D can be obtained from the web site of the EuroQoL Group, http://www.euroqol.org.

6.4.4. **Short Form 6D**

The SF-6D is a utility instrument based on the popular health-related quality of life questionnaire, the Short Form 36 (SF-36) (Brazier *et al.* 2002). The instrument

Table 6.2 Quality of Well-Being classification system

PART 1. Quality of Well-Being/general health policy model: function scales with step definitions and calculating weights

Step no.	Step definition	Weight
	Mobility scale (MOB)	
5	No limitations for health reasons	−0.000
4	Did not drive a car, health related; did not ride in a car as usual for age (younger than 15 years), health related; and/or did not use public transportation, health related; or had or would have used more help than usual for age to use public transportation, health related	−0.062
2	In hospital, health related	−0.090
	Physical activity (PAC)	
4	No limitations for health reasons	−0.000
3	In wheelchair, moved or controlled movement of wheelchair without help from someone else; or had trouble or did not try to lift, stoop, bend over, or use stairs or inclines, health related; and/or limped, used a cane, crutches, or walker, health related; and/or had any other physical limitation in walking, or did not try to walk as far or as fast as other the same age are able, health related.	−0.060

PART 2. Quality of Well-Being/general health policy model: symptom/problem complexes (CPX) with calculating weight

CPX no.	CPX definition	Weight
1	Death (not on respondent's card)	−0.727
2	Loss of consciousness such as seizure (fits), fainting, or coma (out cold or knocked out)	−0.407
3	Burn over large areas of face, body, arms, or legs	−0.387
4	Pain, bleeding, itching, or discharge (drainage) from sexual organs—does not include normal menstrual (monthly) bleeding	−0.349
5	Trouble learning, remembering, or thinking clearly	−0.340
6	Any combination of one or more hands, feet, arms, or legs either missing, deformed (crooked), paralysed (unable to move), or broken—includes wearing artificial limbs or braces	−0.333
7	Pain, stiffness, weakness, numbness, or other discomfort in chest, stomach (including hernia or rupture), side, neck, back, hips, or any joints or hands, feet, arms, or legs	−0.299

No.	Value	Description
1	−0.077	In wheelchair, did not move or control the movement of wheelchair without help from someone else, or in bed, chair, or couch for most or all of the day, health related
		Social activity scale (SAC)
5	−0.000	No limitations for health reasons
4	−0.061	Limited in other (e.g. recreational) role activity, health related
3	−0.061	Limited in major (primary) role activity, health related
2	−0.061	Performed no major role activity, health related, but did perform self-care activities
1	−0.106	Performed no major role activity, health related, and did not perform or had more help than usual in performance of one or more self-care activities, health related

No.	Value	Description
8	−0.292	Pain, burning, bleeding, itching, or other difficulty with rectum, bowel movement, or urination (passing water)
9	−0.290	Sick or upset stomach, vomiting or loose bowel movement, with or without chills, or aching all over
10	−0.259	General tiredness, weakness, or weight loss
11	−0.257	Cough, wheezing, or shortness of breath, with or without fever, chills, or aching all over
12	−0.257	Spells of feeling, upset, being depressed, or of crying
13	−0.244	Headache, or dizziness, or ringing in ears, or spells of feeling hot, nervous, or shaky
14	−0.240	Burning or itching rash on large areas of face, body, arms, or legs
15	−0.237	Trouble talking, such as lisp, stuttering, hoarseness, or being unable to speak
16	−0.230	Pain or discomfort in one or both eyes (such as burning or itching) or any trouble seeing after correction
17	−0.188	Overweight for age and height or skin defect of face, body, arms, or legs, such as scars, pimples, warts, bruises, or changes in colour
18	−0.170	Pain in ear, tooth, jaw, throat, lips, tongue, several missing or crooked permanent teeth—includes wearing bridges or false teeth, stuffy, runny nose; or any trouble hearing—includes wearing a hearing aid

Table 6.2 (*Continued*)

PART 1. Quality of Well-Being/general health policy model: function scales with step definitions and calculating weights

Step no.	Step definition	Weight

PART 2. Quality of Well-Being/general health policy model: symptom/problem complexes (CPX) with calculating weights

CPX no.	CPX definition	Weights
19	Taking medication or staying on a prescribed diet for health reasons	−0.144
20	Wore eyeglasses or contact lenses	−0.101
21	Breathing smog or unpleasant air	−0.101
22	No symptoms or problem (not on respondent's card)	−0.000
23	Standard symptom/problem	−0.257
X24	Trouble sleeping	−0.257
X25	Intoxication	−0.257
X26	Problems with sexual interest or performance	−0.257
X27	Excessive worry or anxiety	−0.257

Note: X indicates that a standardized weight is used.

Adapted from Kaplan and Anderson (1996), Tables 1 and 2.

Table 6.3 Quality of Well-Being scoring formula

	Calculating formulas	
	Formula 1. Point-in-time well-being score for an individual (W): $W = 1 + (CPX wt) + (MOB wt) + (PAC wt) + (SAC wt)$ where wt is the preference-weighted measure for each factor and CPX is symptom/problem complex. For example, the W score for a person with the following description profile may be calculated for 1 day as:	
CPX-11	Cough, wheezing, or shortness of breath, with or without fever, chills, or aching all over	−0.257
MOB-5	No limitations	−0.000
PAC-1	In bed, chair, or couch for most or all of the day, health related	−0.077
SAC-2	Performed no major role activity health related, but did perform self-care	−0.061
	$W = 1 + (-0.257) + (-0.000) + (-0.077) + (-0.061) = 0.605$	
	Formula 2. Well-years (WY) as an output measure: $WY = (\text{No. of persons} \times (CPX wt + MOB wt + PAC wt + SAC wt) \times \text{Time})$	

Adapted from Kaplan and Anderson (1996), Table 1.

was developed, in part, because the SF-36 has been widely used in a large number of studies, and it would be useful to be able to convert the study results to utilities and hence to QALYs. The SF-6D consists of a multi-attribute health status classification system with six attributes (Table 6.6) and a scoring table (Table 6.7). The classification system was developed from the information collected on the SF-36 questionnaire. It uses 11 items from the SF-36 (eight from the SF-12, which is an abbreviated version of the SF-36, and three others from the SF-36 itself). The classification system consists of four to six levels on each of the six attributes for a total of 18 000 unique health states.

The scoring model for the SF-6D was developed based on standard gamble utility measurements on a random sample (n = 836) of the general population of the UK. Each subject provided utilities for six states. A total of 249 different health states were valued. Using econometric modelling on these data the developers investigated a number of different scoring models and recommended a particular one, which is shown in Table 6.7.

To use the SF-6D system, you first must use the SF-36 questionnaire or the SF-12 questionnaire plus the three additional questions to collect the data to classify the patients into the SF-6D classification system. Then you use the scoring table to compute the utilities. The utilities fall on the conventional health utility scale where dead is 0.0 and healthy is 1.0. The worst state in the SF-6D system has a utility of 0.30.

6.4.5. Health Utilities Index

The HUI currently consists of two systems, HUI2 and HUI3 (Furlong *et al.* 2001; Horsman *et al.* 2003). Each includes a health status classification system and a utility

Table 6.4 EQ-5D classification system

Mobility
1. No problems walking
2. Some problem walking about
3. Confined to bed

Self-care
1. No problems with self-care
2. Some problems washing or dressing self
3. Unable to wash or dress self

Usual activities
1. No problems with performing usual activities (e.g. work, study, housework, family or leisure activities)
2. Some problems with performing usual activities
3. Unable to perform usual activities

Pain/discomfort
1. No pain or discomfort
2. Moderate pain or discomfort
3. Extreme pain or discomfort

Anxiety/depression
1. Not anxious or depressed
2. Moderately anxious or depressed
3. Extremely anxious or depressed

Note: For convenience each composite health state has a five-digit code number relating to the relevant level of each dimension, with the dimensions always listed in the order given above. Thus 11223 means

1 No problems walking about
1 No problems with self-care
2 Some problems with performing usual activities
2 Moderate pain or discomfort
3 Extremely anxious or depressed

From Dolan *et al.* (1995), Fig. 1.

scoring formula. In both cases the scoring formula is based on standard gamble utilities measured on the general public, and the scores are on the conventional dead–healthy 0–1 scale.

For most applications, HUI3 should be used as the primary analysis. It has the more detailed descriptive system, it has full structural independence, and population norms are available. HUI2 can be used in a secondary role to provide additional insight. HUI2 has some additional attributes not in the HUI3 that may be useful in specific studies: self-care, emotion with a focus on worry/anxiety, and fertility. HUI2 can also be used as a sensitivity analysis.

Preferences for the HUI2 scoring function were measured on a random sample of parents of schoolchildren in the City of Hamilton, Canada and surrounding district using both a visual analogue technique and a standard gamble instrument.

Table 6.5 EQ-5D scoring formula

Coefficients for TTO tariffs	
Dimension	**Coefficient**
Constant	0.081
Mobility	
level 2	0.069
level 3	0.314
Self-care	
level 2	0.104
level 3	0.214
Usual activity	
level 2	0.036
level 3	0.094
Pain/discomfort	
level 2	0.123
level 3	0.386
Anxiety/depression	
level 2	0.071
level 3	0.236
N3	0.269

From Dolan *et al*. (1995), Table 1.

EuroQol time trade-off scores are calculated by subtracting the relevant coefficients from 1.000. The constant term is used if there is any dysfunction at all. The N3 term is used if any dimension is at level 3. The term for each dimension is selected based on the level of that dimension. The algorithm for computing the tariff is quite straightforward. For example, consider the state 11223:

Full health	= 1.000
Constant term (for any dysfunctional state)	−0.081
Mobility (level 1)	−0
Self-care (level 1)	−0
Usual activities (level 2)	−0.036
Pain or discomfort (level 2)	−0.123
Anxiety or depression (level 3)	−0.236
N3 (level 3 occurs within at least one dimension)	−0.269
Therefore, the estimated value for 11223	= 0.255

Thus, both value and utility functions are available, although the utility function is the one recommended for most applications. States worse than death were identified, but were scored as equal to death. The scoring formula is a multiplicative multi-attribute utility function, with scores that fall on the 0.0 (dead) to 1.0 (perfect health) scale.

Table 6.6 SF-6D classification system

Physical functioning
1. Your health does not limit you in *vigorous activities*.
2. Your health limits you a little in *vigorous activities*.
3. Your health limits you a little in *moderate activities*.
4. Your health limits you a lot in *moderate activities*.
5. Your health limits you a little in *bathing and dressing*.
6. Your health limits you a lot in *bathing and dressing*.

Role limitations
1. You have no problems with your work or other regular daily activities as a result of your physical health or any emotional problems.
2. You are limited in the kind of work or other activities as a result of your physical health.
3. You accomplish less than you would like as a result of emotional problems.
4. You are limited in the kind of work or other activities as a result of your physical health and accomplish less than you would like as a result of emotional problems.

Social functioning
1. Your health limits your social activities *none of the time*.
2. Your health limits your social activities *a little of the time*.
3. Your health limits your social activities *some of the time*.
4. Your health limits your social activities *most of the time*.
5. Your health limits your social activities *all of the time*.

Pain
1. You have no pain.
2. You have pain but it does not interfere with your normal work (both outside the home and housework).
3. You have pain that interferes with your normal work (both outside the home and housework) *a little bit*.
4. You have pain that interferes with your normal work (both outside the home and housework) *moderately*.
5. You have pain that interferes with your normal work (both outside the home and housework) *quite a little bit*.
6. You have pain that interferes with your normal work (both outside the home and housework) *extremely*.

Mental health
1. You feel tense or downhearted and low *none of the time*.
2. You feel tense or downhearted and low *a little bit of the time*.
3. You feel tense or downhearted and low *some of the time*.
4. You feel tense or downhearted and low *most of the time*.
5. You feel tense or downhearted and low *all of the time*.

Vitality
1. You have a lot of energy *all of the time*.
2. You have a lot of energy *most of the time*.
3. You have a lot of energy *some of the time*.
4. You have a lot of energy *none of the time*.

From Brazier *et al.* (2002), Table 1.

Table 6.7 SF-6D utility scoring model

General terms		Physical functioning		Role limitations		Social functioning		Pain		Mental health		Vitality	
Term	Score	Level	Score	Level	Score	Level	Score	Level	Score	Level	Score	Level	Score
C	1.000	PF1	−0.000	RL1	−0.000	SF1	−0.000	PAIN1	−0.000	MH1	−0.000	VIT1	−0.000
MOST	−0.070	PF2	−0.053	RL2	−0.053	SF2	−0.055	PAIN2	−0.047	MH2	−0.049	VIT2	−0.086
		PF3	−0.011	RL3	−0.055	SF3	−0.067	PAIN3	−0.025	MH3	−0.042	VIT3	−0.061
		PF4	−0.040	RL4	−0.050	SF4	−0.070	PAIN4	−0.056	MH4	−0.109	VIT4	−0.054
		PF5	−0.054			SF5	−0.087	PAIN5	−0.091	MH5	−0.128	VIT5	−0.091
		PF6	−0.111					PAIN6	−0.167				

Utility = C + PF + RL + SF + PAIN + MH + VIT + MOST
where Utility = utility on 0–1 dead–healthy scale, C = constant term, PFx = level x on the physical functioning dimension, same for other dimensions, MOST = term to use if any dimension is at its most severe level.

From Brazier et al. (2002), Table 6, Column 5 (Model 10).

The HUI3 classification system was based closely on that of the HUI2. The application-specific attribute, fertility, was dropped. The sensory attribute of HUI2 was expanded in HUI3 into the three attributes: vision, hearing, and speech. The remaining changes were made to increase the structural independence (orthogonality) of the attributes. An attribute is structurally independent of other attributes if it is conceivable for an individual to function at any level on that attribute, regardless of the levels on the other attributes. If all attributes are structurally independent of each other, all combinations of levels in the system are possible. This goal has been achieved in the HUI3. Structural independence is not only useful for the descriptive classification system, but it greatly simplifies the estimation of the scoring function.

Preferences for the HUI3 were measured on a random sample of general population adults living in the City of Hamilton, Canada using both a visual analogue technique and a standard gamble instrument. States worse than death were measured as negative scores on the 0.0 (dead) to 1.0 (perfect health) scale. Both a multiplicative model and a multilinear model have been estimated. The multiplicative model is the one recommended and is the one described below (Feeny *et al.* 2002).

Shown in Tables 6.8–6.11 are the HUI2 classification system (Table 6.8), the HUI2 scoring formula (Table 6.9), the HUI3 classification system (Table 6.10), and the HUI3 scoring formula (Table 6.11). An exercise on calculating HUI scores is provided in Box 6.5.

To use the system, researchers must describe the health states of subjects according to an HUI classification system, and then use the corresponding scoring formula. For clinical studies or population studies, questionnaires have been developed for self-administration or interviewer administration to collect sufficient data to classify the patient or subject into both the HUI2 and the HUI3 systems. The questionnaire takes under 10 minutes for self-administration and only 2–3 minutes for interviewer administration. Questionnaires are available in an increasing number of languages, and can be obtained for a fee from Health Utilities Incorporated, Dundas, Canada, website www.healthutilities.com.

6.4.6. Which system to use?

Having decided to use a preference-based multi-attribute health status system in a study, a researcher must then decide which one to use. While we cannot answer that question for the researcher, we can give some guidance on the considerations.

First, the decision does matter. These systems are far from identical. They differ in the dimensions of health they cover, in the number of levels defined on each dimension, in the description of these levels, and in the severity of the most severe level. In addition, they differ in the population surveyed and in the instruments used to determine the preference-based scoring. Finally, they differ in the theoretical approach taken to modelling the preference data into a scoring formula. For example, although all are multi-attribute systems, only the HUI uses multi-attribute utility theory for the estimation of the utility formula. EQ-5D and SF-6D use econometric modelling. Because of these various differences, it is not surprising that comparative studies show that the same patient groups can score quite differently depending upon the

Table 6.8 Health Utilities Index mark 2 classification system

Attribute	Level	Level description
Sensation	1	Ability to see, hear, and speak normally for age
	2	Requires equipment to see or hear or speak
	3	Sees, hears, or speaks with limitations even with equipment
	4	Blind, deaf, or mute
Mobility	1	Able to walk, bend, lift, jump, and run normally for age
	2	Walks, bends, lifts, jumps, or runs with some limitations but does not require help
	3	Requires mechanical equipment (such as canes, crutches, braces, or wheelchair) to walk or get around independently
	4	Requires the help of another person to walk or get around and requires mechanical equipment as well
	5	Unable to control or use arms and legs
Emotion	1	Generally happy and free from worry
	2	Occasionally fretful, angry, irritable, anxious, depressed, or suffering 'night terrors'
	3	Often fretful, angry, irritable, anxious, depressed, or suffering 'night terrors'
	4	Almost always fretful, angry, irritable, anxious, depressed
	5	Extremely fretful, angry, irritable, anxious, or depressed usually requiring hospitalization or psychiatric institutional care
Cognition	1	Learns and remembers schoolwork normally for age
	2	Learns and remembers schoolwork more slowly than classmates as judged by parents and/or teachers
	3	Learns and remembers very slowly and usually requires special educational assistance
	4	Unable to learn and remember
Self-care	1	Eats, bathes, dresses, and uses the toilet normally for age
	2	Eats, bathes, dresses, or uses the toilet independently with difficulty
	3	Requires mechanical equipment to eat, bathe, dress, or use the toilet independently
	4	Requires the help of another person to eat, bathe, dress, or use the toilet
Pain	1	Free of pain and discomfort
	2	Occasional pain. Discomfort relieved by non-prescription drugs or self-control activity without disruption of normal activities
	3	Frequent pain. Discomfort relieved by oral medicines with occasional disruption of normal activities
	4	Frequent pain, frequent disruption of normal activities. Discomfort requires prescription narcotics for relief
	5	Severe pain. Pain not relieved by drugs and constantly disrupts normal activities
Fertility*	1	Able to have children with a fertile spouse
	2	Difficulty in having children with a fertile spouse
	3	Unable to have children with a fertile spouse

*Fertility attribute can be deleted if not required. Contact developers for details. From Torrance *et al.* (1996a), Table 1.

Table 6.9 Health Utilities Index mark 2 scoring formula

Sensation		Mobility		Emotion		Cognition		Self-care		Pain		Fertility	
x_1	b_1	x_2	b_2	x_3	b_3	x_4	b_4	x_5	b_5	x_6	b_6	x_7	b_7
1	1.00	1	1.00	1	1.00	1	1.00	1	1.00	1	1.00	1	1.00
2	0.95	2	0.97	2	0.93	2	0.95	2	0.97	2	0.97	2	0.97
3	0.86	3	0.84	3	0.81	3	0.88	3	0.91	3	0.85	3	0.88
4	0.61	4	0.73	4	0.70	4	0.65	4	0.80	4	0.64	4	n/a
5	n/a	5	0.58	5	0.53	5	n/a	5	n/a	5	0.38	5	n/a

Formula: $u^* = 1.06(b_1 \times b_2 \times b_3 \times b_4 \times b_5 \times b_6 \times b_7) - 0.06$, where u^* is the utility of the health state on a utility scale where dead has a utility of 0.00 and healthy has a utility of 1.00. Because the worst possible health state was judged by respondents as worse than death, it has a negative utility of −0.03. The standard error of u^* for estimating validation states within the sample is 0.015 for measurement error and sampling error, and 0.06 if model error is also included. x_i is attribute level code for attribute i; b_i is level score for attribute i.

From Torrance et al. (1996a).

Table 6.10 Health Utilities Index mark 3 classification system

Attribute	Level	Level description
Vision	1	Able to see well enough to read ordinary newsprint and recognize a friend on the other side of the street, without glasses or contact lenses
	2	Able to see well enough to read ordinary newsprint and recognize a friend on the other side of the street, but with glasses
	3	Able to read ordinary newsprint with or without glasses but unable to recognize a friend on the other side of the street, even with glasses
	4	Able to recognize a friend on the other side of the street with or without glasses but unable to read ordinary newsprint, even with glasses
	5	Unable to read ordinary newsprint and unable to recognize a friend on the other side of the street, even with glasses
	6	Unable to see at all
Hearing	1	Able to hear what is said in a group conversation with at least three other people, without a hearing aid
	2	Able to hear what is said in a conversation with one other person in a quiet room without a hearing aid, but requires a hearing aid to hear what is said in a group conversation with at least three other people
	3	Able to hear what is said in a conversation with one other person in a quiet room with a hearing aid, and able to hear what is said in a group conversation with at least three other people with a hearing aid
	4	Able to hear what is said in a conversation with one other person in a quiet room without a hearing aid, but unable to hear what is said in a group conversation with at least three other people even with a hearing aid
	5	Able to hear what is said in a conversation with one other person in a quiet room with a hearing aid, but unable to hear what is said in a group conversation with at least three other people even with a hearing aid
	6	Unable to hear at all

Table 6.10 (*Continued*)

Attribute	Level	Level description
Speech	1	Able to be understood completely when speaking with strangers or friends
	2	Able to be understood partially when speaking with strangers but able to be understood completely when speaking with people who know me well
	3	Able to be understood partially when speaking with strangers or people who know me well
	4	Unable to be understood when speaking with strangers but able to be understood partially by people who know me well
	5	Unable to be understood when speaking to other people (or unable to speak at all)
Ambulation	1	Able to walk around the neighborhood without difficulty, and without walking equipment
	2	Able to walk around the neighborhood with difficulty; but does not require walking equipment or the help of another person
	3	Able to walk around the neighborhood with walking equipment, but without the help of another person
	4	Able to walk only short distances with walking equipment, and requires a wheelchair to get around the neighborhood
	5	Unable to walk alone, even with walking equipment. Able to walk short distances with the help of another person, and requires a wheelchair to get around the neighborhood
	6	Cannot walk at all
Dexterity	1	Full use of two hands and ten fingers
	2	Limitations in the use of hands or fingers, but does not require special tools or help of another person
	3	Limitations in the use of hands or fingers, is independent with use of special tools (does not require the help of another person)
	4	Limitations in the use of hands or fingers, requires the help of another person for some tasks (not independent even with use of special tools)
	5	Limitations in use of hands or fingers, requires the help of another person for most tasks (not independent even with use of special tools)
	6	Limitations in use of hands or fingers, requires the help of another person for all tasks (not independent even with use of special tools)
Emotion	1	Happy and interested in life
	2	Somewhat happy
	3	Somewhat unhappy
	4	Very unhappy
	5	So unhappy that life is not worthwhile
Cognition	1	Able to remember most things, think clearly, and solve day-to-day problems
	2	Able to remember most things, but have a little difficulty when trying to think and solve day-to-day problems
	3	Somewhat forgetful, but able to think clearly and solve day-to-day problems

(*Continued*)

Table 6.10 (*Continued*)

Attribute	Level	Level description
	4	Somewhat forgetful, and have a little difficulty when trying to think or solve day-to-day problems
	5	Very forgetful, and have great difficulty when trying to think or solve day-to-day problems
	6	Unable to remember anything at all, and unable to think or solve day-to-day problems
Pain	1	Free of pain and discomfort
	2	Mild to moderate pain that prevents no activities
	3	Moderate pain that prevents a few activities
	4	Moderate to severe pain that prevents some activities
	5	Severe pain that prevents most activities

Table 6.11 Health Utilities Index mark 3 scoring formula

Vision		Hearing		Speech		Ambulation		Dexterity		Emotion		Cognition		Pain	
x_1	b_1	x_2	b_2	x_3	b_3	x_4	b_4	x_5	b_5	x_6	b_6	x_7	b_7	x_8	b_8
1	1.00	1	1.00	1	1.00	1	1.00	1	1.00	1	1.00	1	1.00	1	1.00
2	0.98	2	0.95	2	0.94	2	0.93	2	0.95	2	0.95	2	0.92	2	0.96
3	0.89	3	0.89	3	0.89	3	0.86	3	0.88	3	0.85	3	0.95	3	0.90
4	0.84	4	0.80	4	0.81	4	0.73	4	0.76	4	0.64	4	0.83	4	0.77
5	0.75	5	0.74	5	0.68	5	0.65	5	0.65	5	0.46	5	0.60	5	0.55
6	0.61	6	0.61	6	n/a	6	0.58	6	0.56	6	n/a	6	0.42	6	n/a

Formula (dead–perfect health scale): $u^* = 1.371(b_1 \times b_2 \times b_3 \times b_4 \times b_5 \times b_6 \times b_7 \times b_8) - 0.371$, where u^* is the utility of the health state on a utility scale where dead has a utility of 0.00 and healthy has a utility of 1.00. States worse than dead have negative utilities. x_i is attribute level code for attribute i; b_i is level score for attribute i. For the attribute 'Cognition', the score for level 3 is greater than the score for level 2. This is not a typo, but reflects that level 3 was seen as preferable to level 2.

The standard error of u^*, including model error, is 0.08 for estimating validation states within the sample. For estimating validation states (based on $n = 73$) from an independent sample, the standard error is 0.10 if the states are unweighted, 0.006 if the states are weighted by prevalence excluding the state of perfect health, and 0.004 if the states are weighted by prevalence including the state of perfect health.

From Feeny *et al.* (2002), Table 3.

instrument used (Conner-Spady and Suarez-Almazor 2003; Kopec and Willison 2003; Lubetkin and Gold 2003; O'Brien *et al.* 2003).

In selecting an instrument the researcher should consider a number of factors. In general is the instrument seen as credible? That is, is it an established instrument, like those described above, which has demonstrated feasibility, reliability, validity, and responsiveness in a number of studies? There is a rapidly expanding literature describing applications and measurement characteristics of each of these instruments. For example, the web sites for EQ-5D and HUI each list hundreds of publications on

Box 6.5 **Exercise: Health Utilities Index**

1. In the HU12 system (Table 6.8), the health state of an individual is described as a six- or seven- element vector with each element denoting the level on an attribute. For example, 1321221 would be an individual who was at level 1 sensation, level 3 mobility, level 2 emotion, level 1 cognition, level 2 self-care, level 2 pain, and level 1 fertility. Because the fertility attribute is optional in the system, if only six elements are specified they refer to the first six attributes.

The utility score for a health state is determined using the formula from Table 6.9. If only six elements are specified, b_7 is omitted from the formula (or equivalently, b_7 is set equal to 1).

Determine the HU12 utility scores for the following health states:

(a) 1321221

(b) 2132113

(c) 111111

(d) 112114

(e) 332325

Answers: 0.72, 0.62, 1.00, 0.57, 0.17.

2. In the HU13 system (Tables 6.10 and 6.11) there are more attributes, more levels, and a different scoring formula, but otherwise the notation and the method of calculation is the same.

Determine the HU13 utility scores for the following health states:

(a) 23112211

(b) 11121131

(c) 41131112

(d) 11111451

(e) 66566565

Answers: 0.68, 0.84, 0.58, 0.16, −0.36.

the instrument. Does the health status classification system cover the attributes and the levels of these attributes that are likely to be important to the patient population under study? Has the instrument been used in similar patients and was it responsive? Is the instrument likely to be responsive to the changes expected in the study patients? Does the instrument have ceiling effects or floor effects that will reduce its sensitivity for the patients under study? Only some of the instruments measure states worse than death. Is this likely to be an important aspect of the study? Does the intended audience for the study have any guidance or preference for a particular instrument? For example, the National Institute for Clinical Excellence in the UK specifies that the instrument should be 'a generic and validated classification system for which reliable UK population preference values, elicited using a choice-based method such as the

TTO or standard gamble (but not rating scale), are available' (National Institute for Clinical Excellence 2004, p. 25). They indicate that currently the most appropriate choice in the UK appears to be the EQ-5D, but that other instruments that meet the criteria can be used with justification. If clinicians are an intended audience, do the clinical opinion leaders have a preferred instrument for their field? Is the instrument based on sound theory? How much time is required to complete the questionnaire and is the questionnaire clear and easy to follow. That is, is the patient burden acceptable? And finally, what is the overall cost of using the instrument, including licensing fees, data collection costs, scoring costs, and analysis costs?

If there is not a single obvious instrument for a study, the researcher may wish to consider a pilot study to test several contenders and determine which performs best in the type of patients being studied. The researcher may even wish to use several instruments in the study, designating one as the primary measure and the other(s) as secondary. This can not only provide additional insight into the study findings, but can also be of considerable interest in its own right as a head-to-head comparison of alternative instruments.

One issue that is sometimes raised in instrument selection is the fact that each instrument is scored based on preferences from a particular population, and those preferences may not apply to other populations. For example, the QWB is scored based on the preferences of residents of San Diego, USA, the HUI is scored based on preferences of residents of Hamilton, Canada, and the EQ-5D and SF-6D are scored based on preferences of residents of the UK. The concern is that the scoring may not be appropriate when the instrument is used in other geographic locations. The data, however, suggest that this is not a serious concern. Virtually all of the studies that have replicated health state preference measurements (that is, controlling for method) in different populations have found either no difference or little difference. One of the first such studies was that of Balaban and colleagues who rescored the QWB using the preferences of arthritic patients in the north-east USA (Balaban et al. 1986). The results were not significantly different from the original scoring, which had been based on a general population sample in the south-west USA. Wang et al. (2002) replicated the HUI2 scoring procedure on a separate sample of parents of childhood cancer patients and obtained similar results to the original scoring based on a sample of parents from the general population. Le Gales et al. (2002) replicated the HUI3 scoring procedure on a representative random sample of the French population and obtained results similar to the original scoring based on the Canadian data. These findings are consistent with other studies that have shown that preference scoring does not vary significantly as a function of demographic variables, including race, income, and gender (Kaplan et al. 1988; Kaplan 1994). Similarly they do not vary systematically as a function of prior experience with the rated health state (Balaban et al. 1986; Kaplan 1994; Wang et al. 2002). The evidence, thus, suggests that when preference measurement procedures *are replicated* on different groups of people including different populations in different countries, the results are similar. That is, instrument scores do indeed travel well and are applicable in other geographic locations. Differences that might exist from this geographic factor are small compared to the differences that exist among instruments. Users of studies should be more concerned about the comparability of studies that use different indexes (QWB, EQ-5D, SF-6D, HUI) than about the appropriateness of using an EQ-5D instrument in the USA or a HUI or QWB instrument in Europe.

6.5. Quality-adjusted life-years

One of the key features of conventional CUA is its use of the QALY concept; results are reported in terms of cost per QALY gained.

6.5.1. What is the quality-adjusted life-year concept?

The concept of the QALY was first introduced in 1968 by Herbert Klarman and colleagues in a study on chronic renal failure (Klarman *et al.* 1968). They noted that the quality of life with a kidney transplant was better than that with dialysis, and estimated that it was 25% better. The cost per life-year gained by the different treatment options was calculated with and without this quality adjustment. Although they did not use the term 'quality-adjusted life-year', the concept was identical.

As was first mentioned in Chapter 2, the advantage of the QALY as a measure of health outcome is that it can simultaneously capture gains from reduced morbidity (quality gains) and reduced mortality (quantity gains), and combine these into a single measure. Moreover, the combination is based on the relative desirability of the different outcomes. A simple example is displayed in Fig. 6.6. Without the intervention the individual's health-related quality of life would deteriorate according to the lower path and the person would die at time Death 1. With the intervention the person

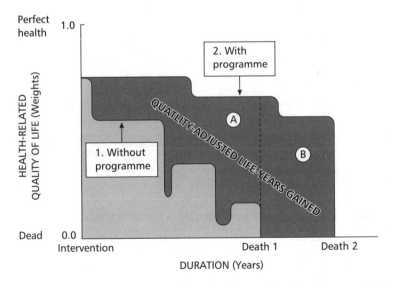

Fig. 6.6 Quality-adjusted life-years gained from an intervention. From Torrance (1996), Fig. 1 and Gold *et al.* (1996), Fig. 4.2.

would deteriorate more slowly, would live longer, and would die at time Death 2. The area between the two curves is the QALY gained by the intervention. For instructional purposes the area can be divided into two parts, A and B, as shown. Part A is the amount of QALY gained due to quality improvement (the gain in health-related quality of life during the time that the person would have otherwise been alive anyhow) and part B is the amount of QALY gained due to quantity improvement (the amount of life extension but factored by the quality of that life extension).

Much more complicated cases can be handled. The paths may cross each other. For example, many cancer treatments cause a QALY loss in the short term in order to achieve a QALY gain in the longer term. The paths may be identical for a long time after the intervention and only diverge in the distant future. An example of this pattern could be a hypertension drug that is well tolerated and has no side-effects but eventually averts serious cardiovascular events. The paths may be uncertain reflecting the variability between apparently similar patients in terms of their prognoses. This uncertainty can be characterized by including a series of alternative paths, with the likelihood of a given patient following each being reflected by a probability. With each path having a QALY value associated with it, the expected (or mean) QALY is calculated as sum of the QALY for each pathway weighted by its respective probability. This is an example of a simple decision analytic model, which will be described in more detail in Chapter 9.

6.5.2. **What are the quality weights?**

To operationalize the QALY concept, as described above, one needs quality weights that represent the health-related quality of life of the health states under consideration. These quality weights are the scale for the vertical axis in Fig. 6.6. The instruments that we have just discussed in Sections 6.3 and 6.4 are used to obtain the required weights.

To satisfy the QALY concept, as described in the previous section, the quality weights must be (1) based on preferences, (2) anchored on perfect health and death, and (3) measured on an interval scale.

The QALY weights for health states should be based on preferences for the health states. This way the more desirable (more preferred) health states receive greater weight and will be favoured in the analysis. Other potential approaches to assigning QALY weights, such as the impact of the health state on earnings, the impact of the health state on health care utilization, the prevalence of the health state in the population, or psychometric scaling techniques are not appropriate for identifying those outcomes that are better or more desirable and differentiating from those that are worse or less desirable.

The scale of QALY weights may contain many points, but two points that must be on the scale are perfect health and death. These two are required because they will both occur in programmes being evaluated with the QALY model, and weights will be required for them. Because these two must always be on the scale, and because they are well specified and understood, they have been selected to be the two anchor points (actually, a better term would be reference points) for the interval scale of QALY weights. This is akin to selecting the freezing point and the boiling point of water to be the anchor points for the interval scale of temperature. To define an interval scale of QALY weights, death and perfect health can be given any two arbitrary values as long as the value for death is smaller than the value for perfect health. The pair of values could be (32, 212), (0, 100), (−5.9, 2.3), (0, 1), or whatever, and the resulting scale would be an interval scale of QALY weights. However, one pair of scores stands out as particularly convenient (death = 0 and perfect health = 1), and this has become the conventional scale for QALY weights. Note that this still allows states worse than death, which would have scores less than zero, and indeed states better than perfect health, if they exist, which would have scores greater than 1.

There are a number of reasons why zero and 1 are particularly convenient scores to assign to death and perfect health respectively. First, take death. Because death is a permanent state, if any score other than zero were used for death, it would mean that in all analyses the (non-zero) death score would be assigned to the state of death for each year off into the future for as long as the death lasted (that is, forever). Thus, the analyses would have streams of numeric outcomes going to infinity—not a pretty picture. Accordingly, zero is the only practical score that can be used for death. Now, take perfect health. The advantage of using 1 for perfect health is that the resulting QALY is then measured in units of 'perfect health years' (that is, 1 year in perfect health = 1 QALY, half a year in perfect health = 0.5 QALY, 1 year in a health state with a QALY weight of 0.5 = 0.5 QALY, and so on). Indeed, at least one agency uses YHL as the term for the concept being described here (see Box 6.6).

Box 6.6 Quality-adjusted life-years and aliases

In the beginning the composite summary outcome measure was not called quality-adjusted life-years. The concept first appeared in 1970 under the term *function years* (Fanshel and Bush 1970). Two years later, in an application to tuberculin testing, the same group mentioned, as an aside, that function years gained are equivalent to 'additional quality-adjusted years of life' (Bush *et al.* 1972). In our early work it was originally called the *index day* (Torrance 1971) and then the *health day* (Torrance *et al.* 1972), and the health status unit day and health status unit year (Torrance 1976*b*). The term *quality-adjusted life-year* with its well-known acronym *QALY* was first popularized by a landmark 1977 paper from Harvard University, published in the *New England Journal of Medicine* (Weinstein and Stason 1977).

Note that all QALYs are not the same. Weights may be based on standard gamble utility measurements, time trade-off value measurements, visual analogue scale value measurements, estimates by physicians or researchers, or preference-weighted systems like the Health Utilities Index, the Quality of Well-Being, or the EuroQol-5D. When weights are based on measured preferences, the preferences may be measured on patients, on the general public, or on some other group. The QALY can be constructed in the conventional way by adding up its parts, or can be determined in a holistic way by measuring utilities for paths of health states.

Quality-adjusted life-years also go by other names. The United States National Centre for Health Statistics use the term years of healthy life (YHL) (Erickson *et al.* 1995), while Statistics Canada uses health-adjusted person-years (HAPY) and health-adjusted life expectancy (HALE) (Berthelot *et al.* 1993).

Scales of measurement can be nominal (for example, colours—red, blue, green), ordinal (for example, size—small, medium, large, extra large, extra extra large), or cardinal (for example, length—in metres, or temperature—in °C). Cardinal scales can be interval (for example, temperature) or ratio (for example, length). The difference between these two is that the ratio scale has an unambiguous zero point that indicates there is absolutely none of the phenomenon being measured. For example, if something has a length of zero, it has no length. However, if something has a temperature of zero, it still has a temperature. A convenient memory aid that lists the types of scales in increasing order of their mathematical properties is the French word for black, noir, standing for *n*ominal, *o*rdinal, *i*nterval, *r*atio.

Because it has an absolute zero, a ratio scale is unique under a positive multiplicative transformation. This means that any ratio scale can be multiplied by any positive constant and the result is still a ratio scale of the same phenomenon, just in different units. This property is used, for example, to convert feet to yards, or metres to miles. Because it has no natural zero, an interval scale is unique under a positive linear transformation. This means that any interval scale x can be transformed to a scale y using a function $y = a + bx$, where a can be any constant and b can be any positive constant. The result will still be an interval scale of the same phenomenon, but in different units and with a different zero. This property is used to convert °F to °C.

An interval scale has the property that ratios of intervals have meaning, but ratios of scale quantities do not. In a ratio scale both types of ratios have meaning. For example, with temperature, the interval scale property means that it is correct to state that the gain in temperature in going from 40°F to 80°F is twice as much as the gain in going from 40°F to 60°F, but it is incorrect to state that 80°F is twice as hot as 40°F. The former statement holds true whether the temperature is measured in °F or °C, while the latter does not. Conversely, in length, it is both correct to state that the gain in length from 40 metres to 80 metres is twice as much as the gain from 40 metres to 60 metres, and that 80 metres is twice as long as 40 metres. Both statements remain true whether the lengths are measured in metres, inches, miles, fathoms, light-years, or any other unit of length.

At first glance it may seem that a scale of health-related quality of life does have a natural zero at death. After all, death represents no health-related quality of life. The problem here is that there can be states worse than death (Torrance *et al.* 1982; Torrance 1984; Patrick *et al.* 1994), and these states require a score for their health-related quality of life. Thus, death is not the bottom of the scale. In fact, there is no well-defined bottom of the scale. Conventionally, as discussed above, death is assigned a zero score and states worse than death take on negative scores. This is akin to the temperature at which water freezes being assigned 0°C and temperatures colder than that are then negative.

Alternatively, it may seem that if you reverse the scale so that perfect health has a score of zero and death has a score of 1, there would be a natural zero at perfect health. Such a scale would represent health-related reductions in quality of life, and numerically would be obtained by taking 1 minus the scale of health-related quality of life. For example, a state with a score of 0.8 on the conventional scale would have a score of 0.2 on the reductions scale. A state worse than death with a score of −0.1 on the conventional scale would have a score of 1.1 on the reductions scale. If perfect health can be considered to be a natural zero for the reductions scale, the reductions scale would qualify as a ratio scale as opposed to an interval scale. This assumption was invoked in the original scaling work of Rosser and colleagues (Rosser and Kind 1978; Rosser and Watts 1978) who used a ratio scaling technique to measure reductions in health-related quality of life. Subjects ranked states in order of severity, and then went down the list comparing each state to the next less severe one. Specifically, for each pair they asked 'how many times more ill is a person described as being in state 2 as compared with state 1? (Rosser and Kind 1978). Finally, the subject was asked to place death on the scale.

Many students of this field have been confused by the seemingly contradictory statements by Rosser and colleagues that the measurements are on a ratio scale and by others like ourselves that the scale is not a ratio scale and the measurements are on an interval scale. The fact is that there are two different scales. The scale of health-related quality of life is an interval scale, and is not a ratio scale. The scale of reductions in health-related quality would be a ratio scale if perfect health is a natural endpoint of the scale at the upper end, and this assumption was invoked in the ratio scaling method of Rosser and colleagues.

Finally, it is useful to note that for economic evaluation an interval scale is required for the QALY weights, but an interval scale is all that is required. First, an interval scale is required because it is important that intervals of equal length on the scale have equal interpretation, and this is the fundamental nature of an interval scale. That is, it is important that a gain from 0.2 to 0.4 on the scale represents the same increase in desirability as a gain from 0.6 to 0.8. This is required because in the QALY calculations those two types of gains will appear equal.

Second, an interval scale is all that is required; there is no need to have a ratio scale. There are two reasons. First, because an interval scale is a type of cardinal scale, all parametric statistical calculations are allowed; for example, mean, standard deviation, t-test, analysis of variance, and so on. Second, because all economic evaluations are comparative, the analysis is always dealing with differences between the programme and the comparator, and all mathematical manipulations on differences (intervals) are valid with an interval scale. That is, it is valid to take ratios of differences (the incremental QALYs gained in programme A compared to its comparator are twice those of programme B compared to its comparator), and to use the differences in other ratios (the incremental cost per incremental QALY for programme A is one-third of that for programme B), as well as to perform the statistical tests (the incremental QALYs gained in programme A are not statistically significantly different from those gained in programme B at the 5% level).

6.5.3. How are quality-adjusted life-years calculated?

Conceptually, the QALY calculation is very straightforward. If both groups start with exactly the same baseline utility, as is the case in Fig. 6.6, the incremental QALYs gained is simply the area under path 2 less the area under path 1. If, on the other hand, there is a difference in baseline utility between the two groups, the area between the two curves must be adjusted to account for this difference. The recommended adjustment method uses multiple regression to estimate the incremental QALY and an associated measure of sampling variability (Manca *et al.* in press). The area under a path can be thought of as the sum of the areas under each component health state on the path, where the area under a health state is the duration of the health state in years, or fraction of a year, multiplied by the quality weight for the health state. This is the QALYs gained without discounting.

Because individuals, and society, generally prefer gains of all types, including health gains, to occur earlier rather than later, future amounts are multiplied by a discount factor to account for this time preference. The technique of discounting, as applied to costs, is described in detail in Chapter 4. The method is the same when applied to QALYs. Essentially the method consists of taking the amounts that will occur in future years and moving them year by year back to the present, reducing the amount each year by r% of the remaining amount, where r% is the annual discount rate.

Examples of QALY calculations with and without discounting are shown in Boxes 6.7 and 6.8.

6.5.4. **Alternatives to quality-adjusted life-years**

The QALY concept is not without controversy. For a sample of the current debate, see the following references (Carr-Hill 1991; Carr-Hill and Morris 1991; Spiegelhalter *et al.* 1992; Broome 1993; Nord 1993; Williams 1995) plus the material in this section. The critics range from those who argue that the QALY approach is needlessly complex and should be replaced by simpler disaggregated measures (Cox *et al.* 1992) to those who claim that the QALY approach is overly simplistic and should be replaced by more complex methods (Mehrez and Gafni 1989, 1991, 1992). Several alternatives to QALYs have been suggested, and the following three are described briefly below: healthy-years equivalents (HYEs), saved-young-life equivalents (SAVEs), and DALYs.

Healthy-year equivalents have been proposed as a theoretically superior alternative to QALYs, but one that is more challenging to execute (Mehrez and Gafni 1989, 1991, 1992). An example of HYE measurement is given in Box 6.9. Essentially, the HYE approach, as proposed by Mehrez and Gafni, differs from the conventional approach to QALYs in two respects. First, it measures the preferences over the entire path (also called profile) of health states through which the individual would pass, rather than for each state alone. Second, it measures the preferences using a two-stage standard gamble measurement procedure that first measures the conventional utility for the path and then measures the number of healthy years that would give the same utility (see Box 6.9).

Variations on the HYE measurement procedure described above are also possible. A simpler variation occurs when the health path consists of only one chronic health state until death (Mehrez and Gafni 1989). Then the result of the two-stage measurement procedure is the HYE for the chronic health state for the duration specified. A more complex variation occurs when the health path is a decision tree; that is, the health path is probabilistic, consisting of multiple branches each with its own probability of occurrence. In this case, the HYE for the probabilistic health path has been called 'extended HYE' (Wakker 1996) and '*ex ante* HYE' (Johannesson 1995*a, b*), and is more complicated to measure (see point 6 below).

Box 6.7 **Exercise: simple quality-adjusted life-year calculations**

The following exercise will give you practice in calculating QALYs in simple cases. Once you have mastered these examples you will be able to handle much more complicated cases by simply following the same principles. In solving these problems you should always begin by sketching a QALY diagram to clarify the calculations required. A QALY diagram is a sketch like Fig. 6.6 which shows the health-related quality of life path taken by the patient with the programme and the path without the programme. The solutions are given in Box 6.8, but try not to look ahead until you have either solved the problems or given up in total frustration.

Questions 1–4 are taken from the first edition of the book. They are still good exercises although the clinical content and the utility scores may be somewhat dated. The only change we made to these questions is to change the discount rate to 5%, which is more consistent with contemporary standards. Questions 5–7 are new in this edition.

In order to calculate QALYs you need two pieces of data: (1) the path of health states and the duration of each health state over the time span for which QALYs are to be calculated, and (2) the preference weights for the health states for the same durations (see Section 6.5.2). The preference weights for questions 1–4 are shown below and came from TTO measurements on a random sample of the general public (Sackett and Torrance 1978). The preference weights for questions 5–7 are shown in Table 6.9 and those for question 8 in Table 6.11.

Part (b) of some questions involves discounting. For discounting methods see Chapter 4. For discounting purposes assume that all health gains or losses that occur throughout a year take place at the beginning of the year.

Preference weights for Questions 1–4

Duration	Health state	Weight
3 months	Hospital dialysis	0.62
3 months	Home confinement for tuberculosis	0.68
8 years	Home dialysis	0.65
8 years	Mastectomy for breast cancer	0.48

1. Sketch the QALY diagram and determine how many QALYs are gained if a person achieves an 8-year life extension on home dialysis,
   (a) assuming no discounting
   (b) assuming discounting at a rate of 5% per annum.

2. Sketch the QALY diagram and determine how many QALYs are gained if a person achieves a 3-month life extension on hospital dialysis,
   (a) assuming no discounting
   (b) assuming discounting at 5% per annum.

Box 6.7 Exercise: simple quality-adjusted life-year calculations *(continued)*

3. Sketch the QALY diagram and determine how many QALYs are gained by preventing a case of tuberculosis that would have been treated at home for 3-months,

   (a) assuming no discounting

   (b) assuming discounting at 5%.

4. Assume a breast-cancer patient will become symptomatic, have a mastectomy, and live an additional 6 years. By screening, you can detect the breast cancer 1 year earlier, perform the mastectomy 1 year earlier, and add two years to the patient's life (that is, she now lives 9 years from the mastectomy instead of 6 years). Sketch the QALY diagram and determine how many QALYs are gained by screening,

   (a) assuming no discounting

   (b) assuming discounting at 5%

5. Sketch the QALY diagram and determine how many QALYs are achieved during the year by a patient in a 1-year clinical trial who has a baseline HUI2 health state of 133114, a 6-month HUI2 health state of 122112, and a 1-year HUI2 health state of 112111. Assume that health status changes between measurements are smooth and gradual over time so that changes in utility scores can be approximated by a straight line.

6. Suppose the patient in Question 5 was the typical patient in the treatment group, and the typical patient in the control group has a baseline HUI2 health state of 133114, a 6-month HU12 health state of 132113 and a 1-year HUI2 health state of 132113. Sketch the QALY diagram for the two patients and determine the QALYs gained over the year for the treatment patient compared to the control patient.

7. In actually implementing the HUI in a clinical trial the patient is asked to think of her health-related quality of life over a defined recall period and to answer the HUI questions accordingly. Redo Questions 5 and 6 assuming the interviews were done precisely at months 0, 6, and 12, the recall period was 4 weeks, and thus the HUI2 score from each interview represents the average health-related quality of life during the recall period.

8. How many QALYs are achieved by each of the following people:

   A lives 20 years in HU13 health state 11111111,
   B lives 20 years in HU13 health state 11113333,
   C lives 20 years in HU13 health state 44444444,

   (a) assuming no discounting

   (b) assuming discounting at 5%.

Box 6.8 **Solutions: simple quality-adjusted life-year calculations**

These are the solutions for the exercises in Box 6.7.

1.

(a) $0.65 \times 8 = 5.2$ QALYs

(b) $0.65 \times (5.7864 + 1.0000) = 4.4$ QALYs

2.

(a) $0.62 \times 0.25 = 0.16$ QALY

(b) $0.62 \times 0.25 = 0.16$ QALY

3.

(a) $(1.00 - 0.68) \times 1/4 = 0.32 \times 1/4 = 0.08$ QALY

(b) $(1.00 - 0.68) \times 1/4 = 0.32 \times 1/4 = 0.08$ QALY

4.

(a) $0.48 \times 2 - (1 - 0.48) \times 1 = 0.96 - 0.52 = 0.44$ QALY

(b) $0.48 \times 0.7107 + 0.48 \times 0.6768 - 0.52 \times 1.00 = 0.67 - 0.52$
$= 0.15$ QALY

Box 6.8 Solutions: simple quality-adjusted life-year calculations (continued)

5.
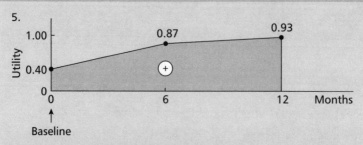

Time	Health state	HUI2 score
0 months	1, 3, 3, 1, 1, 4	0.4016
6 months	1, 2, 2, 1, 1, 2	0.8675
12 months	1, 1, 2, 1, 1, 1	0.9258

$$\text{QALY} = (0.5(0.4016 + 0.8675)6 + 0.5(0.8675 + 0.9258)6)/12$$
$$= 0.766 \text{ QALY}$$

6.
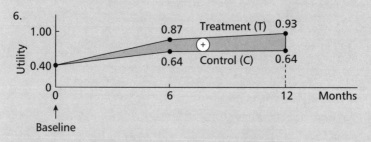

Time	Health state	HUI2 score
Baseline	1, 3, 3, 1, 1, 4	0.4016
6 months	1, 3, 2, 1, 1, 3	0.6439
12 months	1, 3, 2, 1, 1, 3	0.6439

$$\text{QALY(C)} = (0.5(0.4016 + 0.6439)6 + 0.5(0.6439 + 0.6439)6)/12$$
$$= 0.583 \text{ QALY}$$
$$\Delta\text{QALY} = \text{QALY(T)} - \text{QALY(C)} = 0.766 - 0.583 = 0.183 \text{ QALY gained}$$

7.
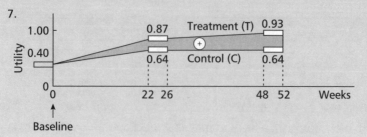

Box 6.8 Solutions: simple quality-adjusted life-year calculations *(continued)*

$$QALY(T) = (0.5(0.4016 + 0.8675)22 + 0.8675 \times 4 + 0.5(0.8675$$
$$+ 0.9258)22 + 0.9258 \times 4)/52$$
$$= 0.786 \; QALY$$
$$QALY(C) = (0.5(0.4016 + 0.6439)22 + 0.6439 \times 4 + 0.5(0.6439$$
$$+0.6439)22 + 0.6439 \times 4)/52$$
$$= 0.593 \; QALY$$
$$\Delta QALY = QALY(T) - QALY(C) = 0.786 - 0.593 = 0.193 \; QALYs \; gained$$

8.

A (a) $1.00 \times 20 = 20$ QALYs.

A (b) $1.00 \times (12.0853 + 1.0000) = 13.1$ QALYs

B (a) $0.5058 \times 20 = 10.1$ QALYs.

B (b) $0.5058 \times (12.0853 + 1.0000) = 6.6$ QALYs

C (a) $-0.2017 \times 20 = -4.0$ QALYs

C (b) $- 0.2017 \times (12.0853 + 1.0000) = -2.6$ QALYs

Box 6.9 **Healthy years equivalents measurement**

This simple example illustrates the measurements process for the HYE (Mehrez and Gafni 1989, 1991, 1992). Consider a health path (also called a health profile) over time as shown below.

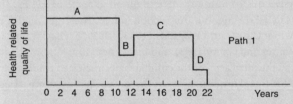

The path can have any length and any pattern. This particular path (path 1) consists of four different health states for different periods of time totalling 22 years, followed by death.

Step 1. Determine utility of path 1

The utility for path 1 is determined using a conventional standard gamble question anchored on perfect health for 22 years and immediate death as shown below. As in any conventional standard gamble, the probability p is varied systematically to find the indifference probability p^*. The result p^* is the NM utility for path 1 on a utility scale where immediate death has a utility of zero and perfect health for 22 years has a utility of 1.

Box 6.9 **Healthy years equivalents measurement** *(continued)*

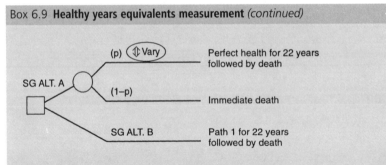

Step 2. Determine HYE for utility of path 1

Step 2 consists of a second standard gamble shown below, which determines the number of healthy years followed by death that would yield the same utility as path 1.

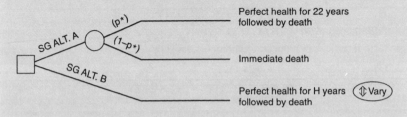

In this standard gamble, H is varied systematically to find the value H^* where the respondent is indifferent between the two alternatives in the standard gamble. Thus, H^* is the number of healthy years followed by death that has a utility of p^*, the same utility as path 1. Thus, H^* is the HYE of path 1.

There has been extensive discussion and debate on all aspects of HYEs. In addition to the references listed throughout this section, other articles on the HYE debate include the following: Culyer and Wagstaff (1993, 1995), Fryback (1993), Gafni and Birch (1993), Mehrez and Gafni (1993), and Bleichrodt (1995). In this book we are not able to go into all the intricacies of the entire debate; interested readers can go to the original sources for that. However, a few of the key points are summarized below.

1. Measuring preferences over a path of health states is theoretically attractive but more difficult in practice. It is theoretically attractive because it is a more general approach to preference measurement, and imposes fewer restrictive assumptions. Thus, it is more likely to capture more accurately the true preferences of the individuals. It is more difficult in practice for two reasons. First, each measurement task is more difficult for the respondent; the certain alternative in the standard gamble is a path of health states rather than a single health state. Because each health state often requires considerable detail to describe appropriately (examples include up to a half page of text, a description of the health status on eight attributes, or even videos to describe a single health state), one may quickly run into cognitive overload with many

subjects. Second, in many practical problems there may be a large number of health paths to be assessed. Indeed, a modest-sized Markov model could easily have eight states and 20 cycles, which would give over 10^{18} unique health paths to be assessed—a daunting task.

2. The concept of measuring preferences over a path of health states is not restricted to HYEs, but could also be used with QALYs, if desired. In such a case, the QALY for a path would be the utility of the path, as measured for example in a single standard gamble, multiplied by the duration of the path. Note that the standard gamble referred to here is identical to step 1 of the HYE procedure (see Box 6.9). Note also that this path-based QALY procedure is just a simple (in concept) variation of the regular QALY procedure. It is just the regular QALY procedure as it would normally be applied to a single chronic state, but with the chronic state replaced in the preference measurement task by the path. Note, finally, that such a path-based QALY is also a utility (see Section 6.6.1), because it is calculated by multiplying a utility by a positive constant.

3. All researchers who have independently evaluated the HYE have concluded that the two-stage standard gamble measurement procedure originally proposed for the HYE is theoretically equivalent to a one-stage TTO procedure (Buckingham 1993; Johannesson et al. 1993; Loomes 1995; Williams 1995; Wakker 1996; Weinstein and Pliskin 1996). This conclusion does not imply that the two measurement procedures will give identical results, but it does imply that if the two procedures differ empirically, there is no theoretical grounds for choosing one over the other. Presumably one would choose the procedure with the least potential for measurement error, which would seem to be the TTO method (Wakker 1996; Weinstein and Pliskin 1996). Note, also, that neither the HYE nor the TTO captures the individual's risk attitude, so neither captures fully the individual's preferences under risk.

4. The HYE is not a utility and is not intended as an alternative to utility theory (Gafni 1996; Wakker 1996). Under von Neumann–Morgenstern utility theory, the appropriate approach for an individual is to solve their decision problem using conventional utility theory. This would involve measuring utilities for each health path (the first standard gamble in the HYE approach), taking expected utilities, and selecting the alternative with the largest expected utility.

5. The HYE may be a useful communication tool for those not trained in decision theory or utility theory. For example, in the case given above, the result could usefully be explained to the decision-maker by converting the expected utility for each alternative into its HYE. This could be done by using a standard gamble like the second one in the HYE approach, except the probability in the gamble alternative of the standard gamble would be based on the expected utility of each decision alternative in the problem, not on the utility of each health path in the problem.

6. As pointed out above in points 3 and 4 the original HYE does not capture an individual's risk attitude and is not a replacement for utility theory. However, an extension to the HYE approach called 'extended HYEs' by Wakker (1996) and 'the certainty–equivalent number of HYEs' or '*ex ante* HYE' by Johannesson (Johannesson 1995a, b) does indeed rank risky health paths according to the individual's preferences. Extended HYEs are defined as the number of healthy years that has the same utility as the gamble rather than the sure thing. More precisely, it is the number of

healthy years that has the same utility as the gamble defined over all possible health paths for the alternative under consideration. For example, a patient facing three treatment options, A, B, and C, would be presented with the full decision tree flowing from option A. This decision tree would take the place of the path in step 1 of the HYE measurement procedure (see Box 6.9). The HYE obtained in step 2 would be the HYE for option A. Similarly, the HYE for each of the other two options would be determined. Then these HYEs would indeed rank the three options according to the patient's preferences. However, the problem with this approach is that as an analytic model it provides no advantage over descriptive empirical reality because it simply replicates the full preference order of the individual. That is, you might just as well have asked the patient to select their preferred option from among A, B, and C, and dispensed with all the measurements. In addition, except in simple problems, the cognitive demands of this approach to measurement would be extremely severe.

An approach using PTOs to determine SAVEs has been suggested as an alternative to the conventional QALY (Nord *et al.* 1993; Nord 1995, 1996, 1999; Green 2001). The basic argument is that the weights for conventional QALYs, and thus the QALYs themselves, reflect an individualistic perspective and not a societal perspective, and thus the conventional QALY does not measure social value. Specifically, it is noted that the weights for conventional QALYs represent an aggregation of preferences and trade-offs that individuals hold for their own health. That is, they represent the trade-offs among various living states and between living states and death that the individuals would want for themselves. In aggregating, all people's preferences are considered equal, although other weighting schemes are possible (Williams 1988), and so the resulting QALY is a particular equity position. Researchers have found that when members of the general public are asked specific PTO questions, like how many patients of type A should be cured to be equivalent in social value to curing 10 patients of type B, the results do not match conventional QALYs (Nord 1995). The reasons often seem to relate to equity considerations (help the sicker people first, treat all equally regardless of capacity to benefit), and perhaps to the 'rule of rescue' (Hadorn 1991) in which life saving is always given the highest priority. The SAVE is the common metric that can be used with the PTO approach. All programmes are converted through PTO measurements to their SAVE value, and programmes are compared on the basis of costs and SAVEs.

Conventional QALYs and SAVEs take different approaches to the definition and measurement of preferences from a societal perspective. In the QALY approach, each member of society is asked what kinds of trade-offs they would like *for themselves*, and the societal decision-making is made consistent with these trade-offs. In the SAVE approach each member of society is asked what kinds of trade-offs they would like *for others*, and this forms the basis for the societal decision-making. It is not clear on theoretical or ethical grounds that one is better than the other. There would be no problem if the two approaches gave similar results, but it appears they do not. The SAVE approach appears to give more emphasis to quantity of life, and less to quality of life. That is, compared to the QALY approach the SAVE approach is less willing to take mortality risks to improve quality of life. This may represent the human tendency, also seen in other fields, of being more conservative when giving advice than when taking it.

The SAVE approach is new and the measurement techniques are still under development (Ubel *et al.* 1996). Indeed, in a review of PTO work to date, Green reports that the technique has limited empirical support and suggests it needs further empirical inquiry (Green 2001).

So, what should an analyst do? Currently, the default method is still the QALY, and generally this should be the primary approach taken by analysts. However, in some studies, or for some decision-makers, analysts may wish also to explore the impact of using a SAVE approach. If the two approaches give dramatically different answers to the resource allocation question, a discussion of the reasons could be quite enlightening for the decision-makers. For further discussion on PTO see Chapter 10.

Disability-adjusted life-years have been developed by the World Health Organization (WHO) for use in their studies; they are conceptually similar to QALYs, but differ in a number of important ways (see Box 6.10). They were first developed for

Box 6.10 How does a disability-adjusted life-year differ from a quality-adjusted life-year?

Disability-adjusted life-years were developed by WHO initially for their Global Burden of Disease and Injury study (Murray and Lopez 1996). Subsequently they have been recommended by WHO for use in generalized cost-effectiveness analysis (Tan-Torres Edejer *et al.* 2003).

Disability-adjusted life-years are conceptually similar to QALYs but differ in the following important ways.

1. The life expectancy used in the QALY depends on the situation. The life expectancy used in the DALY is constant and is set at the greatest reported national life expectancy, that of Japanese women.

2. The disability weights in the QALY are based on preferences, either those of the general public or those of the patients in the study. The disability weights in the DALY are not preferences but are person trade-off scores from a panel of health care workers who met in Geneva in August 1995.

3. Although both sets of disability weights are on the same scale where death has a score of 0 and full health has a score of 1, the QALY weights can take on any value depending upon the health state while the DALY weights, in contrast, can only take on one of seven discrete values. That is, in the DALY system there are only seven health states in addition to dead and healthy.

4. The QALY does not use age weights. The DALY uses age weights that give lower weight to years of the young and the elderly.

The World Health Organization report that they are revising the DALY weights for use in the Global Burden of Disease 2000 study (Tan-Torres Edejer *et al.* 2003). They also report that DALY users should use the age weights in their base case analysis but that a sensitivity analysis can be undertaken without the age weights (Tan-Torres Edejer *et al.* 2003).

use in the Global Burden of Disease and Injury study, sponsored by the World Bank, with the aim of quantifying the burden of disease and injury on human populations (Murray and Lopez 1996). The burden of disease is measured in terms of DALYs lost in comparison to an ideal healthy life with a quality score of 1.0 and a longevity equal to that of the country with the longest life expectancy, Japan. The stated rationale for the standardized life expectancy assumption is that for burden of illness measurements the death of a 40 year old anywhere in the world should count the same; that is, treating like health outcomes as like. This does mean, however, that if the DALY is used for CUA of life-saving interventions in a country with lower life expectancy than Japan, the DALYs gained will be biased upwards. What this does to the rankings of interventions in a given country is not clear. Unlike QALYs, DALYs use age weights. Those in middle age receive extra weight in the DALY system, not because they are more productive but because of their social role whereby they take care of both the young and the elderly. This is a particular equity position that differs from the conventional QALY approach.

More recently WHO has recommended that DALYs be used in generalized CEA (Murray *et al.* 2000; Tan-Torres Edejer *et al.* 2003). Generalized CEA is an approach developed by WHO to evaluate a wide range of possible interventions for chronic diseases and disabling health conditions to identify the optimal package of health care services deliverable within a fixed budget. One of the characteristic features of generalized CEA as proposed by WHO is that each programme is compared not to an alternative programme but to the counterfactual of the null set of the related interventions; that is, the natural history of disease without intervention. The concept is to develop broad general recommendations on the relative cost-effectiveness of various interventions that do not pertain to any specific decision-maker or any local decision constraints.

Since its introduction in 1993 the DALY approach has been heavily debated, and the debate continues. For example, Arnesen and Kapiriri (2004) show that the value choices built into the DALY, notably the age weights, the discount rate, and the disability weights, have a major influence on the rankings of programmes, and yet these value choices are, in part, arbitrary and are far from transparent. They also conclude that the disability weights are of doubtful validity. For another recent review of the DALY approach see Fox-Rushby (2002).

6.6. **Advanced topics**

6.6.1. **Is a quality-adjusted life-year a utility?**

Quality-adjusted life-years are used as the denominator in CUA, so it is natural to think that a QALY is somehow also a utility. In general, it is not.

A utility, in our context here, is an NM utility. So all QALYs that are formed from preferences measured in any way other than with a standard gamble, by definition, cannot be utilities. But what about QALYs formed from preferences for health states measured with a standard gamble? Can they not be utilities? It turns out they can be, but only under quite restrictive assumptions (Weinstein and Fineberg 1980; Torrance and Feeny 1989). The two attributes of quality and quantity must be mutually utility independent (preferences for gambles on the one attribute are independent of the amount of the other attribute); the trade-off of quantity for quality must exhibit the constant proportional trade-off property (the proportion of remaining life that one would trade off for a specified quality improvement is independent of the amount of remaining life), and the single attribute utility function for additional healthy life-years must be linear with time (for a fixed quality level one's utilities are directly proportional to longevity, a property also referred to as risk neutrality with respect to time). These conditions, particularly the latter one, are uncommon in practice, and thus even a utility-weighted QALY is generally not in itself a utility.

However, could a utility-weighted QALY turn out to be a good approximation of a utility? Garber and Phelps (1995) argue that it could, and describe a set of assumptions under which decisions based on cost/QALY would be entirely consistent with welfare economic theory (see also Garber *et al.* 1996). Empirically, it may turn out that QALYs are an adequate approximation of utilities, at least under most situations. So far, there are few data. One study has found that the approximation is not adequate at the individual level, but at the group level it looks promising to use a regression approach to predict path utilities from the utilities of the component states (Kuppermann *et al.* 1997). More research is clearly needed to determine the situations where a QALY is a good approximation of a utility and where it is not.

Finally, does it really matter whether or not a QALY is a utility? Some think not (Culyer 1989). The view is that the QALY is a good basic definition of what we are trying to achieve in health care, and maximizing QALYs is quite an appropriate goal. Because this view is not based on economic welfare theory it has been called the 'extra welfarist' foundation for CUA.

6.6.2. Is it double discounting to discount QALYs?

It is sometimes argued that it is double discounting to discount QALYs if the preference instrument used to measure the QALY weight already incorporated the respondent's time preference (Krahn and Gafni 1993). For example, the TTO method is often said to capture the subject's time preference because it asks time-based questions. So, it would not make sense to discount again, or would it?

To explore this issue we need to look at exactly how a subject's time preference affects the QALY. Time preference in health is normally modelled as a constant discount rate (r) over time (Lipscomb *et al.* 1996). Consider a subject who initially has no time preference ($r = 0$) and rates a state as 0.5 on the TTO. Now, assume the subject suddenly takes on positive time preference ($r > 0$), the normal kind of time preference where we prefer good things to happen earlier and bad things to happen later. The t option in the TTO would now diminish in utility proportionately more than the shorter x option, and to maintain utility indifference the subject would reduce x, thus reducing the TTO score. So, TTO scores would be negatively related to the subject's degree of time preference, but not in direct proportion. For example, if the subject's time preference was 10% per year ($r = 0.1$), this does not mean that the TTO score would reduce by 10%. Large TTO scores would reduce by only a small amount, while small TTO scores would be affected proportionately much more.

Johannesson and colleagues (1994) point out that, at the individual level, depending upon the shape of the individual's utility function, discounted QALYs can lead to programme rankings that violate the individual's preferences. In the special case where the shape of the individual's utility function matches the discounting model with a rate *r*, and the quality weights are being derived using a TTO method, the problem can be avoided by calculating the TTO score by dividing the discounted (at rate *r*) years in full health by the discounted (at rate *r*) years in the index health state. The difficulty, however, for programme evaluation, is that this method only applies at the individual level. Even there it would be complex to implement, probably only applies to a subset of individuals, and would lead to a different discount rate for each individual. In programme evaluation the discount rate reflects the time preference of the decision-maker, not necessarily that of the patients; the discount rate must apply to all patients regardless of their individual rates, and in many applications it applies to outcomes achieved by both current and future patients, thus capturing the intergenerational time preference as well.

Now consider the standard gamble. It incorporates the subject's risk preference, but not time preference. Even though the alternatives of the gamble have time in them, the time is the same in each alternative and if the subject's time preference changes (*r* changes), it affects each alternative proportionally the same, so the utility indifference is not disturbed. Thus, different time preferences do not lead to different scores from the standard gamble. Finally, VAS scores also are not affected by time preference for the same reasons.

So, to summarize, preference scores measured by standard gamble or VAS are not affected by time preference so there is no issue. Preference scores measured by TTO are indeed affected by the subject's time preference, but not in any uniform or proportionate way. Moreover, the subject's time preference may be much different from the modest-sized social rate of discount of 3–5% recommended by most guidelines for economic evaluation (Canadian Coordinating Office for Health Technology Assessment 1997; Gold *et al.* 1996*b*; Torrance *et al.* 1996*b*). Individual time preferences for health have been found to be highly variable, even within subject, and to include both positive and negative rates of discount (Fuchs 1982; Dolan and Gudex 1995). Thus, even with the TTO it is not a simple case that the recommended social rate of discount has been incorporated by the subjects who rated the outcomes. Although a method has been suggested for adjusting TTO scores to account for an individual's time preference (Johannesson *et al.* 1994), it is not clear how this can be used in programme evaluations. It appears to us that more thought and research is needed to clarify this fully, but at the moment our advice would be to continue to discount at the recommended social rate of discount regardless of how the preference weights were obtained.

6.7. Critical appraisal of a published article

Reference: Torrance, G. W., Raynauld, J. P., Walker, V., *et al.* (2001*b*). A prospective, randomised, pragmatic, health outcomes trial evaluating the incorporation of hylan G-F 20 into the treatment paradigm for patients with knee osteoarthritis (Part 2 of 2): economic results. *Osteoarthritis and Cartilage*, **10**, 518–27.

The paper is assessed below using the 10 questions set out in Box 3.1. It is suggested that you locate the article and attempt the exercise before reading the assessment.

1. Was a well-defined question posed in answerable form?

 X YES ___NO ___CAN'T TELL

In this randomized, pragmatic (real-world) trial the authors investigated the costs, effectiveness, cost-effectiveness, and cost-utility of hylan G-F 20 as adjunctive therapy along with appropriate care for the treatment of knee osteoarthritis (p. 519). Specifically they compared appropriate care with hylan G-F 20 to appropriate care alone, from the viewpoint of society (primary viewpoint) and the viewpoint of the health care system (secondary viewpoint). They state that the results should be of decision-making interest to clinicians, particularly those involved in establishing treatment guidelines, and to third-party payers, formulary managers, and fiscal administrators (p. 519).

2. Was a comprehensive description of the competing alternatives given?

___YES X NO ___CAN'T TELL

Although the competing alternatives are clearly stated, they are not comprehensively described in this paper, probably due to page limitations. The authors do, however, reference other papers that provide more details. The primary other paper is the companion clinical manuscript published back to back with this paper: Raynauld, J.-P., Torrance, G. W., Band, P. A., *et al.* (2001). A prospective, randomized, pragmatic, health outcomes trial evaluating the incorporation of hylan G-F 20 into the treatment paradigm for patients with knee osteoarthritis (Part 1 of 2): clinical results. *Osteoarthritis and Cartilage*, **10**, 506–17. In this paper the alternatives are described more fully, and indeed Table II (p. 512) provides the details of the appropriate care provided in each of the alternatives.

Given the research question (real-world effectiveness, cost-effectiveness and cost-utility), the comparator (appropriate care) was appropriate. As the authors state, the comparator was deliberately selected as appropriate care, not usual care, because it was felt that usual care might contain some inappropriate care, and demonstrating that a new treatment is effective and cost-effective compared to inappropriate care is not particularly useful (p. 519). Appropriate care, in this study, was the preferred management strategy of the clinicians encouraged to follow the treatment guidelines (stepped care strategy) published by the American College of Rheumatology and instructed to treat conservatively. Although the guidelines are referenced, they are not reproduced in the paper.

A complete do-nothing alternative (no treatment for osteoarthritis) was not included and, indeed, would not have been ethical given the disease. On the other hand, given that the new treatment (hylan G-F 20) was add-on therapy to appropriate care, the comparator amounted to a do-nothing alternative in this regard; that is, there was no add-on therapy in the comparator arm.

Hylan G-F 20 is not the only viscosupplementation product available for injection into the knee. Additional alternatives that could have been included in this study, but were not, are the other viscosupplementation products. This could have made the results more useful for decision-makers. The broadening of the range of treatment alternatives raises questions over who would fund the relevant clinical trials. However, decision-makers could commission studies using a decision-analytic framework (see Chapter 9) to compare hylan G-F 20 with other treatments.

3. Was there evidence that the programmes' effectiveness had been established?

_X_ YES ___NO ___CAN'T TELL

As the authors state, particularly in the companion clinical paper, the efficacy of hylan G-F 20 had been previously established through several randomized clinical trials, and the product had been approved for use in most countries in the world (p. 518). Accordingly, this study was mounted to investigate the effectiveness, cost-effectiveness, and cost-utility in a real-world setting. To enhance the real-world applicability of the results, the trial was designed to be as pragmatic as possible. The study was conducted in multiple sites with different types of providers, the inclusion/exclusion criteria were liberal, the study was not blinded, the study was 1 year in length, and protocol-driven costs and outcomes were minimized by limiting study-induced clinic visits to baseline and termination (p. 519). For the rest of the year the patients were treated as they would be in regular practice, and data were gathered using telephone interviews.

4. Were all the important and relevant costs and consequences for each alternative identified?

_X_ YES ___NO ___CAN'T TELL

Costs were collected comprehensively for each alternative over the entire 12 months of the study. Costs included physician visits, other health care provider visits, home care visits, emergency room visits, X-rays, tests, procedures, hospitalizations, medications, devices, travel, parking, time loss from work, and time loss from usual activity for those not working. All costs related to health care were collected, although only those costs attributable to osteoarthritis were used in the analysis. Costs were deemed attributable to osteoarthritis if they were caused by osteoarthritis in any joint (not just the treated knee), if they were treatment for osteoarthritis in any joint, or if they were treatment for adverse events related to the treatment of osteoarthritis in any joint. Cost items were identified by the patients in their periodic interviews throughout the study and were verified where possible by comparison with the physician charts. Patients used a diary as a memory aid for recording costs as they occurred. Patients made the initial attribution of cost items to osteoarthritis or not. To enhance consistency across the study, these attributions were reviewed and could be changed first by the local site investigator and second by a blinded adjudication committee for the entire study.

The cost identification and collection in this study was thorough and comprehensive. The decision to limit the analysis of costs to those attributable to osteoarthritis in any joint was a good compromise between the two polar alternatives of limiting costs to those attributable to the treated knee and not limiting costs at all. The problem with the former is that most treatments for osteoarthritis in the knee are systemic, not local.

The problem with the latter is that the cost comparison could be overwhelmed and biased by large random costs not related to the disease and the treatment under study.

Costs were analysed from two viewpoints: the societal viewpoint and the health care system viewpoint. These are the two important viewpoints in the Canadian health care system. The only other viewpoint that the investigators might have considered was the patient/family viewpoint.

Consequences were measured at three levels: osteoarthritis in the study knee, osteoarthritis in all joints, and overall health. Osteoarthritis in the study knee was measured by the Western Ontario McMaster Osteoarthritis Index (WOMAC) instrument, a widely used, well-validated health-related quality of life instrument for this disease, and by the patients' global assessment. Osteoarthritis in all joints was measured by the patients' global assessment. Overall health was measured by the SF-36, a widely used, generic health-related quality of life instrument, and by the HUI, a well-known utility instrument.

Thus a comprehensive range of costs and consequences was identified, consistent with the adoption of a societal viewpoint.

5. Were costs and consequences measured accurately in appropriate physical units?

 _X_ YES ___NO ___CAN'T TELL

All identified items were included in the costs. Costs were reported by patients in physical units not in dollars, except for a few items like parking and travel. For example, patients reported their health care utilization, not its cost. They reported doctor visits, tests performed, pills taken, hospitalizations, and so on. Similarly, patients reported their time off work, not its cost.

Consequences were measured using the units of the instruments: WOMAC, SF-36, HUI, and the patient global assessments. The valuation (scoring) of these instruments is done separately, using the scoring methods provided with the instruments. The use and interpretation of these scores also comes later. For example, the WOMAC score was used in two ways: first as a direct clinical outcome (percentage reduction in pain score), and second as a method to define an 'improved patient' (for example, 20% reduction in pain score).

6. Were costs and consequences valued credibly?

 _X_ YES ___NO ___CAN'T TELL

Costs were valued in 1999 Canadian dollars. Unit costs that were not available for the year 1999 were appropriately adjusted to 1999 using the health and personal care component of the Consumer Price Index. Market prices from the province of Ontario, Canada's largest province, were used for drugs, devices, laboratory services, physician services, and the cost of other health care professionals. Existing costing studies were used as the source of unit costs for emergency room visits and for hospitalizations. In the case of hospitalizations, the costing study (the Ontario Case Costing Project) was a comprehensive study of multiple hospitals and included costs for capital equipment, buildings, and land as well as for operating costs. Time losses, both work time and non-work time, were valued at the Canadian average industrial wage rate.

Consequences were valued in terms of scores improved on outcome instruments (WOMAC, SF-36, HUI3), patients improved, and QALYs gained. The latter two allowed the authors to calculate an incremental cost-effectiveness ratio (cost per additional patient improved) and an incremental cost–utility ratio (cost per additional QALY gained), and were necessary and appropriate to the objectives of the study. The definition of 'patient improved' was based on improvements in the patient's WOMAC score that met or exceeded the pre-determined minimum clinically important difference established in advance by the clinical investigators. The WOMAC score, and hence the CEA, is focused on the index knee. The calculation of QALYs was based on the patient's HUI score, and, thus, represented a measure of the health-related quality of life of the whole patient. The CUA, thus, is focused on the whole patient. The HUI score itself is based on community preferences, and this is consistent with the recommended source of preference weights for use in societal-perspective CUAs.

7. Were costs and consequences adjusted for differential timing?

___YES _X_ NO ___CAN'T TELL

Because this was a 12-month clinical trial, all the costs and consequences occurred within a 1-year period. Accordingly, no discounting was needed. Had the authors gone on to model future costs and effects beyond the 1-year clinical trial period, they would have had to use discounting, but no such modelling was done.

Ideally the analytic horizon in an economic evaluation should be long enough to capture all the significant costs and benefits due to therapy, including long term adverse events and repeat therapy. Thus, the ideal study, in most cases, would follow patients for their lifetime. In this study no modelling or extrapolation was done beyond the 12 months' duration of the trial. The duration of the trial was, however, longer than the average cycle length of 7 months between treatments, so was designed to capture steady state behaviour. The implicit assumption in this study was that continuation of therapy for another similar period of time would produce the same costs and the same effects, that is, steady-state behaviour. This is the implicit assumption when comparing CEAs that use different analytic horizons.

Although it may not be feasible to extend clinical trials over many years, an economic evaluation would, ideally, project costs and benefits into the future. Such a model would be greatly informed by long-term observational studies of patients receiving the therapy, because these could track the maintenance of treatment effect, the need for re-treatment, and the incidence of adverse events.

8. Was an incremental analysis of costs and consequences of alternatives performed?

_X_ YES ___NO ___CAN'T TELL

To determine the cost-effectiveness ratio the authors calculated the incremental (additional) cost per patient of the treatment group versus the control group and divided it by the incremental (additional) probability of the patient being 'improved' in the treatment group versus the control group, thus yielding the incremental cost per additional patient improved. To determine the cost–utility ratio the authors divided the same numerator by the incremental (additional) QALYs per patient in the treatment group versus the control group, thus yielding the incremental cost per additional QALY gained.

9. Was allowance made for uncertainty in the estimation of costs and consequences?

_X_ YES ___NO ___CAN'T TELL

Because the study was based on a clinical trial, as opposed to a modelling study, the authors had stochastic data available, that is, they had individual cost and outcome data on individual patients. They allowed for this uncertainty in data using traditional one-way sensitivity analyses. For costs, they varied the incremental cost to its upper and lower 90% confidence bounds. Similarly, for outcomes they also used the upper and lower 90% confidence bounds. For the CEA they varied the incremental probability of a patient being improved to its confidence bounds. For the CUA they varied the incremental QALYs gained to its confidence bounds. While these methods are appropriate and useful, they are no longer state of the art. With the same data, the authors could have used bootstrap simulation, cost-effectiveness acceptability curves, and/or net benefit statistics.

The authors also allowed for methodological uncertainty. Specifically, they addressed the debate about whether or not to cost lost non-working time by doing it both ways. In the base case analysis, they did not cost such time. In a sensitivity analysis they did.

The sensitivity analyses were interpreted with respect to published decision criteria, that is, would the decision differ or not? Fortunately, the sensitivity analyses made very little difference to the decision that one would reach. Four of the five sensitivity analyses led to the same decision as the base case analysis.

10. Did the presentation and discussion of study results include all issues of concern to users?

___YES ___NO _X_ CAN'T TELL

The authors provided two different indexes, CEA and CUA, each from two different perspectives, societal and health care system. Thus different decision-makers with different needs can select the result that is most appropriate for them. Moreover, clinicians with less interest in the economic evaluation and more in the clinical findings, can go to the clinical article which was published in the same issue of the journal. This approach of publishing a clinical and an economic article back to back is very useful, when it can be done, as it enables more of the information to be published and it enables readers to focus on aspects of particular relevance.

The authors placed their results in context by comparing with other studies. However, they were mindful that indiscriminate use of league tables can be dangerous. Accordingly, they restricted their comparisons in two ways: first, to studies in the same clinical area, and second, to studies that met a minimum standard of methodological quality. The Harvard database of studies, which they used, will be a useful resource for other researchers wishing to make similar restrictions on their league tables.

The authors also placed their results in context by comparing them with published decision criteria. Although these criteria have no official status, they are widely viewed as reasonable, and it is helpful to decision-makers to have the results cast this way.

The authors discussed the generalizability of their findings to other settings, particularly to other countries. They noted that some of the findings would be expected to travel fairly well, notably the clinical findings, the results of the outcome instruments (WOMAC, SF-36, HUI3), and the QALYs. In contrast, the health care utilization and the costs would not be expected to travel well, and would need to be reconsidered in each country based on the specifics of that country's health care system and cost structure.

The authors did not address distributional considerations or ethical issues concerning the treatment. Hylan G-F 20 is registered as a device in Canada, and, accordingly, is not covered under drug plans. Thus, patients in Canada have to fund the purchase from some other source, in some cases from their own pockets. No doubt this has some distributional and ethical implications.

The authors concluded that hylan G-F 20 is cost-effective, that is, that the incremental cost per QALY gained is well below the suggested Canadian threshold for adoption. They did not, however, discuss the implementation issues, particularly who would or should fund the costs.

References

Allais, M. (1991). Cardinal utility history, empirical findings, and applications: an overview. *Theory and Decision*, **31**, 99–140.

Andresen, E. M., Rothenberg, B. M., and Kaplan, R. M. (1998). Performance of a self-administered mailed version of the Quality of Well-Being (QWB-SA) Questionnaire among older adults. *Medical Care*, **36**, 1349–60.

Arnesen, T. and Kapiriri, L. (2004). Can the value choices in DALYs influence global priority-setting? *Health Policy*, **70**, 137–49.

Arrow, K. J. and Debreu, G. (1954). Existence of equilibrium for a competitive economy. *Econometrica*, **22**, 265–90.

Balaban, D., Sagi, P., Goldfarb, N., and Nettler, S. (1986). Weights for scoring the quality of well-being instrument among rheumatoid arthritics: A comparison to general population weights. *Medical Care*, **24**, 973–80.

Bass, E. B., Steinberg, E., Pitt, H., *et al.* (1994). Comparison of the rating scale and the standard gamble in measuring patient preferences for outcomes of gallstone disease. *Medical Decision Making*, **14**, 307–14.

Bell, D. and Farquhar, P. (1986). Perspectives on utility theory. *Operations Research*, **34**, 179–83.

Bennett, K. J. and Torrance, G. W. (1996). Measuring health state preferences and utilities: rating scale, time trade-off and standard gamble techniques. In: *Quality of life and pharmacoeconomics in clinical trials* (2nd edn) (ed. B. Spilker), pp. 253–65. Lippincott-Raven, Philadelphia.

Bennett, K. J., Torrance, G. W., Moran, L. A., Smith, F., and Goldsmith, C. H. (1997). Health state utilities in knee replacement surgery: the development and evaluation of McKnee. *Journal of Rheumatology*, **24**, 1796–1805.

Bennett, K. J., Torrance, G. W., Boyle, M. H., Guscott, R., and Moran, L. A. (2000). Development and testing of a utility measure for major unipolar depression (McSad). *Quality of Life Research*, **9**, 109–120.

Berthelot, J., Roberge, R., and Wolfson, M. (1993). The calculation of health-adjusted life expectancy for a Canadian province using a multi-attribute utility function: a first attempt. In: *Calculation of health expectancies: harmonization, consensus and future perspectives*, (ed. J. M. Robine, C. D. Mathers, M. R. Bone, and I. Romieu), Vol. 226, pp. 161–72. Montrouge, France: John Libbey Eurotext.

Bleichrodt, H. (1995). QALYs and HYEs: Under what conditions are they equivalent? *Journal of Health Economics*, **14**, 17–37.

Bleichrodt, H. (2002). A new explanation for the difference between time trade-off utilities and standard gamble utilities. *Health Economics*, **11**, 447–56.

Bleichrodt, H. and Johannesson, M. (1997). An experimental test of a theoretical foundation for rating scale valuations. *Medical Decision Making*, **17**, 208–16.

Bossert, W. (1991). On intra- and interpersonal utility comparisons. *Social Choice and Welfare*, **8**, 207–19.

Brazier, J., Roberts, J., and Deverill, M. (2002). The estimation of a preference-based measure of health from the SF-36. *Journal of Health Economics*, **21**, 271–92.

Brooks, R. with the EuroQol Group (1996). EuroQol: the current state of play. *Health Policy*, **37**, 53–72.

Broome, J. (1993). QALYS. *Journal of Public Economics*, **50**, 149–67.

Buckingham, K. (1993). A note on HYE (healthy years equivalent). *Journal of Health Economics*, **11**, 301–9.

Buckingham, J. K., Birdsall, J., and Douglas, J. G. (1996). Comparing three versions of the time tradeoff: time for a change? *Medical Decision Making*, **16**, 335–47.

Bush, J., Fanshel, S., and Chen, M. (1972). Analysis of a tuberculin testing program using a health status index. *Socio-Economic Planning Sciences*, **6**, 49–68.

Buxton, M. and Ashby, J. (1988). The time trade-off approach to health state valuation. In: *Measuring health: a practical approach* (ed. G. Teeling Smith), pp. 69–87. John Wiley, Chichester.

Canadian Coordinating Office for Health Technology Assessment (1997). *Guidelines for economic evaluation of pharmaceuticals: Canada, 2nd edition*. Canadian Coordinating Office for Health Technology Assessment, Ottawa (available to download from: http://www.ccohta.ca or email pubs@ccohta.ca).

Carr-Hill, R. (1991). Allocating resources to health care: is the QALY (quality-adjusted life year) a technical solution to a political problem? *International Journal of Health Services. Research*, **21**, 351–63.

Carr-Hill, R. and Morris, J. (1991). Current practice in obtaining the 'Q' in QALYs: a cautionary note. *British Medical Journal*, **303**, 699–701.

Chapman, R. H., Stone, P. W., Sandberg, E. A., Bell, C., and Neumann, P. J. (2000). A comprehensive league table of cost-utility ratios and a sub-table of "Panel-worthy" studies. *Medical Decision Making*, **20**, 451–67.

Churchill, D., Torrance, G., Taylor, D., *et al.* (1987). Measurement of quality of life in end-stage renal disease: The time trade-off approach. *Clinical and Investigative Medicine*, **10**, 14–20.

Cohen, B. J. (1996). Is expected utility theory normative for medical decision making? *Medical Decision Making*, **16**, 1–14.

Conner-Spady, B. and Suarez-Almazor, M. E. (2003). Variation in the estimation of quality-adjusted life-years by different preference-based instruments. *Medical Care*, **41**, 791–801.

Cook, J., Richardson, J., and Street, A. (1994). A cost–utility analysis of treatment options for gallstone disease: methodological issues and results. *Health Economics*, **3**, 157–68.

Cooper, R. and Rappoport, P. (1984). Were the ordinalists wrong about welfare economics? *Journal of Economic Literature*, **22**, 507–30.

Cox, D., Fitzpatrick, R., Fletcher, A., Gore, S., Spiegelhalter, D., and Jones, D. (1992). Quality-of-life assessment: can we keep it simple? *Journal of the Royal Statistical Society Series A*, **155**, 353–93.

Culyer, A. (1989). The normative economics of health care finance and provision. *Oxford Review of Economic Policy*, 5, 34–58.

Culyer, A. J. and Wagstaff A. (1995). QALYs versus HYEs: A reply to Gafni, Birch and Mehrez. *Journal of Health Economics*, 14, 39–45.

Culyer, A. and Wagstaff, A. (1993). QALYs versus HYEs. *Journal of Health Economics*, 11, 311–23.

Currim, I. and Sarin, R. (1992). Robustness of expected utility model in predicting individual choices. *Organizational Behavior and Human Decision Processes*, 52, 544–68.

Dolan, P. and Gudex, C. (1995). Time preference, duration and health state valuations. *Health Economics*, 4, 289–99.

Dolan, P. and Roberts, J. (2002). Modelling valuations for EQ-5D health states: an alternative model using differences in valuation. *Medical Care*, 40, 442–6.

Dolan, P., Gudex, C., Kind, P., and Williams, A. (1995). *A social tariff for EuroQoL: Results from a UK general population survey*, Discussion Paper No. 138. Centre for Health Economics, University of York, York.

Dolan, P., Gudex, C., Kind, P., and Williams, A. (1996a). Valuing health states: a comparison of methods. *Journal of Health Economics*, 15, 209–31.

Dolan, P., Gudex, C., Kind, P., and Williams, A. (1996b). The time trade-off method: results from a general population study. *Health Economics*, 5, 141–54.

Dyer, J. and Sarin, R. (1979). Measurable multi-attribute value functions. *Operations Research*, 27, 810–22.

Dyer, J. and Sarin, R. (1982). Relative risk aversion. *Management Science*, 28, 875–86.

Erickson, P., Wilson, R., and Shannon, I. (1995). *Years of healthy life*, Statistical Notes, No. 7, April 1995. National Center for Health Statistics, Hyattsville, Maryland.

Essink-bot, M., Stouthard, M., and Bonsel, G. (1993). Generalizability of valuations on health states collected with the EuroQol—questionnaire. *Health Economics*, 2, 237–46.

EuroQol Group (1990). EuroQol—a new facility for the measurement of health-related quality of life. *Health Policy*, 16, 199–208.

Fanshel, S. and Bush, J. (1970). A health status index and its application to health services outcomes. *Operations Research*, 18, 1021–66.

Feeny, D., Torrance, G. W., and Labelle, R. (1996). Integrating economic evaluations and quality of life assessments. In: *Quality of life and pharmacoeconomics in clinical trials* (2nd edn) (ed. B. Spilker), pp. 85–95. Lippincott-Raven, Philadelphia.

Feeny, D., Furlong, W., Torrance, *et al.* (2002). Multiattribute and single-attribute utility functions for the Health Utilities Index Mark 3 system. *Medical Care*, 40, 113–28.

Fischer, G. W. (1979). Utility models for multiple objective decisions: Do they accurately represent human preferences. *Decision Sciences*, 10, 451–79.

Fischer, G., Kamlet, M., Fienberg, S., and Schkade, D. (1986). Risk preferences for gains and losses in multiple objective decision making. *Management Science*, 32, 1065–86.

Fishburn, P. and Wakker, P. (1995). The invention of the independence condition for preferences. *Management Science*, 41, 1130–44.

Fox-Rushby, J. (2002). *Disability adjusted life years (DALYs) for decision making? An overview of the literature*. Office of Health Economics, London.

Fryback, D. (1993). QALYs, HYEs, and the loss of innocence (editorial). *Medical Decision Making*, 13, 271–2.

Fuchs, V. R. (1982). Time preference and health: an exploratory study. In: *Economic aspects of health* (ed. V. R. Fuchs), pp. 93–120. University of Chicago Press, Chicago.

Furlong, W., Feeny, D., Torrance, G., Barr, R., and Horsman, J. (1990). *Guide to design and development of health-state utility instrumentation*, Working Paper No. 90–9. McMaster University, Centre for Health Economics and Policy Analysis, Hamilton, Ontario.

Furlong, W. J., Feeny, D. H., Torrance, G. W., and Barr, R. D. (2001). The Health Utilities Index (HUI) system for assessing health-related quality of life in clinical studies. *Annals of Medicine*, **33**, 375–84.

Gafni, A. and Torrance, G. (1984). Risk attitude and time preference in health. *Management Science*, **30**, 440–51.

Gafni, A. (1996). HYEs: Do we need them and can they fulfil the promise? *Medical Decision Making*, **16**, 215–16.

Gafni, A. and Birch, S. (1993). Economics, health and health economics: HYEs versus QALYs. *Journal of Health Economics*, **11**, 325–39.

Garber, A. M. and Phelps, C. E. (1995). *Economic foundations of cost-effectiveness analysis*. National Bureau of Economic Research, Stanford, California.

Garber, A. M., Weinstein, M. C., Torrance, G. W., and Kamlet, M. S. (1996). Theoretical foundations of cost-effectiveness analysis. In: *Cost-effectiveness in health and medicine*. (ed. M. R. Gold, J. E. Siegel, L. B. Russell, and M. C. Weinstein), pp. 25–53. Oxford University Press, New York.

Gerard, K. (1992). Cost–utility in practice: a policy maker's guide to the state of the art. *Health Policy*, **21**, 249–79.

Goel, V. and Detsky, A. (1989). A cost–utility analysis of preoperative total parenteral nutrition. *International Journal of Technology Assessment in Health Care*, **5**, 183–94.

Gold, M. R., Siegel, J. E., Russell, L. B., and Weinstein, M. C. (1996). *Cost-effectiveness in health and medicine*. Oxford University Press, New York.

Gorber, S. (2003). A new classification and measurement system of functional health. *Au Courant (Statistics Canada Catalogue 82–005-XIE)*, **September**, 2–3.

Green, C. (2001). On the societal value of health care: what do we know about the person trade-off technique? *Health Economics*, **10**, 233–43.

Hadorn, D. (1991). Setting health care priorities in Oregon: cost-effectiveness meets the rule of rescue. *Journal of the American Medical Association*, **265**, 2218–25.

Hadorn, D. C. and Uebersax, J. (1995). Large scale outcome evaluation: how should quality of life be measured? I. Calibration of a brief questionnaire and a search for preference subgroups. *Journal of Clinical Epidemiology*, **48**, 607–18.

Hadorn, D. C., Hays, R. D., and Hauber, T. (1992). Improving task comprehension in the measurement of health state preferences. *Journal of Clinical Epidemiology*, **45**, 233–43.

Hall, J., Gerard, K., Salkeld, G., and Richardson, J. (1992). A cost–utility analysis of mammography screening in Australia. *Social Science and Medicine*, **34**, 993–1004.

Hawthorne, G., Richardson, J., and Day, N. A. (2001). A comparison of the Assessment of Quality of Life (AQoL) with four other generic utility instruments. *Annals of Medicine*, **33**, 358–70.

Hey, J. (1979). *Uncertainty in microeconomics*. New York University Press, New York.

Holloway, C. (1979). *Decision making under uncertainty: models and choices*. Prentice-Hall, Englewood Cliffs, New Jersey.

Horsman, J., Furlong, W., Feeny, D., and Torrance, G. (2003). The Health Utilities Index (HUI): concepts, measurement properties and applications. *Health and Quality of Life Outcomes*, **1**, 54 (electronic version available free at http://www.hqlo.com/content/1/1/54).

Howard, R. (1988). Decision analysis: practice and promise. *Management Science*, **34**, 679–95.

Johannesson, M. (1995*a*). Quality-adjusted life years versus healthy-years equivalents—a comment. *Journal of Health Economics*, **14**, 9–16.

Johannesson, M. (1995*b*). The ranking properties of healthy-years equivalents and quality-adjusted life-years under certainty and uncertainty. *International Journal of Technology Assessment in Health Care*, **11**, 40–8.

Johannesson, M., Pliskin, J., and Weinstein, M. (1993). Are healthy-years equivalents an improvement over quality-adjusted life-years? *Medical Decision Making*, **13**, 281–6.

Johannesson, M., Pliskin, J., and Weinstein, M. (1994). A note on QALYs, time trade-off and discounting. *Medical Decision Making*, **14**, 188–93.

Kaplan, R. (1994). Value judgement in the Oregon medicaid experiment. *Medical Care*, **32**, 975–88.

Kaplan, R. M. and Anderson, J. (1988). A general health policy model: Update and applications. *Health Services Research*, **23**, 203–35.

Kaplan, R. M. and Anderson, J. P. (1996). The general health policy model: an integrated approach. In: *Quality of life and pharmacoeconomics in clinical trials* (2nd edn) (ed. B. Spilker), pp. 309–22. Lippincott-Raven, Philadelphia.

Keeney, R. and Raiffa, H. (1976). *Decisions with multiple objectives: preferences and value tradeoffs*. Wiley, New York.

Keeney, R. and Raiffa, H. (1993). *Decisions with multiple objectives: preferences and value tradeoffs* (2nd edn). Cambridge University Press, Cambridge.

Kennedy, W., Reinharz, D., Tessier, G., *et al.* (1995). Cost–utility of chemotherapy and best supportive care in non-small cell lung cancer. *PharmacoEconomics*, **8**, 316–23.

Kind, P. (1996). The EuroQol instrument: an index of health-related quality of life. In: *Quality of life and pharmacoeconomics in clinical trials* (2nd edn) (ed. B. Spilker), pp. 191–201. Lippincott-Raven, Philadelphia.

Klarman, H., Francis, J., and Rosenthal, G. (1968). Cost-effectiveness analysis applied to the treatment of chronic renal disease. *Medical Care*, **6**, 48–54.

Kleindorfer, P., Kunreuther, H., and Schoemaker, P. (1993). *Decision sciences—an integrative perspective*. Cambridge University Press, New York.

Kopec, J. A. and Willison, K. D. (2003). A comparative review of four preference-weighted measures of health-related quality of life. *Journal of Clinical Epidemiology*, **56**, 317–25.

Krahn, M. and Gafni, A. (1993). Discounting in the economic evaluation of health care interventions. *Medical Care*, **31**, 403–18.

Kuppermann, M., Shiboski, S., Feeny, D., Elkin, E. P., and Washington, A. E. (1997). Can preference scores for discrete states be used to derive preference scores for an entire path of events? An application to prenatal diagnosis. *Medical Decision Making*, **17**, 42–55.

Le Gales, C., Buron, C., Costet, N., Rosman, S., and Slama, G. (2002). Development of a preference-weighted health status classification system in France: the Health Utilities Index. *Health Care Management Science*, **5**, 41–51.

Lenert, L. A. (2001). The reliability and internal consistency of an Internet-capable computer program for measuring utilities. *Quality of Life Research*, **9**, 811–817.

Lipscomb, J., Weinstein, M. C., and Torrance, G. W. (1996). Time preference. In: Cost-effectiveness in health and medicine (ed. M. R. Gold, J. E. Siegel, L. B. Russell, and M. C. Weinstein), pp. 214–46. Oxford University Press, New York.

Loomes, G. (1991). Evidence of a new violation of the independence axiom. *Journal of Risk and Uncertainty*, **4**, 91–108.

Loomes, G. (1995). The myth of the HYE. *Journal of Health Economics*, **14**, 1–7.

Lubetkin, E. I. and Gold, M. R. (2003). Areas of decrement in health-related quality of life (HRQL): comparing the SF-12, EQ-5D, and HUI3. *Quality of Life Research*, **12**, 1059–67.

Luce, R. (1992). Where does subjective expected utility fail descriptively? *Journal of Risk and Uncertainty*, **5**, 5–27.

Luce, R. and Raiffa, H. (1957). *Games and decisions*. Wiley, New York.

Manca, A., Hawkins, N., and Sculpher, M. (in press). Estimating mean QALYs in trial-based cost-effectiveness analysis: the importance of controlling for baseline utility. *Health Economics*, **13**.

Martin, A. J., Glasziou, P. P., Simes, R. J., and Lumley, T. A. (2000). Comparison of standard gamble, time trade-off, and adjusted time trade-off scores. *International Journal of Technology Assessment in Health Care*, **16**, 137–47.

Mehrez, A. and Gafni, A. (1989). Quality-adjusted life years, utility theory, and healthy-years equivalents. *Medical Decision Making*, **9**, 142–9.

Mehrez, A. and Gafni, A. (1990). Evaluating health-related quality of life: An indifference curve interpretation for the time trade-off technique. *Social Science in Medicine*, **31**, 1281–3.

Mehrez, A. and Gafni, A. (1991). The healthy-years equivalents: how to measure them using the standard gamble approach. *Medical Decision Making*, **11**, 140–6.

Mehrez, A. and Gafni, A. (1992). Preference based outcome measures for economic evaluation of drug interventions: quality adjusted life years (QALYs) versus healthy years equivalents (HYEs). *PharmacoEconomics*, **1**, 338–45.

Mehrez, A. and Gafni, A. (1993). Healthy-years equivalents versus quality-adjusted life years: in pursuit of progress. *Medical Decision Making*, **13**, 287–92.

Miyamoto, J. M. (1988). Generic utility theory: measurement foundations and applications in multiattribute utility theory. *Journal of Mathematical Psychology*, **32**, 357–404.

Murray, C. J. L. and Lopez, A. D. (1996). *The global burden of disease: a comprehensive assessment of mortality and disability from diseases, injuries, and risk factors in 1990 and projected to 2020*. Harvard University Press, Cambridge.

Murray, C. J. L., Evans, D. B., Acharya, A., and Baltussen, R. M. P. M. (2000). Development of WHO guidelines on generalized cost-effectiveness analysis. *Health Economics*, **9**, 235–52.

National Institute for Clinical Excellence (2004). *Guide to the methods of technology appraisal*, April 2004. London: UK National Health Service, National Institute for Clinical Excellence.

Nease, R. F. (1996). Do violations of the axioms of expected utility theory threaten decision analysis? *Medical Decision Making*, **16**, 399–403.

Nord, E. (1993). Toward quality assurance in QALY calculations. *International Journal of Technology Assessment in Health Care*, **9**, 37–45.

Nord, E. (1995). The person-trade-off approach to valuing health care programs. *Medical Decision Making*, **15**, 201–8.

Nord, E. (1996). Health status index models for use in resource allocation decisions: A critical review in the light of observed preferences for social choice. *International Journal of Technology Assessment in Health Care*, **12**, 31–44.

Nord, E. (1999). *Cost-value analysis in health care: making sense out of QALYs*. Cambridge University Press, Cambridge.

Nord, E., Richardson, J., and Macarounas-Kirchmann, K. (1993). Social evaluation of health care versus personal evaluation of health states. *International Journal of Technology Assessment in Health Care*, **9**, 463–78.

O'Brien, B. J., Torrance, G. W., and Moran, L. A. (1994). *A practical guide to health state preference measurement: a video introduction*, Working Paper No. 95–2. Centre for Health Economics and Policy Analysis, McMaster University, Hamilton, Ontario.

O'Brien, B., Spath, M., Blackhouse, G., Severens, J. L., Dorian, P., and Brazier, J. (2003). A view from the bridge: agreement between the SF-6D utility algorithm and the Health Utilities Index. *Health Economics Letters*, **7**, 9–15.

O'Leary, J. F., Fairclough, D. L., Jankowski, M. K., and Weeks, J. C. (1995). Comparison of time trade-off utilities and rating scale values of cancer patients and their relatives: evidence for a possible plateau relationship. *Medical Decision Making*, **15**, 132–7.

Oldridge, N., Furlong, W., Feeny, D., *et al.* (1993). Economic evaluation of cardiac rehabilitation soon after acute myocardial infarction. *American Journal of Cardiology*, **72**, 154–61.

Patrick, D. and Erickson, P. (1993). *Health status and health policy: quality of life in health care evaluation and resource allocation*. Oxford University Press, New York.

Patrick, D., Bush, J., and Chen, M. (1973). Methods for measuring levels of well-being for a health status index. *Health Services Research*, **8**, 228–45.

Patrick, D., Starks, H., Cain, K., Uhlmann, R., and Pearlman, R. (1994). Measuring preferences for health states worse than death. *Medical Decision Making*, **14**, 9–18.

Raiffa, H. (1968). Decision analysis: introductory lectures on choices under uncertainty. Addison-Wesley, Reading, Massachusetts.

Raynauld, J.-P., Torrance, G. W., Band, P. A., *et al.* (2001). A prospective, randomised, pragmatic, health outcomes trial evaluating the incorporation of hylan G-F 20 into the treatment paradigm for patients with knee osteoarthritis (Part 1 of 2): clinical results. *Osteoarthritis and Cartilage*, **10**, 506–17.

Read, J., Quinn, R., Berwick, D., Fineberg, H., and Weinstein, M. (1984). Preferences for health outcomes—Comparisons of assessment methods. *Medical Decision Making*, **4**, 315–29.

Robinson, A., Loomes, G., and Jones-Lee, M. (2001). Visual analogue scales, standard gambles and relative risk aversion. *Medical Decision Making*, **21**, 17–27.

Ross, P. L., Littenberg, B., Fearn, P., Scardino, P. T., Karakiewicz, P. I., and Kattan, M. W. (2003). Paper standard gamble: a paper-based measure of standard gamble utility for current health. *International Journal of Technology Assessment in Health Care*, **19**, 135–47.

Rosser, R. and Kind, P. (1978). A scale of valuations of states of illness: is there a social consensus. *International Journal of Epidemiology*, **7**, 347–58.

Rosser, R. and Watts, V. (1978). The measurement of illness. *Journal of Operational Research Society*, **29**, 529–40.

Russell, R. and Wilkinson, M. (1979). *Microeconomics: a synthesis of modern and neoclassical theory*. Wiley, New York.

Rutten-van Molken, M. P. M. H., Bakker, C. H., van Doorslaer, E. K. A., and van der Linden, S. (1995). Methodological issues of patient utility measurement: experience from two clinical trials. *Medical Care*, **33**, 922–37.

Sackett, D. and Torrance, G. (1978). The utility of different health states as perceived by the general public. *Journal of Chronic Diseases*, **31**, 697–704.

Schoemaker, P. (1991). Choices involving uncertain probabilities—tests of generalized utility models. *Journal of Economic Behavior and Organization*, **16**, 295–317.

Schoemaker, P. (1992). Subjective expected utility theory revisited: a *reductio ad absurdum* paradox. *Theory and Decision*, **33**, 1–21.

Sen, A. (1991). Utility: ideas and terminology. *Economics and Philosophy*, **7**, 277–83.

Sinclair, J., Torrance, G., Boyle, M., Horwood, S., Saigal, S., and Sackett, D. (1981). Evaluation of neonatal intensive care programs. *New England Journal of Medicine*, **305**, 489–94.

Sintonen, H. (2001). The 15D instrument of health-related quality of life: properties and applications. *Annals of Medicine*, **33**, 328–36.

Spiegelhalter, D., Gore, S., Fitzpatrick, R., Fletcher, A., Jones, D., and Cox, D. (1992). Quality-of-life measures in health care. III: Resource allocation. *British Medical Journal*, **305**, 1205–9.

Spilker, B. (1996). *Quality of life and pharmacoeconomics in clinical trials* (2nd edn). Lippincott–Raven, Philadelphia.

Stiggelbout, A., Kiebert, G., Kievit, J., Leer, J., Stoter, G., and de Haes, J. (1994). Utility assessment in cancer patients: adjustment of time tradeoff scores for the utility of life years and comparison with standard gamble scores. *Medical Decision Making*, **14**, 82–90.

Streiner, D. L. and Norman, G. R. (1989). *Health measurement scales: a practical guide to their development and use*. Oxford University Press, Oxford.

Tan-Torres Edejer, T., Baltussen, R., *et al.* (2003). *Making choices in health: WHO guide to cost-effectiveness analysis*. Geneva, World Health Organization.

Torrance, G. W. (1971). *A generalized cost-effectiveness model for the evaluation of health programs* (doctoral dissertation). State University of New York at Buffalo, Buffalo.

Torrance, G. W. (1976a). Social preferences for health states: An empirical evaluation of three measurement techniques. *Socio-Economic Planning Sciences*, **10**, 129–36.

Torrance, G. W. (1976b). Health status index models: A unified mathematical view. *Management Science*, **22**, 990–1001.

Torrance, G. W. (1984). Health states worse than death. In: *Proceedings of Third International Conference on Systems Science in Health Care* (ed. W. V. Eimeren, R. Engel-brecht, and C. D. Flagle), pp. 1085–9. Springer, Berlin.

Torrance, G. W. (1986). Measurement of health-state utilities for economic appraisal: a review. *Journal of Health Economics*, **5**, 1–30.

Torrance, G. W. (1996). Designing and conducting cost–utility analyses. In: *Quality of life and pharmacoeconomics in Clinical Trials: Second Edition* (ed. B. Spilker), pp. 1105–11. Lippincott-Raven, Philadelphia.

Torrance, G. W. and Feeny, D. (1989). Utilities and quality-adjusted life years. *International Journal of Technology Assessment in Health Care*, **5**, 559–75.

Torrance, G. W., Thomas, W., and Sackett, D. (1972). A utility maximization model for evaluation of health care programs. *Health Services Research*, **7**, 118–33.

Torrance, G. W., Boyle, M. H., and Horwood, S. P. (1982). Application of multi-attribute utility theory to measure social preferences for health states. *Operations Research*, **30**, 1043–9.

Torrance, G. W., Furlong, W. J., Feeny, D. H., and Boyle, M. (1995). Multi-attribute preference functions: health utilities index. *PharmacoEconomics*, **7**, 503–20.

Torrance, G. W., Feeny, D. H., Furlong, W. J., Barr, R. D., Zhang, Y., and Wang, Q. (1996a). Multi-attribute utility function for a comprehensive health status classification system: health utilities index mark 2. *Medical Care*, **34**, 702–22.

Torrance, G. W., Blaker, D., Detsky, *et al.* (1996b). Canadian guidelines for economic evaluation of pharmaceuticals. *PharmacoEconomics*, **9**, 535–59.

Torrance, G. W., Feeny, D., and Furlong, W. (2001*a*). Visual analog scales: do they have a role in the measurement of preferences for health states? *Medical Decision Making*, **21**, 329–34.

Torrance, G. W., Raynauld, J. P., Walker, V., *et al.* (2001*b*). A prospective, randomised, pragmatic, health outcomes trial evaluating the incorporation of hylan G-F 20 into the treatment paradigm for patients with knee osteoarthritis (Part 2 of 2): economic results. *Osteoarthritis and Cartilage*, **10**, 518–27.

Torrance, G. W., Furlong, W., and Feeny, D. (2002). Health utility estimation. *Expert Review of Pharmacoeconomics and Outcomes Research*, **2**, 99–108.

Torrance, G. W., Keresteci, M. A., Casey, *et al.* (2004). Development and initial validation of a new preference-based disease-specific health-related quality of life instrument for erectile function. *Quality of Life Research*, **13**, 349–59.

Tversky, A. and Kahneman, D. (1992). Advances in prospect theory: cumulative representation of uncertainty. *Journal of Risk and Uncertainty*, **5**, 297–323.

Ubel, P. A., Loewenstein, G., Scanlon, D., and Kamlet, M. (1996). Individual utilities are inconsistent with rationing choices: a partial explanation of why Oregon's cost-effectiveness list failed. *Medical Decision Making*, **16**, 108–16.

von Neumann, J. and Morgenstern, O. (1944). *Theory of games and economic behaviour*. Princeton University Press, Princeton, New Jersey.

Wakker, P. (1996). A criticism of healthy years equivalents. *Medical Decision Making*, **16**, 207–14.

Wakker, P., Erev, I., and Weber, E. (1994). Comonotonic independence: the critical test between classical and rank-dependent utility theories. *Journal of Risk and Uncertainty*, **9**, 195–230.

Wang, Q., Furlong, W., Feeny, D., Torrance, G., and Barr, R. (2002). How robust is the Health Utilities Index Mark 2 utility function? *Medical Decision Making*, **22**, 350–8.

Weinstein, M. and Fineberg, H. C. (1980). *Clinical decision analysis*. Saunders, Philadelphia.

Weinstein, M. and Pliskin, J. (1996). Perspectives on healthy years equivalents (HYEs): What are the issues? *Medical Decision Making*, **16**, 205–6.

Weinstein, M. and Stason, W. (1977). Foundations of cost-effectiveness analysis for health and medical practices. *New England Journal of Medicine*, **296**, 716–21.

Williams, A. (1988). Ethics and efficiency in the provision of health care. In: *Philosophy and Medical Welfare* (ed. M. Bell and S. Mendux), pp. 111–26. Cambridge University Press, Cambridge.

Williams, A. (1995). Economics, QALYs and medical ethics—A health economist's perspective. *Health Care Analysis: Journal of Health Philosophy and Policy*, **3**, 221–6.

Wolfson, A. D., Sinclair, A. J., Bombardier, C., and McGeer, A. (1982). Preference measurements for functional status in stroke patients: inter-rater and inter-technique comparisons. In: *Values and long term care* (ed. R. Kane and R. Kane), pp. 191–214. D.C. Heath, Lexington.

Annex 6.1. **Simulated interview**

The following example and exercise is provided to give some feeling for how the main preference measurement instruments described in Sections 6.3.1, 6.3.2, and 6.3.3 are actually used in practice. This example is unchanged from the first edition of the book. The example is still valid, but note that now it is considered better technique to use a converging ping-pong strategy for changing the probabilities offered in the standard gamble, or the times offered in the time trade-off (Furlong *et al.* 1990). In addition, we now recommend that if a visual analogue scale (feeling thermometer) instrument is used, it should precede the standard gamble or time trade-off.

Consider the following simulated interview between an interviewer (I) and a subject (S) to measure the preference scores for three chronic health states (A, B, C) and three temporary states (D, E, F). The preference scale is the conventional one anchored by dead = 0 and healthy = 1. In this example each state is measured three times, by three different techniques: standard gamble, time trade-off, and category scaling. The task is to determine the 18 preference scores (six states, three techniques) (answers in Table 6.12).

Hint: In the standard gamble and the time trade-off methods you must determine the subject's 'indifference point'. This is the point at which the subject is indifferent between (cannot decide between) choice 1 and choice 2. If the subject switches their choice on two adjacent questions, the indifference point is taken to be halfway between. If the subject expresses indifference on a particular question, that is taken as the indifference point.

Notation: I = Interviewer, S = Subject, A > B means A is preferred to B.

1. **Chronic health states**
    I: Thank you for agreeing to participate. On each of these three sheets is a description of a chronic condition. Each sheet is labelled A, B, or C. (*Note to reader*: the conditions can be quite disparate, like kidney dialysis, blind, mental retardation.) Please imagine that you will have to spend the rest of your life in one of these conditions. Rank the conditions in order of preference, and relative to 'healthy' and 'dead'. That is, if any of the conditions are better than being healthy or worse than being dead, please indicate.
    S: Alright, healthy > A > B > C > dead.
    I: Good. Now I have a device here called a probability wheel (see Torrance 1976*a*, p. 131; Torrance 1986, p. 20). The wheel is divided into two sectors; a blue sector and a yellow sector. First let us adjust the wheel so it is half blue and half yellow. Now consider the following choices; which do you prefer, choice 1 or choice 2? In choice 1 you get chronic condition C for the rest of your life. In choice 2 you get either 2a or 2b described below depending on the outcome of the spin of this pointer on the wheel. That is, if you choose 2, I am going to spin this pointer on the wheel and if it stops on blue you get 2a but if it stops on yellow you get 2b. 2a is healthy for the rest of your life, 2b is immediate death. Now which do you choose, 1 or 2?
    S: Well C is pretty bad, I think I'd take my chances and select choice 2.
    I: Alright. Now I am going to adjust the wheel so it is only 40% blue and 60% yellow. Now the pointer has a greater chance of stopping on yellow in which case you get 2b, immediate death. Would you still select choice 2?
    S: Yes.
    I: OK, now I'll adjust the wheel again so it is 30% blue, 70% yellow. Would you still select choice 2?
    S: No, I don't think so. That's too risky now, I'd take choice 1.
    I: OK, that's the end of that one, thank you. Now, imagine a new situation. Here you again have two choices, and I want to know which you prefer. Choice 1 is

condition B for the rest of your life. Choice 2 is the same as before. Let's reset the wheel to 50% blue and 50% yellow. Now, which choice do you prefer?

S: I think I'd take choice 1.

I: OK, now I'll adjust the wheel to 60% blue, 40% yellow. Now, how do you feel about the choices?

S: Oh, that makes choice 2 more attractive. I think I'll switch to it.

I: Fine, thank you. Now we have another new situation. This time choice 1 is condition A for the rest of your life. Choice 2 is the same as before. Let's reset the wheel to 50/50, now which do you prefer?

S: Choice 1 definitely.

I: OK, now I'll adjust the wheel to 60% blue, 40% yellow. Now what do you think?

S: Still choice 1.

I: OK, let's move the wheel to 70% blue, and 30% yellow.

S: Still choice 1.

I: OK, let's move the wheel to 80% blue, 20% yellow.

S: Now, that makes it difficult to decide. I think choice 1 and choice 2 now seem about the same to me. I really don't much care which I get.

I: OK, fine thank you. Now I have a new type of question for you. Given your age, your remaining life expectancy is another 40 years. I am going to give you some choices and ask you which you prefer. Choice 1 is to live your remaining 40 years in condition C. Choice 2 is to live a shorter time, but healthy. For example, let's say in choice 2 you get to live only 20 more years, but healthy. Which would you take, choice 1 or choice 2?

S: I'd say choice 2, because C is really pretty bad.

I: OK, what if choice 2 was only 15 years, but still healthy.

S: Oh, that's getting pretty tough, but I think I'd still take choice 2.

I: OK, what if choice 2 is only 14 years?

S: That's about my limit. Any less than 14 years I'll switch to choice 1. Fourteen years is right on the knife edge, I could go either way.

I: OK, fine thank you. Now a new situation. Choice 1 is condition B for your remaining 40 years. In choice 2 you will have only 20 years to live, but they will be healthy years.

S: Well that's pretty hard to choose. I think those two choices are about the same.

I: Fine. Now for the last situation concerning these chronic states. Choice 1 is condition A for your remaining 40 years. In choice 2 your will have only 20 years to live but they will be healthy years.

S: Well, I think this time I would take choice 1.

I: OK, let's make choice 2, 25 years, all healthy.

S: I'd still take choice 1.

I: OK, let's make choice 2, 30 years, all healthy.

S: I'd still take choice 1.

I: OK, let's make choice 2, 35 years, all healthy.

S: OK, this time I would take choice 2.

I: Fine, thank you. Now for the last type of question relating to these health states, I have here a device we call a 'feeling thermometer' (see Torrance 1982, p. 40). As you can see it is a thermometer-shaped 0–100 scale on a felt board, with 0 labelled 'least desirable' and 100 labelled 'most desirable'. I also have these five narrow foam sticks pointed at each end labelled respectively healthy, dead, A, B, and C. I want you to select the foam stick that represents the most desirable way to spend the rest of your life and place it on the felt board beside the thermometer at 100. Similarly, please select the least desirable and place it at 0. Now place the other sticks somewhere between the top and the bottom of the thermometer depending on how you feel about spending the rest of your life in each condition. If you feel the same about two sticks just put them on top of each other. The distance between the sticks should all be relative to each other. For example, if you feel that the difference in desirability between healthy and A is twice as great as the difference between A and B, the spacing between the sticks healthy and A should be adjusted to be twice that between A and B.

S: OK, I think that's it.

I: Thinking it over, are there any changes you would like to make?

S: No, I think not.

I: Fine, now please read out the sticks and the thermometer values they are beside.

S: OK, Healthy 100, A 80, B 52, C 35, Dead 0.

I: Fine, thank you very much, that completes this phase of the interview.

2. Temporary health states

I: Here are three different sheets. Each sheet describes a temporary dysfunctional health condition, which you would have for 3 months. At the end of the 3 months you will be completely recovered. Each sheet is labelled D, E, or F. (*Note to reader*: The conditions can be quite disparate like mononucleosis for 3 months, hospital confinement with kidney dialysis for 3 months for the treatment of temporary kidney failure, clinical depression for 3 months.) Imagine that you will have to spend the next 3 months in one of these conditions. Please rank them in order of preference.

S: OK, I'd say D > E > F.

I: Good, now I'm going to get out the probability wheel and give you some choices again. For this first situation imagine that, unfortunately, you have only 3 months to live. Choice 1 is to spend these 3 months in condition F. In choice 2 you get either 2a or 2b depending on the spin of the pointer on the wheel; blue gives you 2a, yellow 2b. 2a is healthy for the 3 months, 2b is immediate death. With the wheel at 50% blue, 50% yellow, which would you choose?

S: F is pretty bad, I'll take choice 2.

I: OK, 40% blue, 60% yellow.

S: That's about my indifference point. Any less blue and I'll switch for sure.

I: Fine, now here's a completely new situation, that fortunately does not involve dying. This time you will always completely recover at the end of the 3 months. Choice 1 is condition E for the 3 months. Choice 2 is either 2a (if blue) or 2b (if yellow) depending on the outcome of the spin. 2a is immediate cure, 2b condition F for 3 months. With the wheel at 50% blue, 50% yellow which would you choose?

S: Choice 1.

I: OK, 60% blue, 40% yellow.

S: Choice 2.

I: Good, thanks. Now for a similar question. Choice 1 is condition D for 3 months followed by cure. Choice 2 is a spin leading to 2a (blue), immediate cure and 2b (yellow), condition E for 3 months followed by cure. With the wheel at 50/50 which would you choose?

S: Choice 2.

I: OK, 40% blue, 60% yellow?

S: Still choice 2.

I: OK, 30% blue, 70% yellow?

S: OK, now I'll switch to choice 1.

I: Good, thanks. That completes the probability wheel questions. Now, here's a new question. Unfortunately, in this question we must again assume you have only 3 months to live. Choice 1 is to spend this last 12 weeks in condition F. In choice 2 you live for a shorter period of time, but healthy. Let's say 6 weeks.

S: I'd take Choice 2.

I: OK, what if it was only 5 weeks?

S: That's about my indifference point.

I: Good, now we'll change the situation so you no longer die. Now, you will be completely cured at the end of the temporary condition. Which would you prefer: choice 1, 12 weeks of E; choice 2, 6 weeks of F?

S: Choice 1.

I: OK, what if choice 2 is only 5 weeks?

S: OK, now I'd take choice 2.

I: Good, now for the last situation. Again the choices are followed by complete cure. Choice 1, 12 weeks of D, choice 2, 6 weeks of E.

S: Choice 2.

I: OK, what if choice 2 is 7 weeks?

S: I'd still take it.

I: What if it is 8 weeks?

S: Now I can't tell. That's my indifference point. Any longer than that and I'd switch to choice 1.

I: Good, that completes these questions. Now we just have the feeling thermometer to do again and then we're finished. This time the five sticks are labelled healthy, dead, D, E, and F. Furthermore, this time we must assume that you have only 3 months to live. Please place the five sticks on the feeling thermometer following the same instructions as the last time. When you're ready please read them out to me.

S: OK, here they come: Healthy 100, D 81, E 75, F 41, Dead 0.

I: OK, terrific. That completes the interview. Thank you very much. You have been very helpful.

Table 6.12 Calculation of health state preference scores from the simulated interview

	Standard gamble	Time trade-off	Rating scale (thermometer)
Chronic states (lifetime)			
Healthy	1.00	1.00	1.00
A	0.80	0.81	0.80
B	0.55	0.50	0.52
C	0.35	0.35	0.35
Dead	0.00	0.00	0.00
Temporary states (3 months)			
Healthy	1.00	1.00	1.00
D	0.82	0.82	0.81
E	0.73	0.73	0.75
F	0.40	0.42	0.41
Dead	0.00	0.00	0.00

Calculations

$C = 14/40 = 0.35$
$B = 20/40 = 0.50$
$A = 32.5/40 = 0.81$

$F = 0.40$
$E = 0.55 \times 1.00 + 0.45 \times 0.40 = 0.73$
$D = 0.35 \times 1.00 + 0.65 \times 0.73 = 0.82$

$F = 5/12 = 0.42$
$E = 1 - (1 - 0.42)(5.5/12) = 0.73$
$D = 1 - (1 - 0.73)(8/12) = 0.82$

Chapter 7

Cost–benefit analysis

7.1. Some basics

The feature that distinguishes among techniques of economic evaluation is the way in which the consequences of health care programmes are valued. Cost–benefit analysis (CBA) requires programme consequences to be valued in monetary units, thus enabling the analyst to make a direct comparison of the programme's incremental cost with its incremental consequences in commensurate units of measurement, be they dollars, pounds, or yen. In this chapter we briefly examine the theoretical underpinnings of CBA and clarify the ways in which CBA differs from cost-effectiveness analysis (CEA) and cost–utility analysis (CUA). Recent texts giving more detailed exposition of the theory and practice of CBA in health care include Johansson (1995) and Johannesson (1996a). Perhaps not surprisingly, the major portion of this chapter is given over to measurement issues concerning how consequences of health care programmes can be valued in terms of money. We trace a brief history of money valuation for health outcomes and lay out the advantages and disadvantages, conceptual and practical, of different approaches.

7.1.1. Cost–benefit analysis: an approach or an analysis?

In casual conversation it might be reasonable to refer to all the evaluation techniques in this book as being 'cost–benefit analysis'. Indeed, in an influential early article, Williams (1974) used the phrase the 'cost–benefit approach' as a generic description of the way of thinking that economics brings to health care evaluation, where the problem is framed in terms of a production relationship between resource inputs and health outputs. But in defining CBA as a specific technique of evaluation we need to be much more precise with the use of language. As shown in Box 7.1, CBA compares the discounted future streams of incremental programme benefits with incremental programme costs; the difference between these two streams being the net social benefit of the programme. In simple terms, the goal of analysis is to identify whether a programme's benefits exceed its costs, a positive net social benefit indicating that a programme is worthwhile. Although, as we will discuss below, the precise decision rule for CBA will depend upon the context of the evaluation and specifically if one is allocating resources within a fixed budget or not (Pauly 1995). An alternative formulation considers whether the ratio of benefit to cost is greater than unity, although this formulation is generally regarded as problematic because the location of items in numerator or denominator can easily change the ratio (see Birch and Donaldson 1987 and Box 2.4).

Box 7.1 **Cost–benefit analysis: a formulation in search of data**

Given $i = 1, \ldots I$ possible investments

$$\text{NSB}_i = \sum_{t=1}^{n} \frac{b_i(t) - c_i(t)}{(1 + r)^{t-1}}$$

NSB_i = net social benefit of project i (discounted)

$b_i(t)$ = benefits (in money terms) derived in year t

$c_i(t)$ = costs (in money terms) in year t

$1/(1 + r)$ = discount factor at annual interest rate r

n = lifetime of project

The primary goal of CBA is to identify projects where NSB >0. It will also be useful, for allocation within a fixed budget, to rank projects according to their NSB. The major issue for health care CBA is the valuation of health outcomes in money $b_i(t)$.

Cost–benefit analysis is a form of full economic evaluation because programme outputs must be measured and valued. However, there is significant mislabelling of studies in the health care literature with studies that compare only programme costs (that is, partial evaluation) using the term 'cost–benefit analysis'. In a literature review, Zarnke *et al.* (1997) found that 60% of studies claiming to be CBA were actually cost comparisons where no attempt had been made to value benefits in monetary terms. As illustrated in Box 7.2, such restricted cost comparison formulations of CBA can be misleading for resource allocation because only programmes that generate cost savings would be seen as worthwhile.

7.1.2. **The cost–benefit analysis question: is the programme worthwhile?**

As we have seen in previous chapters, CEA and CUA are well suited to the task of allocating a fixed budget to competing programmes so as to maximize the selected effectiveness measure (for example, life-years saved, quality-adjusted life-years (QALYs) gained, healthy-years equivalents (HYEs) gained). However, to do so requires both complete and comparable data on all alternatives and requires a formal periodic budget allocation process during which all programmes are assessed simultaneously—both of these requirements seldom exist in health care. More commonly, programmes are discussed one at a time, or a few at a time, and decisions are required without the luxury of complete data on all alternatives. Arguably, in this one-at-a-time decision-making, CBA has an advantage over CEA/CUA.

Given the difficulties in attaching money values to health outcomes, which we describe below, it is useful to outline some of the key differences between CBA and the

Box 7.2 **Cost comparisons labelled as cost–benefit analysis: pertussis vaccination**

In this study by Koplan *et al.* (1979), of pertussis vaccination, costs were measured as the resource cost of the vaccine, the treatment of complications resulting from the vaccine, and the treatment of cases of pertussis that resulted despite being vaccinated. These were called the costs with the programme. Benefits were defined as the savings in medical care costs by preventing pertussis and its sequelae. These were called the costs without the programme. The authors computed the following ratio:

$$\frac{\text{costs without programme}}{\text{cost with programme}} = \frac{\$1\,866\,153}{\$720\,862} = 2.6 : 1$$

This means that the benefits outweighed the costs incurred by 2.6 times. But this formulation does not meet a contemporary definition of CBA because no attempt was made to value, in money terms, the health consequences of the vaccination programme. Benefits have only been defined as cost savings. Consider what would happen if the above ratio had been less than 1, that is, the programme is cost increasing but it provided health benefits. Using this type of partial evaluation we would only implement programmes that were cost saving.

techniques of CEA and CUA. As we have seen, in non-dominance circumstances where the new programme produces better outcomes at additional costs, both CEA and CUA tell us the price of achieving a particular goal whether it is the incremental cost of a life-year gained, a case of disease detected, or a QALY gained. What CEA/CUA cannot tell us, is whether such a goal is *worth* achieving given the social opportunity costs of all the resources consumed. Hence, to *make decisions* using CEA/CUA we must invoke some external criterion of value, either through the use of implied values from cost per QALY league tables, the opportunity cost associated with a specific budget constraint, or published threshold values, which are often arbitrary (see Chapter 10). Ultimately, although both CEA and CUA avoid money valuation of health outcomes *as part of the analysis*, to make any resource allocation decision using CEA/CUA data a decision-maker (implicitly or explicitly) must place a money value on the health outcomes and any other programme benefits. Ideally the decision-maker should know the social opportunity costs (that is, forgone benefits to society) of the programme that would be displaced.

The fact that both CEA/CUA and CBA ultimately require money valuation of health outcomes has led some authors (Phelps and Mushlin 1991) to argue that the techniques are nearly equivalent. However, there is a fundamental philosophical difference. Following Sugden and Williams (1979), CEA/CUA is based on a 'decision-making' philosophy where elected or appointed decision-makers review results and decide on the relative values assigned to competing programmes and goals. In contrast, the philosophical foundation of CBA is in principles of welfare economics where the relevant source of values is believed to be individual consumers. A basic tenet of CBA therefore is that individual consumers are deemed to be the relevant source of monetary values for programme outcomes. This issue is explored further in Chapter 10.

7.1.3. Cost–benefit analysis has broader scope than cost-effectiveness analysis/cost–utility analysis

In many respects CBA is broader in scope than CEA/CUA. Because CBA converts all costs and benefits to money it is not restricted to comparing programmes within health care but can be used (although not without problems) to inform resource allocation decisions both within and between sectors of the economy (Drummond and Stoddart 1995). Some analysts have attempted to use willingness-to-pay (WTP) to compare health and non-health programmes (Olsen and Donaldson 1997). Indeed, in public sector economic evaluation in areas such as transport and environment, the application of CBA has a long history (Sugden and Williams 1979) and is the most widely used form of economic evaluation. In contrast CEA/CUA is necessarily restricted to the comparison of health care programmes that produce similar units of outcome such as QALYs. Cost-effectiveness analysis/cost–utility analysis address mainly questions of *production efficiency* with outcomes restricted to health benefits. In contrast, CBA is broader in scope and able to inform questions of *allocative efficiency*, because it assigns relative values to health and non-health related goals to determine which goals are worth achieving, given the alternative uses of resources, and thereby determining which programmes are worthwhile.

Some researchers have attempted to quantify some of the non-health benefits that consumers derive from health care programmes such as 'reassurance value' arising from knowledge of a test or procedure. This source of value has been called 'process utility' (as distinct from the utility of health outcomes) by Donaldson and Shackley (1997) and an application to quantify the monetary value of reassurance and information can be found in Donaldson et al. (1995) and Donaldson et al. (1997a). The analysis of WTP by pregnant women for additional (non-diagnostic) ultrasound could also be framed in this way (Berwick and Weinstein 1985). Another perspective on this point, however, is that if a person exhibits anxiety because they are not reassured in the process of care, then such anxiety could be measured as impairment of their psychological well-being and hence be a measurable component of health-related quality of life or utility.

Another contrasting feature of CEA/CUA and CBA is that the former techniques are typically more narrowly client focused. For example, in a clinical evaluation the focus of a CEA would typically be the expected health outcome for the patients treated. As argued by Labelle and Hurley (1992), the standard CEA/CUA framework does not usually capture effects that spill over to other persons—which can be positive or negative—known as externalities in economics. (In theory, it is possible to capture such effects in CEA/CUA, but in practice, this is rarely done. In one such example, Ades et al. (1999) considered the health outcomes for both mother and infant in an evaluation of ante-natal HIV screening. In addition, there are some studies that consider caregivers' utility, but only as part of an evaluation of services for caregivers, as opposed to the patients themselves (Drummond *et al.* 1991). Also, in a study primarily designed to explore the differences between preference-based instruments, Neumann *et al.* (2000) report health state preference values for both Alzheimer's disease patients and their carers.)

In contrast, as will be discussed later, using techniques of WTP the CBA framework can quantify a broad range of effects. For example, the total societal willingness-to-pay for a new AIDS drug is the sum of the value accruing directly to the patients but also the value that others (current non-patients) attach to the new treatments. However, in a review of the literature, Olsen and Smith (2001) suggest that in many respects WTP studies in health care fail to live up to this image in practice. Out of 71 studies, only 17 described the health outcomes in terms of more than one health dimension, although studies with a deliberate focus on attributes beyond health outcomes offered a more comprehensive and understandable description of these benefits. They conclude that a separate scenario description prior to the valuation exercise is required, and furthermore that the preferences be elicited by face-to-face interviewing.

7.2. Assigning money values to health outcomes

There are three general approaches to the monetary valuation of health outcomes: (1) human capital, (2) revealed preferences, and (3) stated preferences of WTP (known as *contingent valuation*). We discuss each of these approaches and review both theoretical and practical strengths and weaknesses. As illustrated by the quotations in Box 7.3, the whole topic of attempting to assign money values to health outcomes explicitly as part of CBA has been, and remains, controversial. What is often overlooked, however, is that such valuations occur—often implicitly—every day when decisions are made by both individuals and societies that trade-off health objectives against other benefits.

7.2.1. The human capital approach

The utilization of a health care programme can be viewed as an investment in a person's human capital. In measuring the pay-back on this investment the value of the

---

Box 7.3 **The rhetoric of assigning money values to health**

'The major disadvantage of the benefit–cost framework is the requirement that human lives and quality of life be valued in monetary units. Many decision-makers find this difficult or unethical or do not trust analyses that depend upon such valuations.' (Weinstein and Fineberg 1980, p. 240)

'To be trained in medicine, nursing or one of the other "sharp end" disciplines and then be faced with some hard-nosed, cold-blooded economist placing money values on human life and suffering is anathema to many.' (Mooney 1992)

'Cost–benefit analysis's primary valuation method is *willingness-to-pay* (WTP), an approach whose difficulty lies in its intrinsic favoring of programs and diseases of the affluent over those of the poor.' (Gold *et al.* 1996)

healthy time produced can be quantified in terms of the person's renewed or increased production in the market-place. Hence the human capital method places monetary weights on healthy time using market wage rates and the value of the programme is assessed in terms of the present value of future earnings. This human capital method of valuing health status has been used for many years (for an early application see Mushkin 1978). We can distinguish between two uses of the human capital concept: (1) as the *sole* basis for valuing all aspects of health improvements, and (2) as a method of valuing *part* of the benefits of health care interventions, using earnings data as a means of valuing productivity changes only. For an illustration of the human capital approach to health care CBA, consider the rubella vaccination example in Box 7.4.

There are a number of measurement difficulties with the human capital approach. First, although in theory wage rates reflect the marginal productivity of a worker there are often imperfections in labour markets and wage rates may reflect, *inter alia*, inequities such as discrimination by race or gender. Second, if the study is from a societal perspective the analyst would need to consider the value of healthy time gained that is not sold for a wage. This raises a general class of problems of how economists place shadow prices on non-marketed resources. For example, suppose a homemaker receives some treatment and is now able to return to their duties looking after the children, whereas previously they could not. There are two methods for attaching a shadow price to this time. (1) An *opportunity cost of time* argument would be that the value of this production in the home must be *at least* as great as what could be earned in the labour market, otherwise the homemaker would choose to enter the labour market. Hence, the time would be valued according to the wage rate forgone. (2) A *replacement cost* approach would attempt to quantify how much it would cost to replace the homemaker in the home with services from the market (for example, cleaning, child minding, and so on). Both of these approaches have been used to value homemakers' time in studies; see Klarman *et al.* (1968) for the opportunity cost and Weisbrod (1964) for the replacement cost approaches.

Box 7.4 **Cost–benefit analysis using human capital method: rubella vaccination**

This study examined the costs and consequences of providing rubella vaccination. The consequences were conceptualized as those costs that would be avoided with the vaccination programme. Consequences included not only the averted medical costs associated with acute rubella and congenital rubella syndrome, but also the reduced economic productivity that results from a disability or premature death. In order to place a monetary value on reduced productivity, the authors computed average lifetime earnings and estimated the amount of earnings that would be lost if no rubella vaccination programme were in effect. They found that the costs of the programme totalled $28 937 400 and the value of lost productivity totalled $9 521 200 for both medical conditions (Schoenbaum *et al.* 1976).

7.2.2. **Human capital and welfare economics**

In addition to some of the practical measurement problems of using the human capital approach, it came under attack in the 1970s by economists who argued that this production-based method for valuing health improvements was not consistent with the theoretical foundation of CBA from welfare economics. The most notable contribution to this debate was by Mishan (1971).

Although this book is intended for a practical audience of persons who wish to use economic evaluation, it is useful to spend a few sentences explaining some of the welfare economics underpinnings of CBA (for a more detailed conceptual approach, see Johansson 1995). First, welfare economics is a branch of economics that can address *normative* questions because it embodies certain value judgements. In contrast, most of economics is *positive* because it makes predictions without value judgements (for example, raising the price of a product *will* reduce its demand). What do we mean by a value judgement in this context? Examine Box 7.5 for the two key value judgements of welfare economics. The proposition (and judgement) is that social welfare *should* comprise individuals' welfare and that individuals *should* be considered the best source of information on their own welfare. Further, it is assumed that resource allocation is proceeding by the forces of a competitive market that is in equilibrium and that current (that is, pre-programme) income distribution is appropriate. These

---

Box 7.5 **Pareto principles in brief**

Vilfredo Pareto was a nineteenth-century sociologist who is best known for his thoughts on the general principles of economic policy evaluation. He worked in the efficiency tradition of utilitarianism with its focus on the 'greatest good of the greatest number', with less attention to distributional or equity issues. The general question he sought to answer was 'How would we judge whether society as a whole was better off from a policy or programme?'

Key assumptions

1 Social welfare is made up from the welfare (or utilities) of each individual member of society.

2 Individuals are the best judges of their own welfare (consumer sovereignty).

Principles

1 *Actual Pareto improvement.* A policy that makes one or more persons better off and makes no person any worse off.

2 *Potential Pareto improvement.* (Kaldor–Hicks criterion.) A policy that creates gainers and losers in welfare, but if the gainers *could* compensate the losers and remain better off themselves after the change, then society as a whole has benefited. Because compensation does not actually have to be paid, this principle raises some equity issues about who gains and who loses.

propositions form the foundation for the Pareto principles in Box 7.5, which are central to CBA. Specifically, it is the contemporary reinterpretation of the Pareto principles by British economists Nicholas Kaldor (Kaldor 1939) and Sir John Hicks (Hicks 1939, 1941) that forms the basis for CBA to be operationalized, with programme benefits being valued using a compensation test and the principles of WTP.

Returning to the critique of the human capital approach, Mishan (1971) pointed out that the valuation method was not consistent with the principles of welfare economics (see Box 7.5) because it offers a narrow view of the utility consequences of a project restricted to impacts on labour productivity. The more fundamental and relevant notion of value embedded in welfare economics is what consumers who gain from the programme are willing to *sacrifice* to have the programme in question. It is this collective willingness-to-pay (that is, willingness to sacrifice other goods and services) that is the focus of CBA, recognizing that not all consumers will benefit and some may lose and require compensation. Mishan's contribution was to shift the focus of the debate and practical measurement toward contemplating what monetary compensation individuals required for reduced health, or how much they would be willing to pay for improved health.

Advocates of this Pareto school of compensation test were also quick to point out that study should focus on an individual's health–money decisions *under uncertainty* rather than certainty (Jones-Lee 1976). Under a certainty scenario a person might (quite reasonably) request infinite compensation for, say, loss of life, which would make CBA intractable. Rather, the argument was that valuations should be made on money versus health risk trade-offs. Based on this notion of valuing a so-called statistical life rather than an actual life, two types of enquiry emerged. The first was revealed preference studies looking at wage-risk trade-offs. The second was stated preference studies examining hypothetical scenarios and WTP. This second type of survey method has become known as contingent valuation.

7.2.3. Revealed preference studies

A number of wage–risk studies have been published, in which the goal is to examine the relationship between particular health risks associated with a hazardous job and wage rates that individuals require to accept the job (Marin and Psacharopoulos 1982). This approach is consistent with the welfare economics framework just discussed, because it is based on individual preferences regarding the value of increased (decreased) health risk, such as injury at work, as a trade-off against increased (decreased) income, which represents all other goods and services the person might consume. An example of the wage–risk approach is given in Box 7.6.

The strength of the wage–risk approach is that it is based on actual consumer choices involving health versus money, rather than hypothetical scenarios and preference statements. However, a weakness of the approach is that estimated values have varied widely and estimation seems to be very context and job specific. Using observed data there is always the problem of disentangling the many factors that will confound the relationship between wage and health risk. Furthermore, for use in a specific CBA of a treatment programme it is necessary to observe an occupational

Box 7.6 **Value of a statistical life**

Wage-risk example

'Suppose jobs A and B are identical except that workers in job A have higher annual fatal injury risks such that, on average, there is one more job-related death per year for every 10 000 workers in job A than in job B, and workers in job A earn $500 more per year than those in job B. The implied value of statistical life is then $5 million for workers in job B who are each willing to forgo $500 per year for a 1-in-10 000 lower annual risk.' (Fisher *et al.* 1989)

choice where the relevant health outcome is the focus of compensation or payment. A more fundamental concern is that the observed risk–money trade-offs may not reflect the kind of rational choice revealing preferences that economists believe, because of the many imperfections intervening in labour markets and limitations in how individuals perceive occupational risks. It is not possible to review comprehensively the volume of work that has been done in this area but the interested reader should consult Viscusi (1992) for a good review.

It is worth noting at this point that there is another valuation principle that might also be referred to as revealed preference but is not based on individual consumers. This approach is a review of past decisions, such as court awards for injury compensation, to elicit the minimum value that society (or its elected representatives) places on health outcomes (Mooney 1977). In practice, however, many such legal awards are actually based on human capital calculation of discounted earnings streams. Shifting the focus slightly, one might also be tempted to review previous government health care funding decisions as a source of revealed preference to determine dollar values assigned to health outcomes. But the danger here is one of circularity because we would use previous decisions in future analyses in the belief that some rational process had truthfully revealed societal values for health outcomes in the prior decision.

7.2.4. **Contingent valuation studies**

As the name suggests, contingent valuation studies use survey methods to present respondents with hypothetical scenarios about the programme or problem under evaluation. Respondents are required to think about the *contingency* of an actual market existing for a programme or health benefit and to reveal the *maximum* they would be willing to pay for such a programme or benefit. Why are we interested in the maximum WTP? Consider a simple consumer decision to buy a chocolate bar. A measure of how much the consumer values the chocolate bar is the maximum that they would be willing to pay. The difference between this value and the price they have to pay in the market is known as consumer surplus. Of course, for products like chocolate bars one does not need to hire high-priced economists to do a formal CBA; each consumer does this calculation in their own head. However, the logic carries over to contingent valuation studies for non-marketed goods such as a health care programme where we are trying to estimate value in relation to cost for purposes of collective funding. Hence in contingent valuation studies consumers are asked to consider what they would be willing to pay, and thereby sacrifice in terms of other commodities, for the programme benefits if they were in the market-place.

Here we take health programme benefits to be broadly defined; some may be improvements in health status while others may be attributes such as the value of being better informed about one's health or the value associated with the process of care (Donaldson and Shackley 1997). It is the aggregation of this consumer surplus—which can be large, small, positive, or negative—across individuals that forms the basis of the cost–benefit calculus. In many ways, therefore, CBA studies based on contingent valuation and statements of WTP can be thought of as attempts to replace missing markets, albeit hypothetically, in an attempt to measure underlying consumer demand and valuation for non-marketed social goods such as health care programmes.

Before reviewing the use of contingent valuation methods in health care it is important to recognize that the need to value health gains and losses for inclusion in CBA has arisen in other public sectors such as transport and environment. Indeed, much of the pioneering work on contingent valuation methods was undertaken in transport CBA by economists such as Jones-Lee (1976). An example of a contingent valuation question to estimate a money value for loss of life in the context of road safety is given in Box 7.7. As can be seen, an important advantage of this example is its realism, because it involves an easily understood choice that many people have faced—albeit with a little less precision on the risk of death! Hence in this example the contingency is not difficult to imagine because actual markets for cars do exist where price is related to safety features (for example, inclusion/exclusion of air bags). Indeed, with this example one can even compare stated preferences with revealed preferences from actual market data.

Another set of conceptual distinctions are shown in Box 7.8. Studies can use either the utility concept of compensating or equivalent variation and can ask questions of WTP or willingness-to-accept (WTA), depending upon whether a programme is being introduced or removed. For example, in Box 7.8 under the concept of compensating variation and for the introduction of a programme for an individual who gains from this programme, we would wish to find out the maximum amount that must be taken from the gainer to maintain them at the current (before-programme) level of utility. This would be the maximum they would be willing to pay for the project to go ahead. In contrast, equivalent variation for the same individual would be the minimum amount that must be paid to this *potential* gainer to forgo the gain and to make their utility equal to what it would have been after the change. Hence the equivalent variation is the minimum the individual would be willing to accept in compensation to forego the project. A more rigorous derivation and discussion of these concepts can be found in Johansson (1995), and this text also gives a discussion of the circumstances under which these concepts yield the same money values. Reviews of studies conducting money valuations of health programme benefits indicate that the majority of studies use WTP in the context of programme introduction and compensating variation (Diener *et al.* 1998).

> ## Box 7.7 **Value of a statistical life: road safety contingent valuation example**
>
> 'Suppose that you are buying a particular make of car. You can, if you want, choose to have a new kind of safety feature fitted to the car at an extra cost. The next few questions will ask about how much extra you would be prepared to pay for some different types of safety feature. You must bear in mind how much you personally can afford.
>
> As we said earlier, the risk of a car driver being killed in an accident is 10 in 100 000. You could choose to have a safety feature fitted to your car which would halve the risk of the car driver being killed, down to 5 in 100 000. Taking into account how much you can personally afford, what is the most that you would be prepared to pay to have this safety feature fitted to the car?' (Jones-Lee *et al.* 1985)
>
> ### Hypothetical example
>
> Current risk of death without safety feature = 10 in 100 00
>
> New risk with safety feature = 5 in 100 000
>
> Reduction in risk (dR) = 5 in 100 000
>
> Maximum (for example) premium willing to pay (dV) = £50
>
> Implied value of life = dV/dR
>
> $$= £50/5 \times 10^{-5}$$
>
> $$= £1 \text{ m}$$

7.2.5. **Contingent valuation studies in health care**

In recent years there has been rapid growth in the number of contingent valuation studies published in the health care literature. In Box 7.9 we give some examples of these studies and the diversity of clinical areas that have been studied, ranging from arthritis to depression to *in vitro* fertilization (IVF). (See Smith (2003) for a comprehensive list of studies published between 1985 and 2001.) It should be noted, however, that most of the published health care contingent valuation studies are experimental in nature, attempting to explore measurement feasibility issues rather than being full programme evaluations using CBA. This cautious embrace of contingent valuation is partly due to some of the inherent difficulties in measuring WTP and partly to some ongoing conceptual debates concerning what questions should be asked of whom in health care contingent valuation studies. To review and summarize some of these issues, the next section considers some of the theoretical and practical considerations that face the analyst seeking to design a contingent valuation study to value the benefits of a health care programme.

Box 7.8 Use of willingness-to-pay and willingness-to-accept questions in the contexts of compensating variation and equivalent variation

Temporal perspective and Programme status:		Does this consumer gain or lose in utility from before–after change?	Compensating variation (CV)	Equivalent variation (EV)
Before	After		$+/− required *after* the change to make utility same as before the change	$+/− required *before* the change to make utility the same as after the change
	Project A	Gain	A₁ WTP: maximum amount that must be taken from gainer to maintain at current (before) level of utility	A₃ WTA: minimum amount that must be paid to *potential* gainers to forgo the gain and make utility equal to what it would have been after the change
No programme	Programme	Loss	A₂ WTA: minimum amount that must be paid to loser to maintain at current (before) level of utility	A₄ WTP: maximum amount that must be taken from *potential* loser to forgo the loss and make utility level equal to what it would have been after the change
	Project B	Loss	B₁ WTA: minimum amount that must be paid to loser to maintain at current (before) level of utility	B₃ WTP: maximum amount that must be taken from *potential* loser to forgo the loss and make utility level equal to what it would have been after the change
Programme	No programme	Gain	B₂ WTP: maximum amount that must be taken from gainer to maintain at current (before) level of utility	B₄ WTA: minimum amount that must be paid to *potential* gainers to forgo the gain and make utility equal to what it would have been after the change

From O'Brien and Gafni (1996).

Box 7.9 **Health care contingent valuation studies**

Here are some examples of published contingent valuation studies in health care. Most of them are feasibility or pilot studies of WTP and not full CBA studies.

Thompson (1986)	New arthritis drug
Appel *et al.* (1990)	Non-ionic contrast media
Donaldson (1990)	Care of the elderly
Berwick and Weinstein (1985)	Ultrasound with pregnancy
Johannesson and Jönsson (1991)	Hypertension/cholesterol lowering
Neumann and Johannesson (1994)	*In vitro* fertilization
O'Brien and Viramontes (1994)	Chronic obstructive pulmonary disease
O'Brien *et al.* (1995)	New antidepressant drug
Ryan *et al.* (1997)	Ante-natal care
Wagner *et al.* (2000)	Mammography
Dalmau-Matarradona (2001)	Home care services in day case surgery
Shackley and Donaldson (2002)	Programmes for cancer, heart disease, and community care
Dranitsaris *et al.* (2004)	Treatments for ovarian cancer

7.3. **What might we mean by willingness-to-pay?**

It is important to keep in mind that WTP is a measurement technique, and it is how and why this technique is applied that determines its usefulness for CBA. Reviews of WTP studies in health care have revealed wide variation in what questions are being asked, of whom, and how (O'Brien and Gafni 1996). There is disagreement therefore concerning how WTP should be measured and how such measures can be incorporated into CBA.

In this section we explore different ways in which the concept of WTP can be defined and measured for inclusion in a health care CBA. A simple framework is presented in Box 7.10, which distinguishes between improvements in health *per se* and other sources of benefit, all of which could, in theory, be valued by WTP. For the health component we also consider the nature of the commodity defined in a WTP study with particular emphasis on the role of uncertainty. We describe and illustrate this framework in the following sections.

7.3.1. **Global versus restricted willingness-to-pay**

There are three broad categories of benefits that can arise from a health care programme: (1) intangible benefits, which are the value of improved health *per se* to the individual consumer of a programme; (2) future health care costs avoided; (3) increased productive output due to improved health status. One 'restricted' perspective on WTP is that it would be used only to value those components of benefit for which no money values existed from other market sources. In this approach, WTP estimates are restricted to quantifying the money value of changes in health *per se*, with future health care cost savings and production gains being valued using market prices. (This distinction was discussed earlier in Chapter 2.)

An alternative 'global' perspective on this measurement task is to argue that the purpose of the contingent valuation study is to learn about how the individual consumer would value a specific health care programme in a world where private markets and price signals for all goods and services were operational. However, in this free market scenario for contingent valuation, consistency also calls for us to ask the respondent to consider in their valuation the future health care costs that they individually would sustain in the private market world and also work-related income effects as a consequence of ill health or treatment. As an example, consider a decision to buy a more expensive but more effective cold medication over the counter from a pharmacy. A consumer's decision (and willingness-to-pay) would be driven not only by anticipated health benefits but also, in part, by cost offsets from other medications they may no longer need to purchase if they bought the more expensive cold medications. They might also include the costs associated with work absence in deciding whether or not to buy the more expensive medications. Therefore in this simple private market consumer purchase example, as individual's willingness-to-pay for a medication is a function not only of the health benefits but also of future out-of-pocket cost savings and income effects from work absence. By analogy this thought process can be transferred to contingent markets for health care programmes that are covered by insurance or taxation.

As discussed above and illustrated in Box 7.10, the concept of contingent markets is very powerful and can be used to assign money values to all aspects of benefit arising from a health care programme, not simply the value of health itself. While these global and restricted strategies are alternative ways to proceed, great caution needs to be exercised in how respondents are being questioned and whether there is potential

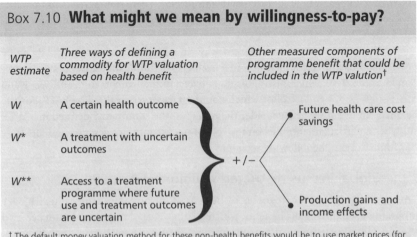

Box 7.10 **What might we mean by willingness-to-pay?**

WTP estimate	Three ways of defining a commodity for WTP valuation based on health benefit	Other measured components of programme benefit that could be included in the WTP valution[†]
W	A certain health outcome	Future health care cost savings
W*	A treatment with uncertain outcomes	
W**	Access to a treatment programme where future use and treatment outcomes are uncertain	Production gains and income effects

$+/-$

† The default money valuation method for these non-health benefits would be to use market prices (for example, wage rates for production). However, in theory, the contingent valuation scenario could be a purely private market for all goods and services, requiring the respondent to state a global WTP based on all consequences of the programme.

for double-counting of some programme benefits. For example, when assessing an individual's willingness-to-pay for a new antihypertensive medication the respondent needs to be told explicitly whether they should be considering income effects due to work absence arising from the disease or its treatment. Double-counting would arise if the individual had considered income effects in answering the WTP questions but the analyst also valued attributable production gains using wage rate data (that is, a human capital calculation).

7.3.2. What good or service is being valued?

Even if we focus on the restricted form of WTP based on health benefits, as shown in Box 7.10, there are at least three ways in which a good or service for valuation can be defined: (1) find the WTP for a certain health outcome (W); (2) find the WTP for a treatment with uncertain health outcomes (W^*); (3) find the WTP for access to a treatment programme where future use and treatment outcomes are both uncertain (W^{**}). Consistent with the welfare economics of health care market failure as outlined by Arrow (1963), the main distinction between these three definitions of the good or service being valued is uncertainty. The difference between W and W^* is the inclusion of uncertainty on the supply side with respect to outcomes for a given treatment. In moving to W^{**} we also include uncertainty on the demand side, because individuals are being asked about their willingness-to-pay for a health care programme given they are uncertain whether they need or will demand this service in the future.

Here we review these three definitions of the goods or service being valued, as illustrated in Box 7.10.

1. *Valuing a certain health outcome (W)*. Authors such as Pauly (1995) have suggested that finding the 'shadow price' for a QALY may be a useful bridge between CUA and CBA. Some empirical work on the relationship between health status measures and WTP has also been undertaken (Reed-Johnson *et al.* 1994). Studies that fall in this first use of WTP to value certain health outcomes would include the early work of Thompson (1986), where persons with arthritis were asked open-ended questions for the maximum they would be willing to pay to achieve a cure of their arthritis.

2. *Valuing a treatment with uncertain outcomes (W*)*. As indicated by authors such as Gafni (1991), a limitation of basing WTP estimates on certain health outcomes is that the consequences of health care programmes are inherently uncertain. Under W^* therefore, the goal of measurement is to determine the maximum the respondent would be willing to pay to consume a treatment programme with outcomes that are not certainties but have specified probabilities. Although one can multiply certain health values (h) by probabilities to devise expected money values for the programme, the values collected directly on uncertain prospects (W^*) will only be the same as the expected values if individuals are risk neutral with respect to income and health.

3. *Valuing access to a treatment programme (W**)*. In most developed countries we observe that health care services are funded and delivered on the basis of insurance or tax contributions. This reflects an important characteristic of the health care market,

which is that illness and the demand for health care is uncertain. The consequence of such insurance or tax arrangements would be that persons do not bear the full cost (if any) of the service at the point of delivery. Hence it has been argued by Gafni (1991) that WTP questions should be framed in a way that incorporates this demand side uncertainty. Specifically, in Box 7.10 we characterize W^{**} as being the maximum an individual would be willing to pay for access to a treatment programme where both future use and treatment outcomes are uncertain. For example, this hypothetical choice might use the payment vehicle of increased insurance premiums or taxation to ensure a programme is made available. A distinction is therefore made between an *ex post* perspective such as W^* where the individual undertaking the valuation knows that they are a consumer of the treatment and that the only uncertainty is on the probability of outcomes, versus an *ex ante* perspective such as W^{**} where the individual's valuation needs to incorporate the probability of sustaining the illness and needing the service in question.

In Box 7.11 we illustrate the difference between the *ex post* and *ex ante* perspectives using an example of IVF from Neumann and Johannesson (1994). This was a population-based survey where the authors explored WTP for IVF services using both

---

Box 7.11 Willingness-to-pay for *in vitro* fertilization

This study illustrates two different approaches estimates to forming contingent valuation questions. The *ex post* or user based approach estimates how much you will pay at the point of consumption. The *ex ante* or insurance based approach estimates how much you will pay for insurance coverage.

Ex post perspective (user based)
- assume you are infertile and want children
- IVF has 10% chance of being successful if purchased
- mean WTP of $17 730 (if 10% chance of success)
- $28 054 (if 25% chance of success)
- $43 576 (if 50% chance of success)

Ex ante perspective (insurance based)
- assume you have 10% chance of being infertile
- IVF has 10% chance of success
- you can buy one-time insurance premium for IVF coverage
- mean WTP of $865

Implied WTP per statistical baby
- $177 730(user based)
- $1.8m (insurance based)

From Neumann and Johannesson (1994).

an *ex post* scenario (assuming infertility, what would you pay out-of-pocket) and an *ex ante* scenario (where the individuals are asked to assume they have a 10% chance of being infertile and they can buy insurance coverage for IVF). What is notable from Box 7.11 is that the implied value per statistical baby is much higher for the *ex ante* or insurance-based approach ($1.8 m) than the *ex post* or user-based approach ($0.17 m). This is because in the insurance-based setting persons are now also incorporating their risk aversion into the valuation of access to the programme.

As a further illustration of how such *ex ante* insurance-based questions can be asked in practice, Box 7.12, taken from a study by O'Brien *et al.* (1998), shows how respondents who were enrolees in a health maintenance organization (HMO) in the

---

Box 7.12 **Example of *ex ante* insurance-based willingness-to-pay**

Option A: your HMO plan covers chemotherapy

◆ Assume that your chance of getting cancer over the next 5 years is 1 in 100.

◆ You continue to pay your current monthly insurance premium for health care.

If you get cancer

◆ You get chemotherapy but not GCSF.

◆ Over six cycles of chemotherapy your chance of neutropenic fever is

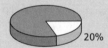

◆ You cannot buy GCSF or get it covered by another plan.

Option B: your HMO plan covers chemotherapy and GCSF

◆ Assume that your chance of getting cancer over the next 5 years is 1 in 100.

◆ You pay a monthly supplement to cover GCSF in addition to your current insurance premium for health care.

If you get cancer

◆ You get chemotherapy with GCSF.

◆ Over six cycles of chemotherapy your chance of neutropenic fever is

◆ You cannot buy GCSF or get it covered by another plan.

If GCSF was not currently covered by your HMO plan (Option A), would you consider paying an increased premium for coverage of GCSF (Option B)?
From O'Brien *et al.* (1998).

USA were asked whether they were willing to upgrade their insurance coverage to include a new supportive drug used in cancer chemotherapy known as GCSF. The benefit of this drug is that it reduces the risk of neutropenic fever following chemotherapy; in the example in Box 7.12 the reduction in risk is from 20% to 10% over the six cycles of chemotherapy. A bidding algorithm was used (see below) to find the maximum additional monthly premium persons would pay to have the new drug covered.

7.3.3. Connecting the *W*s

The *W*s in Box 7.10 are clearly connected, and the nature of the relationship depends, *inter alia*, upon the risk preferences of the respondents. For example, one could measure money values for certain health outcomes (W) and multiply these by their probabilities of arising to calculate the expected money value of a treatment programme. However, this expected value would only correspond with the measured *ex ante* value W^* to the extent that individuals were risk neutral (with respect to income and health) in their preferences. As was described in Chapter 6, we generally observe that individuals are risk averse and therefore the *ex ante* value would be less than the expected value. This risk preference relationship is also true for W^* in relation to W^{**}, and this has been analyzed recently by Johannesson (1996*b*).

We have already discussed the relationship between the restricted concept of WTP (W, W^*, or W^{**} in this framework), with its primary focus on the value of health benefits, and the more global concept of WTP where a respondent is required to value all health and non-health benefits in money terms. It is this concept of global or overall WTP that was labelled as W', back in Fig. 2.1. In practice it is unlikely that many studies will attempt to measure W', but in theory it could be done.

7.3.4. Other sources of utility for money valuation

As we discussed earlier, the work of Donaldson and Shackley (1997) has emphasized the role of non-health benefits (for example, information) for inclusion in WTP. Depending upon the programme there may be significant non-health sources of (dis)utility to capture.

Another important source of private health care market failure, identified by Arrow (1963), is due to spillovers or externalities. The concept of externality in the consumption of health care is best explained using the example of an infectious disease where one person might be willing to pay for another person to receive treatment so as to reduce the risks of disease transmission to themselves or others. More generally, there might also be humanitarian spillovers in that one person derives utility from the knowledge that others can gain access to needed health care services. The implications of externalities for WTP studies is that the sampling frame for inquiry must extend to all persons whose utility is impacted by the introduction of the programme. For example, in assessing WTP for an (elective) new vaccination programme for an infectious disease one would need to draw survey samples from all persons who would benefit from the programme, including the direct benefit to those who vaccinate and the indirect benefit of those not vaccinating but are now at lower risk.

7.3.5. **A simple example**

To illustrate how WTP data might be used in a CBA, consider the decision context of an HMO trying to decide whether to place a new drug on its formulary. Let us suppose a WTP survey similar to that described in O'Brien *et al.* (1998)—the GCSF study described in Boxes 7.12 and 7.13—has been undertaken on a sample of HMO enrolees. The WTP scenario was the maximum additional insurance that respondents would pay to have the drug covered over a 5-year period. The first task would be to forecast the total WTP (for the HMO population) from the sample using multiple regression analysis based upon known characteristics of the sample and population. Suppose the (discounted) total WTP over the 5 years is $10 m. The cost of the programme is a function, in part, of how many persons will receive the treatment, over the same time period, and this must also be forecast. Suppose the estimated cost is $7 m with an estimated $2 m in cost savings from health care resources not consumed by persons who receive the treatment for a net cost (discounted) of $5 m. For simplicity, assume that there are no productivity losses or that gains and losses cancel out. Using these data the programme has a positive net benefit of $5 m (that is, $10 m − $7 m + $2 m). How this information can be used to inform resource allocation depends upon a number of things but particularly whether one is allocating resources within a fixed or non-fixed budget setting.

Box 7.13 **Bidding algorithms used in the GCSF willingness-to-pay study**

Bid level	Insurance-based bid scale ($)	Bid algorithm #1	Bid algorithm #2
1	1		
2	5		
3	10		
4	15		
5	25		
6	50		
7	100		

Y = willing to pay this bid; N = not willing to pay this bid.

Persons accepting bid level 7 were then asked an open-ended question for the maximum they were willing to pay. From O'Brien *et al.* (1998).

In a non-fixed budget scenario, the HMO might decide to add the new programme and actually raise insurance premiums, thus increasing its budget. In a competitive market, if these marginal adjustments to coverage, which could be up or down, do not reflect consumers' values then consumers (or their employers) may elect to switch to other plans. The second scenario for WTP-based CBA is with a fixed budget. In this circumstance, knowledge that the new programme has a positive net benefit is of partial value for resource allocation and prioritizing services. To implement the new programme without expanding the budget, efficiency criteria would argue for a rank ordering of existing programmes by the size of their net benefit to facilitate comparison with the new programme. Efficiency would require us to replace programmes with small net benefit by programmes with larger net benefits. The practical difficulty with this scenario is that it is data hungry and works by comparison of net benefit; having data on the new programme is a necessary but not sufficient condition for making resource-allocation decisions.

7.4. Pragmatic measurement issues

7.4.1. Issues of bias and precision

The goal of the contingent valuation measurement task is to obtain precise and unbiased estimates of WTP. To pose such a question in a way that is both believable and clear to a respondent is not a trivial undertaking and is at least as complex (probably more so) as the utility measurement tasks described in Chapter 6. There are two types of general question format: open ended and closed ended. Open-ended questions pose a difficult cognitive task for most respondents because we are typically not used to thinking about the *maximum* we would pay for something. Experience with this approach suggests that although it may produce unbiased estimates of WTP because the respondent is not prompted, it is very imprecise with widely varying responses and many non-responses or protest responses (Johannesson 1996a); also see Donaldson et al. (1997b) on evaluation of open-ended question formats.

Closed-ended question formats have been used in health care contingent valuation studies in two general formats: bidding games to find within-person maximum value and so-called 'take-it-or-leave-it' between-person surveys. Bidding games use a predetermined search algorithm to bid the respondent up or down, conditional upon how they respond to a prompted monetary value. Much like an auction, if you say 'yes' to $50 we will ask you a higher amount; 'no', and we will ask you a lower amount; for example, see the study by O'Brien and Viramontes (1994). While the bidding game improves upon open-ended questions for the precision of the estimated maximum WTP, it may do so at the expense of introducing a bias in the form of starting point bias. This bias is a form of framing effect where the respondents' answers are influenced by the first numbers presented in the bidding game. Although a number of non-health and health care studies have found evidence of starting point bias (Stalhammer 1996), this result is not conclusive because others have used bidding games and found no evidence of starting point bias, even though it was explicitly tested for (O'Brien and Viramontes 1994; O'Brien et al. 1998).

To illustrate this concept, we show in Box 7.13 the bidding game used in the same GCSF study mentioned in Box 7.12 from O'Brien *et al.* (1998). Respondents received one of two bid algorithms and analysis showed that the hypothesis of no starting point bias could not be rejected.

The second type of closed-ended question format is an approach used widely in environmental economic evaluation where surveys of large numbers of persons are typically undertaken to elicit values for some environmental programme or problem. (A controversial environmental example where contingent valuation methods have been used is the valuation of natural resources destroyed by the Exxon Valdez oil spill in Prince William Sound.) The essence of this approach is that each respondent is only asked one question ('take-it-or-leave-it'); for example, 'would you be willing to pay an extra $50 per month on your taxes for this programme—yes or no'? The money amount each person is asked is randomly selected from a range. So, for example, the next person might be asked if they are willing to pay $100, and so on. The data are then analysed using econometric techniques such as probit analysis to identify a bid curve—that is, the quantitative relationship between the proportion of persons accepting or rejecting the bid at different levels of the bid. By mathematically integrating for the area under this bid curve one can determine the mean WTP, or, alternatively, identify the median WTP. For a discussion of this approach in health care see Johannesson (1996*a*).

The 'take-it-or-leave-it' categorical approach has been used in health care contingent valuation studies by Johannesson (1996*b*) with some success. The difficulties with this approach are in identifying the relevant range from which to sample bids and also in the large sample size one needs for precise estimation. A variant of this approach, which increases precision, is to ask another (random) bid question of each respondent, but the direction being conditional on the answer to the first question. In the future it is likely that interviews will be computer based so that random bid selection (first or subsequent) is easy to achieve. However, there is still some residual risk of bias because the analyst must choose the *range* from which bids are sampled.

Some studies compare more than one method of eliciting WTP (Frew *et al.* 2003; Frew *et al.* 2004; Whynes *et al.* 2003; Ryan *et al.* 2004). Ryan *et al.* (2004) compared the payment card (bidding approach) with the dichotomous choice (take-it-or-leave-it) approach. They found that the dichotomous choice method consistently gave higher estimates of WTP. Whynes *et al.* (2003) showed that range bias was prevalent in payment-scale WTP formats.

7.4.2. Validation of willingness-to-pay by tests of scope

Is it possible to validate the findings of a WTP study? The 'gold standard' against which we would like to compare predicted WTP from compensating variation (CV) surveys is what consumers would *actually* pay. Unfortunately, for most of the health programme benefits studied by CV methods, actual market may not exist so *criterion validity* cannot easily be established. However, there are some useful tests of *construct validity* that can be examined in WTP studies. The logic of construct validation in this setting is to determine whether the data are consistent with theoretical constructs that should be present if the WTP responses are measuring the value we intend.

There are two simple propositions ('constructs') from economic theory that can be tested. First, most goods have what is known as a positive income elasticity meaning that, other things being equal, higher respondent incomes should be associated with higher WTP. Second, the more of a positively valued good that is supplied by a hypothetical programme, the greater should be a persons' WTP, although the marginal utility of additional units of benefit is likely to decline.

This second principle was strongly endorsed by official guidelines for WTP studies for environmental damage assessment (National Oceanic and Atmospheric Administration (NOAA) 1993). The NOAA panel termed these validation techniques 'scope tests' because the proposition is that WTP should vary with the scope of the benefit (or damage) arising from the hypothetical programme. Scope tests are an important part of WTP validation and have been recommended by European guidelines on health care WTP studies where, for example, the magnitude of a treatment effect or other health benefit can be varied in the survey (Johannesson et al. 1996). For examples of scope tests in health care WTP studies see Kartman et al. (1996), Stalhammer and Johannesson (1996), and O'Brien et al. (1998).

7.4.3. Payments and health care settings

One of the key difficulties with contingent valuation studies is making the scenario realistic for the respondent. Even if we adopt an *ex ante* insurance-based perspective, most consumers will not be familiar with purchasing access to individual health care programmes. It is likely that these forms of payment scenarios will work better in some health care systems such as in the USA where consumers are used to paying more directly for health care than in other health care systems such as in the UK, which has a system of social provision based on taxation contributions. In the environmental economic evaluation literature it has been customary to characterize the decision problem as whether to vote in favour of or against a proposal to have a programme implemented that would have an associated tax contribution. In this kind of format the respondent has their mind focused on the idea of a referendum rather than an actual purchasing decision. In some settings this may be more realistic for the respondent than to consider insurance contributions.

7.4.4. Research into willingness-to-pay methods

Willingness-to-pay methods have attracted considerable interest from health economist researchers. Reviews of the literature (Diener et al. 1998; Klose 1999; Olsen and Smith 2001; Smith 2003; Bayoumi 2004) come to slightly different conclusions on the overall quality of the literature and whether it is improving over time. Smith (2003) argues that further research is required in several areas, including scenario development and presentation, payment vehicle (for example, out-of-pocket payment or insurance), expression of risk, time period of valuation, and survey administration. Researchers are responding to this challenge, although a comprehensive review of this literature is beyond the scope of this book.

7.5. **Exercise: designing a contingent valuation survey for a new treatment for ovarian cancer**

Scenario

The government is trying to decide whether they should reimburse a new therapy for ovarian cancer. Design a WTP survey for a CBA of this new treatment for ovarian cancer. Assume that among women who receive this therapy there is a 5% rate of complete cure from the cancer, but the majority will sustain some side-effects from the treatment. Data suggest there are productivity gains with more women in the treated group being able to return to work. There are also cost offsets with treated women receiving fewer health care services in the future.

Specific questions

1 Which components of benefit arising from this treatment programme would you value using WTP? Consider the pros and cons of using a 'global' WTP estimate for valuing all programme benefits versus a 'restricted' WTP for health benefits and market prices for other components of benefit.

2 How would you define the commodity that the respondent is being asked to pay for? Consider the alternative formulations of W, W^*, and W^{**} discussed in this chapter. What kind of payment vehicle is 'believable' for each of these formulations?

3 The draft study proposal is to interview a sample of women with ovarian cancer. Would you include other subjects in the survey, and why?

Solutions/ideas

1. Using the 'global approach' discussed in this chapter we would frame a WTP scenario for the individual for the contingent market for the new therapy, where future attributable costs and employment effects were a personal responsibility and to be met out-of-pocket. If one used this approach and made it explicit that the respondent should consider these attributes in their valuation then it would not be appropriate to use market prices to value future health care cost savings or wage rates to value productivity effects. To do so would be double-counting because the individual has been asked to consider these in a private market scenario where they are the responsibility of the individual. In practice this global approach may be a difficult cognitive task for the respondent. An easier route may be to use market prices for the future costs and productivity effects but use the WTP approach only for the benefit of the health effects, that is, the 'restricted' approach to WTP. If this approach is adopted, however, it is still important to state explicitly to the respondent that they should not consider income effects associated with work absence or future costs associated with the disease in their valuation.

2. The key difference between the three Ws is the incorporation of uncertainty into the valuation tasks. Perhaps the simplest task would be to estimate money values for the (certain) health states arising in the evaluation. More generally, however, it would be more desirable to include uncertainty with respect to outcomes such that individuals were being asked to value the treatment with probabilities of therapeutic benefit but also probabilities of harm. One of the difficulties here is the extent to which the multiple attributes of outcome and associated probabilities can be presented to

respondents in a manner that will be comprehensible. The payment vehicle one might adopt for this type of money valuation could be additional out-of-pocket expense at the point of consumption (for example, a variable co-payment on a medication). A difficulty with this payment vehicle format is that it may not be believable to respondents if the therapy is a major medical procedure that would normally be covered by a health care system at zero cost to the patient. The consequence of such a question framing might be a number of protest responses from respondents.

Formulating the valuation question to estimate W^{**} is more complex yet. Now the respondents need to be presented with information both on the uncertain outcomes of therapy but also on probability of needing this therapy themselves in some future time period. How one frames a payment vehicle to address W^{**} is also complex and will be conditional upon the system of health care financing that the respondent is familiar with. For example, in a predominantly private insurance system it may be most meaningful to ask the respondent to consider additional insurance premiums that they would be willing to pay to gain coverage and access to the treatment programme. In a predominantly tax-financed health care system it may be necessary to frame the question in terms of additional tax contributions (either national or local) that would facilitate the availability of the new treatment programme.

3. While it may be of interest to interview women with ovarian cancer in the estimation of W or W^{*}, the total societal WTP will necessitate a broader sampling. For example, to estimate W^{**} one would need to also interview women who do not currently have ovarian cancer but are at risk of this disease. These individuals may be willing to preserve the option of having this programme available should they need it in the future. More generally, there is also the issue of externality or spillover benefits to other members of the population who are not at current or future risk of ovarian cancer (that is, men). Men may be willing to pledge additional insurance or tax dollars to cover the ovarian cancer treatment programme either through a self-interested motivation (that is, wives and daughters at risk) or through a general humanitarian or altruistic motivation where they are expressing a statement of value for women more generally.

7.6. **Conjoint analysis and discrete choice experiments**

The survey method of data collection and analysis known as conjoint analysis was developed in mathematical psychology and marketing and has close links to the approach known as multiattribute utility theory described in Chapter 6. Conjoint analysis is based on the premises that any good or service can be described by its characteristics (or attributes) and the extent to which an individual values a good or service depends on the levels of these characteristics.

Good introductions to the use of ranking and rating conjoint analysis and discrete choice experiments (DCEs) are provided by Ryan and Farrar (2000), and Ryan and Gerard (2003). Due to its grounding in random utility theory, economists tend to prefer the methodology of DCEs rather than the ranking and rating methodologies of the conjoint analysis method. They point out that the technique can be used to show individuals are willing to trade between the characteristics of treatments or services, to estimate the relative importance of different characteristics, to estimate whether a characteristic or attribute is important, and to predict the demand for a given good or service with given characteristics. The particular relevance in the context of CBA is that the payment vehicle of 'cost' can be included as one of the attributes. Then, the ratio (or marginal rate of substitution) of any given attribute to the absolute parameter on the cost attribute shows how much money the individual is willing to pay for a unit change in that attribute.

There are several key steps in undertaking a conjoint analysis. First, the characteristics of the treatment or service must be identified. These may often be pre-defined, but can also be obtained from literature reviews or focus group discussions with health professionals or patients. In the case of a treatment, the characteristics are likely to relate to the main dimensions of efficacy and the major adverse events. A review of the literature (Ryan and Gerard 2003) suggested that four to six attributes was acceptable, in relation to the respondents' ability to complete the choice task.

Second, levels need to be assigned to the characteristics. These may be cardinal (for example, cure after 1 day being twice as good as cure after 2 days), ordinal (for example, severe pain being worse than moderate pain), or categorical, where there is no natural ordering (for example, one adverse event versus another).

Third, scenarios need to be drawn up that describe all possible configurations of the characteristics and levels chosen. Clearly, the major issue here is that the potential number of scenarios is dependent on the number of characteristics and levels defined. Because it is usually impossible to include all the scenarios in any given survey (full factorial design), experimental designs are used to reduce the number to a manageable level whilst maintaining orthogonality (fractional factorial design). Because the design property of orthogonality precludes collinearity between attributes, this enhances statistical efficiency. Designs should also allow for the nature of the attributes (for example, ordinal or categorical), be orthogonal-in-differences, allow for interactions where relevant, and have minimal overlap of levels. For a summary of these design criteria see Louviere et al. (2000) and Huber and Zwerina (1996). Also, Carlsson and Martinsson (2003) provide a concise review of design techniques for stated preference discrete choice methods in health economics including random designs and optimal design strategies.

Fourth, preferences for the scenarios need to be elicited using discrete choices. Respondents are presented with a number of choices and, for each, asked to choose their preferred one. Possible responses include stating that either A or B is preferred (where one option may also be a fixed 'status quo'), that A or B is preferred on a graded scale, that indifference is preferred, or that the 'non participation or neither' option is preferred. These different elicitation formats each have advantages and disadvantages. However, it is important to identify the appropriate elicitation format for the question being addressed. For example, where a non-participation option (inclusion of a 'prefer neither' option) is incorrectly excluded, this may give rise to overestimation of any values obtained (Morey et al. 1993). (An example of a graded elicitation format with an opt-out option is shown in Box 7.14.)

Finally, the data need to be analysed. Usually this is done using econometric techniques, where, for a binary response format, the utility function is specified in

Box 7.14 **Estimating trade-offs that individuals are willing to make between location of treatment and waiting time in the provision of orthodontic services**

The policy question determined that treatment location (that is, local clinic or hospital) and waiting time were the main attributes individuals would be concerned about. In total 16 scenarios were possible, considering first and second appointments and four levels of waiting time. Fifteen discrete choices were constructed by comparing the current service to all alternatives. An example of one of these choices is given below.

	(a) Current			(b) Alternative			Which option would you choose? (please tick one box for each choice)				
	First appoint- ment	Second appoint- ment	Waiting time (months)	First appoint- ment	Second appoint- ment	Waiting time (months)	Definitely (a) current	Probably (a) current	No preference	Probably (b) alternative	Definitely (b) alternative
Choice1	Hospital	Hospital	8	or Local	Local	12					
Choice2	Hospital	Hospital	8	or Hospital	Hospital	16					
Choice3	Hospital	Hospital	8	or Local	Local	16					

A random effects ordered probit model was fitted thus:

$$\Delta B = B_1 \, \mathrm{LOC}_1 + B_2 \, \mathrm{LOC}_2 + B_3 \, \mathrm{WAIT}.$$

Seventy three (out of 160) individuals gave consistent responses.

Variable	Coefficient	p value
LOC_1	$-0.77(B_1)$	<0.001
LOC_2	$-0.91(B_2)$	<0.001
WAIT	$-0.59(B_3)$	<0.001

The interpretation is the benefit of the service is significantly associated with lower waiting times and first and second appointments in a local clinic. Individuals are willing to wait an extra 1.3 months ($B_1/B_3 = 0.77/0.59$) to have their first appointment in a local clinic. From Ryan and Farrar (2003).

additive form: $\Delta U = \beta_1 X_1 + \beta_2 X_2 + \beta_3 X_3 + \ldots + \beta_n X_n$, where ΔU is the change in utility in moving from treatment A to B, X_j ($j = 1, 2, \ldots, n$) are the differences in attribute levels A and B, and β_j ($j = 1, 2, \ldots, n$) are the coefficients of the model to be estimated. The method of analysis depends upon the elicitation format; for instance, when a non-participation option is included this may require analysis using a nested logit model.

Discrete choice experiments are becoming increasingly popular in the health care field. Examples include examination of individuals' preferences for service provision (for example, out-of-hours care provided by general practitioners)

(Scott *et al.* 2003) and for treatment characteristics (for example, therapies for osteoarthritis and prostate cancer) (Ratcliffe *et al.* 2004; Sculpher *et al.* 2004). (See Ryan and Gerard (2003) for a review of the literature.) This approach has many of the advantages of contingent valuation, in that it enables non-health characteristics, or attributes related to process utility, to be included. One major additional advantage is that, whilst WTP tells us about the valuation of the whole 'bundle' of characteristics, DCEs help us understand the relative valuations of, or the trade-offs between, various attributes. This would be of particular relevance to a health planner considering options for provision of a particular service, or a clinical researcher wanting to understand the relative valuation of the outcomes, side-effects, or other characteristics of a particular therapy (for example, how much is an oral formulation of a drug valued relative to administration by injection?) (see Box 7.15).

As with standard WTP estimations by contingent valuations, DCEs raise a number of methodological issues. (See Louviere *et al.* (2000) for a full discussion.) Many of these are already being addressed in the literature, including internal validity and consistency (Ryan *et al.* 1998; McIntosh and Ryan 2002) and test–retest reliability (Bryan *et al.* 2000). However, one issue of particular importance to CBA deserves special mention, namely, the inclusion of a cost attribute in order to estimate WTP. Ratcliffe (2000) argues that this should be viewed with caution as the level at which the cost attribute is set can influence the WTP estimates for the levels of other attributes and hence the total WTP value inferred for that individual to receive their chosen intervention. Also, in an empirical study using a large dataset, Skjoldborg and Gyrd-Hansen (2003) found that the cost range applied in DCEs, and the inclusion of a dummy variable to represent the utility associated with payment *per se*, could affect the WTP values. Morey *et al.* (1993) and Mitchell and Carson (1989) outline the importance of modelling the participation decision when estimating welfare estimates using DCEs. Morey *et al.* (1993) note that DCE WTP values are sensitive to the valuation model employed and that modelling the participation decision is crucial in obtaining accurate estimates. Finally, weighting the values by the probability of choosing each alternative should also be carried out using a multiple alternative DCE study (Lancsar and Savage 2004; Bennett and Blamey 2001).

In summary, DCEs represent an interesting development in economic evaluation and facilitate estimates of value that cannot be obtained by other methods. However, many normative and methodological issues remain to be resolved (Bryan and Dolan 2004). A research agenda is set out by Ryan and Gerard (2003), who argue that the growing enthusiasm by health economists to use DCEs must be balanced by the need to follow a paced development that both draws from, and builds on, knowledge from other disciplines.

7.7. Willingness-to-pay estimates and health policy decisions

Although several imperfections in the methodology of WTP studies have been identified, the approach is now firmly established within the research community. However, is the methodology sufficiently refined to enable health policy decisions to

Box 7.15 **Patients' preferences for the management of non-metastatic prostate cancer**

Several situations exist where patients face trade-offs between the risks and benefits of alternative therapies. Sculpher *et al.* (2004) explored men's trade-offs in the field of non-metastatic prostate cancer, where different treatments, whilst increasing life expectancy, have various side-effects including diarrhoea, hot flushes, ability to maintain an erection, breast swelling or tenderness, and loss of physical energy and sex drive. Also, in settings where patients have to pay for medication, or incur other expenses in obtaining care, there could also be impacts on out-of-pocket expenses.

Some results from their discrete choice experiment are shown in Table 1. The coefficients for the attributes were all statistically significant from zero. Negative values indicate that the more severe the problem, the less likely the patient is to prefer that scenario. (The negative value for out-of-pocket expenses indicates that the higher the costs, the less likely the patient is to prefer that scenario.) The positive value for life expectancy indicates that the greater the life expectancy the more likely the patient is to prefer that scenario.

Table 1 Results of second part of discrete choice exercise

Variable	Coefficient (95% confidence interval)	Standard error	*P*-value
Diarrhoea	−0.4193 (−0.5454 to −0.2931)	0.0644	<0.001
Hot flushes	−0.1225 (−0.2162 to −0.0287)	0.0479	0.010
Breast tenderness	−0.4329 (−0.6147 to −0.2512)	0.0927	<0.001
Out-of-pocket expenses	−0.0016 (−0.0025 to −0.0007)	0.0004	0.001
Life expectancy	0.2329 (0.1827 to 0.2832)	0.0256	<0.001
Constant	0.1278 (0.0262 to 0.2294)	0.0618	0.014
Number of observations	992; 164.35; P < 0.0001*		

* χ^2-test.

Table 2 shows the marginal rates of substitution between life expectancy and the other attributes—that is, how much life expectancy the men were willing to trade off to achieve an improvement by one level in one of the other attributes. For example, men are willing to trade off 1.8 months of life expectancy to change diarrhoea from a moderate to mild level, or from mild to absent.

Box 7.15 **Patients' preferences for the management of non-metastatic prostate cancer** *(Continued)*

Table 2 Patients' marginal rates of substitution between life expectancy and other attributes

Attribute	Life expectancy willing to forgo (months)	Single-level improvement
Diarrhoea	1.8	From moderate to mild or from mild to absent
Hot flushes	0.5	From moderate to mild or from mild to absent
Breast swelling	1.9	From present to absent
Loss of libido	1.3	From present to absent
Problems in maintaining an erection		
Aged <70 years	1.8	From moderate to mild or from mild to absent
Aged >70 years	0.9	From moderate to mild or from mild to absent
Lack of energy or 'pep'	3.0	From present to absent

be based on WTP estimates or the results of CBAs? Olsen and Smith (2001) express considerable disappointment, commenting that 'after this (attempted) careful review, these authors have the distinct feeling of a huge mismatch between the theoretical glory of WTP and the usefulness for public health policy of the majority of surveys which have applied this method'.

There appear to be two main issues. First, the estimates obtained can vary by the elicitation method used and are sometimes inconsistent. For example, Stewart *et al.* (2002) found that the reported WTP for three health care programmes varied within a single survey, depending on the order in which the programmes were presented. Also, in two other studies (Shackley and Donaldson 2002; Olsen *et al.* 2004), inconsistencies were found between respondents' willingness-to-pay for health programmes and the ordinal ranking they placed on the programmes. Because the main purpose of applying WTP in this context is to elicit public preferences for how policy makers should allocate health care resources, these findings do cast some doubt on its application.

Second, it is important that the WTP estimates obtained are relevant to the decision-making context concerned. In the case of the study of GCSF discussed earlier, it was relevant to ask enrolees of an HMO whether they would pay more to have the drug covered, because in reviewing their options for health insurance, individuals could conceivably compare plans in terms of the premiums charged and the range of coverage given.

However, many economic evaluations are undertaken to inform decisions undertaken by public policy makers and the relevance of WTP studies needs to be considered in this context. For example, in a study undertaken in eight Canadian provinces, Dranitsaris *et al.* (2004) found that a patient surrogate sample of 80 oncology pharmacists and nurses were willing to pay a mean of 64 Canadian dollars extra per chemotherapy cycle for docetaxel as an alternative to paclitaxel. Because this estimate was marginally lower than the incremental cost of docetaxel ($87 per cycle) the authors argue that both options should be offered to patients.

However, as Olsen and Smith (2001) point out, the fact that patients (or their surrogates) are willing to sacrifice the alternative *private* consumption that their WTP would have purchased, suggests that the only justifiable source of funding is private income. In order to inform the decisions of public decision-makers operating under a (relatively) fixed budget, one has to make sure that the opportunity cost, in terms of benefits forgone in the deferred public programme(s), is less than the WTP. We cannot tell this without valuing the programmes to be deferred. The problem is that most WTP studies value just one programme and do not present these choices. This issue is discussed further in Chapter 10.

Nevertheless, WTP studies can provide information to policy makers on the intensity of individuals' preferences for particular health programmes, even if they do not provide the whole basis for the decision. Also, WTP surveys can provide useful information in situations where there are close substitute therapies for a given condition.

7.8. **Conclusions**

As we have indicated in this chapter, CBA is, at least in theory, the most powerful of the techniques for economic evaluation because it can directly address questions of allocative efficiency which the other techniques cannot. But this advantage comes only after the analyst has overcome a number of difficulties associated with assigning a monetary value to programme benefits. Much of this chapter has focused on this thorny issue and we have described how experience with contingent valuation techniques has given rise to new enthusiasm for implementing WTP in health care programme evaluation. Whether the promise held out by these approaches is fulfilled remains to be seen. We noted that although a number of feasibility and pilot studies have appeared in the literature, there are very few complete CBA studies that use WTP as the basis for valuing all outcomes.

Conjoint analysis, and more specifically DCEs, represent another useful way of exploring the valuations individuals place on the attributes of health care interventions and treatments. These approaches can also be used to estimate WTP, but some commentators suggest that this should be pursued with caution.

The further development of CBA in health care will be helped by careful use of language and definitions. Numerous published studies are termed CBA yet only offer a partial evaluation, comparing direct costs with and without the programme. A consistent use of the label for this technique will help focus the minds of analysts and consumers of CBA studies on the precise issues of theory and empiricism that continue to challenge this approach.

References

Ades, A. E., Sculpher, M. J., Gibb, D. M., Gupta, R., and Ratcliffe, J. (1999). Cost-effectiveness analysis of antenatal HIV screening in United Kingdom. *British Medical Journal*, **319**, 1230–4.

Appel, L. J., Steinberg, E. P., Powe, N. R., Anderson, G. F., Dwyer, S. A., and Faden, R. R. (1990). Risk reduction from low osmolality contrast media. What do patients think it is worth? *Medical Care*, **28**, 324–34.

Arrow, K. (1963). Uncertainty and the welfare economics of medical care. *American Economic Review*, **53**, 941–73.

Bayoumi, A. M. (2004). The measurement of contingent valuation for health economics. *PharmacoEconomics*, **22**, 691–700.

Bennett, J. and Blamey, R. (2001). *The choice modelling approach to environmental valuation.* Edward Elgar, Cheltenham.

Berwick, D.M. and Weinstein, M.C. (1985). What do patients value? Willingness-to-pay for ultrasound in normal pregnancy. *Medical Care*, **23**, 881–93.

Birch, S. and Donaldson, C. (1987). Applications of cost benefit analysis to health care departures from welfare economic theory. *Journal of Health Economics*, **6**, 211–25.

Bryan, S. and Dolan, P. (2004). Discrete choice experiments in health economics: for better or for worse? *European Journal of Health Economics*, **5**, 199–202.

Bryan, S., Gold, L., Sheldon, R., and Buxton, M. (2000). Preference measurement using conjoint methods: an empirical investigation of reliability. *Health Economics*, **9**, 385–95.

Carlsson, P. and Martinsson, P. (2003). Design techniques for stated preference methods in health economics. *Health Economics*, **12**, 281–94.

Dalmau-Matarradona, E. (2001). Alternative approaches to obtain optimal bid values in contingent valuation studies and to model protest zeros: estimating the determinants of individuals' willingness to pay for home care services in day case surgery. *Health Economics*, **10**, 101–18.

Diener, A., O'Brien, B., and Gafni, A. (1998). Health care contingent valuation studies: a review and classification of the literature. *Health Economics*, **7**, 313–26.

Donaldson, C. (1990). Willingness to pay for publicly-provided goods: a possible measure of benefit? *Journal of Health Economics*, **6**, 103–18.

Donaldson, C. and Shackley, P. (1997). Does 'process utility' exist? A case study of willingness to pay for laparoscopic cholecystectomy. *Social Science and Medicine*, **44**, 699–707.

Donaldson, C., Shackley, P., Abdalla, M., and Miedzybrodzka, Z. (1995). Willingness to pay for antenatal carrier screening for cystic fibrosis. *Health Economics*, **4**, 439–52.

Donaldson, C., Mapp, T., Farrar, S., Walker, A., and Macphee, S. (1997a). Assessing community values in health care: is the 'willingness to pay' method feasible? *Health Care Analysis*, **5**, 7–29.

Donaldson, C., Thomas, R., and Torgerson, D. J. (1997b). Validity of open-ended and payment scale approaches to eliciting willingness to pay. *Applied Economics*, **29**, 79–84.

Dranitsaris, G., Elia-Pacitti, J., and Cottrell, W. (2004). Measuring treatment preferences and willingness to pay for docetaxel in advanced ovarian cancer. *PharmacoEconomics*, **22**, 375–87.

Drummond, M. F. and Stoddart, G. L. (1995). Economic evaluation of health-producing technologies across different sectors: Can valid methods be developed? *Health Policy*, **33**, 219–31.

Drummond, M. F., Mohide, E. A., Tew, M., Streiner, D. L., Pringle, D. M., and Gilbert, J. R. (1991). Economic evaluation of a support programme for caregivers of demented elderly. *International Journal of Technology Assessment in Health Care*, 7, 209–19.

Fisher, A., Chestnut, L. G., and Violette, D. M. (1989). The value of reducing risks of death: A note on new evidence. *Journal of Policy and Management*, 8, 88.

Frew, E. J., Whynes, D. K., and Wolstenholme, J. L. (2003). Eliciting willingness to pay: comparing closed-ended with open-ended and payment scale formats. *Medical Decision Making*, 23, 150–9.

Frew, E. J., Wolstenholme, J. L., and Whynes, D. K. (2004). Comparing willingness-to-pay: bidding game format versus open-ended and payment scale formats. *Health Policy*, 68, 289–98.

Gafni, A. (1991). Using willingness-to-pay as a measure of benefits: What is the relevant question to ask in the context of public decision-making? *Medical Care*, 29, 1246–52.

Gold, M. R., Siegel, J. E., Russell, L. B., and Weinstein, M. C. (ed.) (1996). *Cost-effectiveness in health and medicine*. Oxford University Press, New York.

Hicks, J. R. (1939). The foundation of welfare economics. *Economic Journal*, 49, 696–712.

Hicks, J. R. (1941). The four consumer surpluses. *The Review of Economic Studies*, 11, 31–41.

Huber, J. and Zwerina, K. (1996). The importance of utility balance in efficient choice set designs. *Journal of Marketing Research*, 33, 307–17.

Johannesson, M. (1996a). *Theory and methods of economic evaluation of health care*. Kluwer, Dordrecht.

Johannesson, M. (1996b). *Ex ante* versus expected willingness-to-pay. *Social Science and Medicine*, 42, 305–11.

Johannesson, M. and Jönsson, B. (1991). Economic evaluation in health care: Is there a role for cost–benefit analysis? *Health Policy*, 17, 1–23.

Johannesson, M. and Jönsson, B. (1991). Willingness to pay for antihypertensive therapy results of a Swedish pilot study. *Journal of Health Economics*, 10, 461–74.

Johannesson, M. and Jönsson, B., and Karlsson, G. (1996). Outcome measurement in economic evaluation. *Health Economics*, 5, 279–96.

Johansson, P. O. (1995). *Evaluating health risks*. Cambridge University Press, Cambridge.

Jones-Lee, M. W. (1976). *The value of a life: an economic analysis*. University of Chicago Press, Chicago.

Jones-Lee, M. W., Hammerton, M., and Phillips, P. R. (1985). The value of safety: Results of a national sample survey. *Economic Journal*, 95, 49–72.

Kaldor, N. (1939). Welfare propositions of economic and interpersonal comparisons of utility. *Economic Journal*, 49, 549–52.

Kartman, B., Andersson, F., and Johannesson, M. (1996). Willingness to pay for reductions in angina pectoris attacks. *Medical Decision Making*, 16, 246–53.

Klarman, H. E., Francis, J. O. S., and Rosenthal, G. (1968). Cost-effectiveness analysis applied to the treatment of chronic renal disease. *Medical Care*, 6, 48–54.

Klose, T. (1999). The contingent valuation method in health care. *Health Policy*, 47, 97–123.

Koplan, J. P., *et al.* (1979). Pertussis vaccine—an analysis of benefits, risk and costs. *New England Journal of Medicine*, 301, 906–11.

Labelle, R. and Hurley, J. (1992). Implications of basing health care resource allocations on cost–utility analysis in the presence of externalities. *Journal of Health Economics*, 11, 259–77.

Lancsar, E. and Savage, E. (2004). Deriving welfare measures from discrete choice experiments: inconsistency between current methods and random utility and welfare theory. *Health Economics Letters*, **13**, 901–7.

Louviere, J. J., Henscher, D. A., and Swait, J. D. (2000). *Stated choice methods. Analysis and application.* Cambridge, Cambridge University Press.

Marin, A. and Psacharopoulos, G. (1982). The reward for risk in the labour market: Evidence from the United Kingdom and a reconciliation with other studies. *Journal of Political Economy*, **90**, 827–53.

McIntosh, E. and Ryan, M. (2002). Using discrete choice experiments to derive welfare estimates for the provision of elective surgery: implications of discontinuous preferences. *Journal of Economic Psychology*, **23**, 367–82.

Mishan, E. J. (1971). Evaluation of life and limb: a theoretical approach. *Journal of Political Economy*, **79**, 687–706.

Mitchell, R. C. and Carson, R. T. (1989). *Using surveys to value public goods: the contingent valuation method.* Resources for the Future, Washington DC.

Mooney, G. (1977). *The valuation of human life.* MacMillan, London.

Mooney, G. (1992). Economics, medicine and health care. Wheatsheaf, Hemel Hempstead.

Morey, E. R., Rowe, R. D., and Watson, M. (1993). A repeated nested logit model of atlantic salmon fishing. *American Journal of Agricultural Economics*, **75**, 578–92.

Mushkin, S. (1978). Cost of disease and illness in the United States in the year 2000. *Public Health Reports*, **93**, 493.

National Oceanic and Atmospheric Administration. (1993). Natural resource damage assessments under the oil pollution act of 1990. Notice of proposed rules. *Federal Register*, **58**, R4612.

Neumann, P. and Johannesson, M. (1994). The willingness-to-pay for *in vitro* fertilization: A pilot study using contingent valuation. *Medical Care*, **32**, 686–99.

Neumann, P. J., Sandberg, E. A., Araki, S. S., Kuntz, K. M., Feeny, D., and Weinstein, M. C. (2000). A comparison of HU12 and HU13 utility scores in Alzheimer's disease. *Medical Decision Making*, **20**, 413–22.

O'Brien, B. and Gafni, A. (1996). When do the 'dollars' make sense? Toward a conceptual framework for contingent valuation studies in health care. *Medical Decision Making*, **16**, 288–99.

O'Brien, B. and Viramontes, J. L. (1994). Willingness-to-pay: A valid and reliable measure of health state preference? *Medical Decision Making*, **14**, 289–97.

O'Brien, B. J., Novosel, S., Torrance, G., and Streiner, D. (1995). Assessing the economic value of a new antidepressant: A willingness-to-pay approach. *PharmacoEconomics*, **8**, 34–45.

O'Brien, B., Goeree, R., Gafni, A., *et al.* (1998). Assessing the value of a new pharmaceutical: a feasibility study of contingent valuation in managed care. *Medical Care*, **36**, 370–84.

Olsen, J. A. and Donaldson, C. (1997). Helicopters, hearts and hips: using willingness to pay to set principles for public sector health care programmes. *Social Science and Medicine*, **46**, 1–12.

Olsen, J. A. and Smith, R. D. (2001). Theory versus practice: a review of 'willingness-to-pay' in health and health care. *Health Economics*, **10**, 39–52.

Olsen, J. A., Kidholm, K., Donaldson, C., and Shackley, P. (2004). Willingness to pay for public health care: a comparison of two approaches. *Health Policy*, **70**, 217–18.

Pauly, M. V. (1995). Valuing health care benefits in money terms. In: *Valuing health care* (ed. F.A. Sloan), pp. 99–124. Cambridge University Press, Cambridge.

Phelps, C. E. and Mushlin, A. (1991). On the (near) equivalence of cost-effectiveness and cost–benefit analyses. *International Journal of Technology Assessment in Health Care*, **7**, 12–21.

Ratcliffe, J. (2000). The use of conjoint analysis to elicit willingness to pay. Proceed with caution? *International Journal of Technology Assessment in Health Care*, **16**, 270–90.

Ratcliffe, J., Buxton, M., McGarry, T., Sheldon, R., and Chancellor, J. (2004). Patients' preferences for characteristics associated with treatments for arthritis. *Rheumatology*, **43**, 337–45.

Reed-Johnson, F., Fries, E. E., and Banzhaf, H. S. (1994). *Valuing morbidity: an integration of the willingness-to-pay and health status literatures*, Working Paper No. T-G401, Triangle Economic Research, North Carolina.

Ryan, M. and Farrar, S. (2000). Using conjoint analysis to elicit preferences for health care. *British Medical Journal*, **320**, 1530–3.

Ryan, M. and Gerard, K. (2003). Using discrete choice experiment to value health care programmes: current practice and future research reflections. *Applied Health Economics and Health Policy*, **2**, 55–64.

Ryan, M., McIntosh, E., and Shackley, P. (1998). Methodological issues in the application of conjoint analysis in health care. *Health Economics*, **7**, 373–8.

Ryan, M., Ratcliffe, J., and Tucker, J. (1997). Using willingness to pay to value alternative models of antenatal care. *Social Science and Medicine*, **44**, 371–80.

Ryan, M., Scott, D. A., and Donaldson, C. (2004). Valuing health care using willingness to pay: a comparison of the payment card and dichotomous choice methods. *Journal of Health Economics*, **23**, 237–58.

Schoenbaum, S. C., Hyde, J. N., Bartoshesky, L., and Crampton, K. (1976). Benefit–cost analysis of rubella vaccination policy. *New England Journal of Medicine*, **294**, 306–10.

Scott, A., Watson, M. S., and Ross, S. (2003). Eliciting preferences of the community for out-of-hours care provided by general practitioners: a stated preference discrete choice experiment. *Social Science and Medicine*, **50**, 804–14.

Sculpher, M. J., Bryan, S., Fry, P., de Winter, P., Payne, H., and Emberton, M. (2004). Patients' preferences for the management of non-metastatic prostate cancer: discrete choice experiment. *British Medical Journal*, **328**, 382.

Shackley, P. and Donaldson, C. (2002). Should we use willingness to pay to elicit community preferences for health care? New evidence from the 'marginal' approach. *Journal of Health Economics*, **21**, 971–91.

Skjoldborg, U. S. and Gyrd-Hansen, D. (2003). Conjoint analysis. The cost variable: an Achille's heel? *Health Economics*, **12**, 479–91.

Smith, R. D. (2003). Construction of the contingent valuation market in health care: a critical assessment. *Health Economics*, **12**, 609–28.

Stalhammer, N. O. (1996). An empirical note on willingness-to-pay and starting-point bias. *Medical Decision Making*, **16**, 242–7.

Stalhammer, N. O. and Johannesson, M. (1996). Valuation of health changes with the contingent valuation method: a test of scope and question order effects. *Health Economics*, **5**, 531–41.

Stewart, J. M., O'Shea, E., Donaldson, C., and Shackley, P. (2002). Do ordering effects matter in willingness-to-pay studies of health care? *Journal of Health Economics*, **21**, 585–99.

Sugden, R. and Williams, A. H. (1979). *The principles of practical cost–benefit analysis*. Oxford University Press, Oxford.

Thompson, M. S. (1986). Willingness-to-pay and accepts risks to cure chronic disease. *American Journal of Public Health*, **76**, 392–6.

Viscusi, K. P. (1992). *Fatal trade-offs*. Oxford University Press, Oxford.

Wagner, T. H., Hu, T.-W., Duenas, G. V., and Pasick, R. J. (2000). Willingness to pay for mammography: item development and testing among five ethnic groups. *Health Policy*, **53**, 105–21.

Weinstein, M. C. and Fineberg, H. V. (1980). *Clinical decision analysis*. Saunders, Philadelphia.

Weisbrod, B. A. (1964). Collective consumption services of individual consumption goods. *Quarterly Journal of Economics*, **78**, 471–7.

Whynes, D. K., Frew, E. J., and Wolstenholme, J. L. (2003). A comparison of two methods for eliciting contingent valuations of colorectal cancer screening. *Journal of Health Economics*, **22**, 555–74.

Williams, A. (1974). The cost–benefit approach. *British Medical Bulletin*, **30**, 252–6.

Zarnke, K. B., Levine, M. A. H., and O'Brien, B. J. (1997). Cost–benefit analysis in the health care literature: don't judge a study by its label. *Journal of Clinical Epidemiology*, **50(7)**, 813–22.

Chapter 8

Economic evaluation using patient-level data

8.1. Introduction

In this chapter we review some general principles concerning economic evaluation using patient-level data, which usually means the collection of data alongside *randomized controlled trials*. Many of the issues covered are also pertinent, however, when an observational study is used as a vehicle for economic evaluation (for example, analysis of patient records or charts). The intent of the chapter is to examine general issues that are common to all the techniques of economic evaluation. The discussion of specific issues, such as the collection and analysis of utility or willingness-to-pay data, can be found in earlier chapters. Undertaking economic evaluation based on the secondary analysis of data using the approach of decision analytic modelling is considered in Chapter 9. The emphasis here is to illustrate different *analytic strategies* that face a researcher embarking upon a new study involving primary data collection. Previous chapters have indicated what information needs to be collected, at least in theory, for economic evaluation. This chapter addresses two pragmatic empirical questions: (1) How do I collect relevant data? (2) How do I analyse the data when I have them? A particularly important aim of the chapter is to describe, in non-technical terms, some of the important developments in the statistical analysis of patient-level data collected in trial-based cost-effectiveness studies.

8.2. Randomized trials and economic evaluation

8.2.1. The 'piggyback' economic evaluation

For health care interventions such as new pharmaceuticals, many countries have formal requirements for provision of safety and efficacy data prior to product licensing. The accepted standard for the collection of such data is the randomized controlled trial. Given that these trials are typically a necessary condition for the successful licensing of a pharmaceutical, it is reasonable to assess whether economic data could also be collected within the same study and thus facilitate a trial-based economic evaluation. That is, can economic evaluation simply be 'piggybacked' on to an existing clinical trial? The advantages of having economic evaluation data collected prospectively as part of the trial are that (1) having patient-specific data on both costs and outcomes is potentially attractive for analysis and internal validity; (2) given the (typically) large fixed costs incurred in collecting clinical data, the marginal cost of collecting economic data may be modest.

There are, however, numerous issues and problems that researchers face when conducting economic evaluation as part of a trial that has been designed primarily for clinical purposes (for example, licensing). We have already touched on one philosophical issue concerning the timing of data availability. Particularly for pharmaceuticals, it may not be possible to collect 'real-world' data, ideally required for economic evaluation, before the drug is in the marketplace. A number of other potential limitations are considered below.

1. *Choice of comparison therapy*. A threat to the external validity of any cost-effectiveness study (that is, its generalizability to patients other than those in the trial) exists when the comparison therapy is not the most relevant for the policy question being addressed. In many countries, a placebo comparison plays an important role in regulatory approval of new medicines. For economic evaluation, the relevance of a placebo-controlled study depends upon whether the new drug is intended as *adjunctive* therapy or as a *substitute* for an existing therapy that is the current standard of care. For example, in assessing the cost-effectiveness of a new antiemetic drug, ondansetron, Buxton and O'Brien (1992) made comparison (using published trials) against a widely used and effective existing therapy, metoclopramide (Rusthoven *et al.* 1992). Trials comparing against placebo, as a proxy for no therapy (Cubeddu *et al.* 1990; Beck *et al.* 1993) would not be a relevant comparison for the economic question because they do not reveal the incremental impact of the new therapy on population health.

In some circumstances, placebo comparison data may be appropriate for economic studies; this is typically the case where the new drug will not be a substitute for another but will be a new *adjunctive* therapy. An example would be the placebo-controlled trials of misoprostol for prophylaxis against gastrointestinal complications in persons taking anti-inflammatory drugs; a number of economic studies were undertaken using these trial data (Drummond *et al.* 1992). Here the placebo is a close approximation to no additional therapy.

In circumstances where the relevant comparison is an existing therapy and head-to-head comparative trials have been done, the active comparison used in the trial(s) may not be the most relevant for the economic analysis. For example, in Canada, the approval of the first low-molecular-weight heparin (enoxaparin) for prophylaxis against deep-vein thrombosis (DVT) following orthopaedic surgery was based on trial comparisons against standard heparin. Although the cost-effectiveness of enoxaparin versus standard heparin was studied (Anderson *et al.* 1993) this may not have been the most relevant economic comparison because survey evidence suggested that low-dose warfarin was the most widely used drug for this indication in North America (Paiment *et al.* 1987). However, a revised economic analysis, based on decision analysis but comparing enoxaparin and warfarin (O'Brien *et al.* 1994*a*), had a weaker inferential base for efficacy because no head-to-head trials of these drugs had been published.

In some circumstances, the cost-effectiveness of a new intervention will have to be assessed against a number of alternative new options as well as existing therapies. An example was a recent economic evaluation of new treatments for epilepsy in adults where six new therapies were compared with each other and two older interventions (Wilby *et al.* 2003).

2. *Gold standard measurement of outcomes.* Randomized trials often employ measurements for outcomes that are more detailed, invasive, or frequent than is customary in usual care. For example, in comparing alternative acid suppressant drugs, the outcome of duodenal ulcer recurrence is usually determined in clinical trials by endoscopy of all patients at fixed follow-up times (Walt *et al.* 1984); but outside of a trial, the management of such patients would be based largely upon symptoms. For an economic analysis to relate to routine practice, it must reflect the fact that some persons without symptoms will have ulcer recurrence (although silent) and some persons with symptoms may not have ulcer recurrence. This might require the analyst to attempt some adjustment of trial-based ulcer recurrence rates based on the proportion that are symptomatic and would be observed in clinical practice. (This issue was discussed in Chapter 5.)

Another example is the diagnosis of DVT in clinical trials of low-molecular-weight heparin. The gold standard measurement in such studies is venography—an invasive, relatively expensive, often painful test involving injection of contrast media. But in routine clinical practice if venography is not universally and routinely used as the first-line test for DVT, how useful is this knowledge of the 'truth' for economic evaluation? In the study of enoxaparin referred to above (O'Brien *et al.* 1994*a*), the true rates of DVT (by venography) were used from the trial as the prior probabilities of disease for treatment and control, in a decision analytic model which incorporated the conditional likelihood and costs of these DVTs being detected by a routine diagnostic algorithm based on clinical signs and symptoms and ultrasound. Such a model includes the costs and outcomes of errors in diagnosis that will happen in routine practice but were not part of the trial because the physician will not generally use costly and invasive tests as first-line therapy. Such 'adjustments' to efficacy data are necessary to make data appropriate for decision-making, but they also require some non-trial data inputs, for example, on the sensitivity and specificity of clinical diagnosis and ultrasound.

3. *Intermediate versus final health outcomes.* Some interventions are expected to have a beneficial impact on health outcomes but not for many years. Pharmaceuticals with such a feature have often been assessed in trials that have been designed to detect differences in one or more intermediate biomedical markers. If there is considered to be reasonable evidence that the intermediate marker is predictive of the ultimate measure of health gain such as reduced long-term mortality, then showing difference in the intermediate endpoint may be sufficient for the product to be licensed. The early trials of cholesterol-lowering drugs are a good example where the outcome is the measured change in total blood cholesterol or some subfraction (O'Brien 1991).

For decisions about resource allocation, however, knowing that an intervention has a positive impact on an intermediate marker is not sufficient to show cost-effectiveness, and the impact on *final* health outcomes such as mortality and morbidity will have to be indirectly quantified. As mentioned in Chapter 5 and discussed more fully in Chapter 9, this quantitative link is often made using decision modelling based on epidemiological data. In the case of cholesterol-lowering drugs, for example, data from cohort studies such as the Framingham study were used with models to predict changes in final outcomes (for example, deaths and myocardial infarctions) from changes in risk factors such as blood serum cholesterol (Morris *et al.* 1997). Over the longer term, trials may emerge that seek to confirm the link between the intermediate and final outcomes by directly measuring the impact of an intervention on changes in health. In the case of cholesterol-lowering therapies, for example, this was the case with the 4S Study (Scandinavian Simvastatin Survival Study Group 1994) and Heart Protection Study (Heart Protection Study Collaborative Group 2002) both of which had a follow-up period of several years. These 'outcome trials' have supported economic evaluations that will inform future resource use decisions (Johannesson *et al.* 1997), but this sort of trial is typically unavailable when therapies are launched.

4. *Inadequate patient follow-up or sample size.* A feature of many clinical trials is that patient follow-up and data collection often terminate abruptly when the patient experiences one of the clinical outcome 'events' of interest. From the perspective of the economic analyst this can be frustrating as the cost-effectiveness of an intervention may be dependent on the patient's prognosis subsequent to the event. Many examples can be found in cardiovascular therapy where events such as stroke or myocardial infarction are recorded but with no indication of their longer-term implications for health outcomes and costs.

Another important issue regarding economic evaluation alongside clinical trials is whether the sample size is appropriate for economic analysis. Over the last decade, there has been considerable development in methods for the statistical analysis of economic data as part of trials. In part, this has included consideration of the extent to which standard hypothesis testing, which predominates in the clinical evaluation literature, is also relevant to economic analysis. If so, there would be clear implications for the methods used to select sample sizes for economic evaluations based on randomized trials. These issues are discussed further in Section 8.3.2.

5. *Protocol-driven costs and outcomes.* A problem with basing cost estimates on data gathered as part of a trial designed for clinical evaluation is the extent to which one is capturing resource use associated with the trial *per se* (that is, including the costs of doing the research) rather than the costs of providing the therapy. These so-called *protocol-driven costs* can arise in a number of different ways. For example, to preserve blinding in their comparison of oral gold (auranofin) versus placebo, Thompson *et al.* (1989) required regular blood tests for patients randomized to placebo; in the analysis they excluded these costs from the placebo control group. However, excluding these protocol-driven costs may not be the only factor requiring adjustment because there may also be some form of ascertainment bias in that patients in both groups were seeing a physician more regularly for tests than in routine practice and therapy may have been modified based on observations that would not occur outside the trial. The point to stress is that, at the outset of any clinical trial where an economic question is also being addressed, it is important to establish the extent to which patient management and resource use reflects regular practice.

As experience with economic evaluation alongside clinical trials increases, there will be more subtle protocol biases to consider. For example, the requirement in many trials that the physician be blind to the treatment assigned to a patient may have a bearing upon the way that patient is managed in the trial. In routine practice, *knowing* that the patient is receiving a given treatment may make the physician less cautious in terms of frequency of observation or test-ordering; this therefore poses a threat to the external validity of the cost data collected within the trial (Freemantle and Drummond 1997).

Another central feature of clinical trials is the emphasis of conforming to the rules mandated by the protocol, the principle of compliance by physicians and patients. Great efforts are typically made in the conduct of a clinical trial to ensure that patients consume their prescribed medications and that physicians prescribe such drugs according to protocol. Outside of the trial, when the drug is used in routine practice, there are no such guarantees. To the extent that patients do not comply with the prescribed therapy, there may be a dilution of the treatment effect originally observed in the trial. For example, the Lipid Research Clinics Coronary Primary Prevention Trial (Lipid Research Clinics Programme 1984) demonstrated a clear association between compliance with the study drug (cholestyramine for cholesterol lowering) and outcomes. This leads one to speculate by how much any observed treatment effect will be diluted when the drug is being prescribed outside the strictures of a trial, when compliance may drop even further. Hughes *et al.* (2001) provide a good review of the issues related to patient compliance in economic evaluation.

8.2.2. Pragmatic trials for economic evaluation

Rather than attempting to 'piggyback' economic evaluation questions on to an existing clinical trial designed to address safety and efficacy questions, an alternative option is to design trials specifically as a vehicle for economic evaluation. Using the distinction between the 'explanatory' orientation (that is, can the intervention work?) versus the 'pragmatic' orientation (that is, does the intervention work?), introduced by Schwartz and Lellouch (1967), the focus of an economic trial would be pragmatic. The intention is to offer some compromise between the goals of internal and external validity (that is, avoiding bias and maximizing generalizability); the pragmatic trial retains the concept of subjects being randomly allocated to treatments to minimize bias, but offers fewer restrictions in how patients are recruited and followed after randomization, thus increasing external validity or generalizability.

The aim of pragmatic trials is to evaluate the effectiveness or cost-effectiveness of an intervention under the real-world conditions that would prevail once the intervention was in routine use (Schwartz and Lellouch 1967; Buxton *et al.* 1997). The main design features of such studies are that

(1) patients typical of the normal caseload are enrolled;

(2) the therapy of interest is compared with current care;

(3) the settings and physicians involved are fairly representative of the totality;

(4) physicians and patients are not blind to the therapy (in order to take into account all the advantages or disadvantages of therapy);

(5) all enrolled patients are followed under routine conditions;

(6) a wide range of endpoints is measured (efficacy, feasibility, tolerance, quality of life, resource use, and so on).

As an example of a pragmatic trial that examined economic endpoints, Oster *et al.* (1995, 1996) compared two strategies for lowering elevated cholesterol in a pragmatic trial based in a health maintenance organization in California. They assessed cost, clinical outcome (in post-treatment total serum cholesterol), and patient satisfaction with the Health Maintenance Organisation's current regimen (stepped care with niacin followed by other agents) compared with first-line therapy with lovastatin. Every attempt was made to make the trial reflect real-world practice and delivery of care; physicians determined the frequency of follow-up visits and the dose of the drug. Furthermore, patients incurred some expenses for their medications as they would in regular practice. (Another good example of a pragmatic trial is the FIRST study; see Schulman *et al.* 1996.)

Despite examples of successful pragmatic randomized trials for economic evaluation, they retain some of the general problems associated with using trials as a vehicle for economic evaluation. These include the difficulty of comparing more than two or three options and the problems of long-term follow-up. Such considerations have led to the view that modelling in economic evaluation is 'an unavoidable fact of life' (Buxton *et al.* 1997). The limitations of trial-based economic evaluation and the role of decision analytic modelling is discussed in Chapter 9.

8.2.3. **Data collection issues**

When collecting resource use data as part of a clinical trial, we have already discussed the need to identify and minimize resource consequences that are due to the research protocol and do not characterize the delivery of care in the normal setting. But how does one actually collect the resource quantities associated with therapy as part of the evaluation? The first point is that, to the extent possible, it makes sense to build upon the research infrastructure that will be already in place for collecting the clinical data. For example, many clinical trials of hospital-based acute therapies would collect data using a case report form (CRF) designed for completion by a study nurse. To facilitate collection of resource quantities associated with therapy, one can add pages to the same CRF and extend the responsibility of data collection by the study nurse to include key items of resources. Studies will obviously vary in the amount of detail and precision needed in the collection of resource quantities. At a minimum, for a hospital-based study, it would be desirable to know the total length of stay in hospital, the length of stay in high-cost areas such as intensive care, and major diagnostic or therapeutic procedures such as computed tomography scans or surgery. As we discussed in Chapter 3, depending upon the intervention being evaluated, the precision of costing may need to be much greater. For example, if one is comparing two alternative treatments in the intensive care unit, much more detailed information on the resources consumed in the intensive care unit would obviously be appropriate.

In addition to the resource quantities associated with the initiation of therapy, it is also necessary to capture downstream resource consequences of the treatment or the disease. Typically these downstream costs could be an exacerbation of the problem warranting re-admission to hospital, or a mild complication resulting in consultation with a family physician or attendance at an emergency room. Capturing these data is more problematic for a number of reasons. First, if a person is re-hospitalized at a hospital that is not part of the clinical trial, then knowledge of this re-hospitalization and access to information on resource consumption from that hospital may be limited. To facilitate information retrieval it may be necessary to ensure that patients have given approval for such data gathering as part of the informed consent documentation. The monitoring of such events can be achieved either by patient recall or, depending upon local circumstances, it may be possible to use computerized databases of physician reimbursement claims or hospital discharges.

In many trials, ambulatory physician visits are often recorded using patient recall. For example, are the patients asked whether they have seen a family doctor in the past 3 months for a reason associated with their hypertension or its treatment? As with any survey technique, the reliability of patient recall comes into question, particularly when one is studying population groups where recall may be a problem (for example, the elderly). Also, the method of follow-up contact could be by mail survey or telephone follow-up, and depending upon the patient group being studied there are advantages and disadvantages of both methods. Readers who are interested in more detailed discussion of principles of data collection for economic data as part of trials and design of CRFs should consult Mauskopf *et al.* (1996) and Glick *et al.* (2001).

8.3. **Statistical analysis of patient-level data**

Increased use of trial-based economic evaluation has led to a greater focus on issues of statistical analysis. This is because such studies provide data on resource use, treatment effect and, in many cases, utility for all or a subsample of patients in the study. This provides an opportunity to consider the uncertainty around estimates of costs and (in most cases) cost-effectiveness in the patient *population* or subpopulation of interest based on the *sample* data in the trial.

Hence the presence of sampled patient-level data on costs and effects offers the opportunity to move from *deterministic* to *stochastic* analysis for trial-based economic evaluation. Deterministic economic analysis is where cost and effect variables are analysed as point estimates. In the context of trials, this could be because there has been a focus solely on mean estimates, with the precision of those estimates ignored. If we consider a treatment that is both more costly and more effective than control, the economic comparison was illustrated in the top right quadrant of the cost-effectiveness plane (see Box 3.1). The slope of the line extending from the origin (the control) through our study estimate, point A, represents the incremental cost-effectiveness of the treatment relative to control. In the absence of any data on sampling variation for costs or effects, some form of sensitivity analysis would then be used to determine plausible ranges that may contain the true cost-effectiveness ratio.

As discussed in Chapter 3 (and more fully in Chapter 9), there are three major limitations with sensitivity analysis.

1 The analyst has discretion as to which variables and what alternative values are included in the sensitivity analysis, creating the potential for a form of selection bias (conscious or otherwise).

2 Interpretation of a sensitivity analysis is essentially arbitrary because there are no guidelines or standards as to what degree of variation in results is acceptable evidence that the analysis is 'robust'.

3 Variation of uncertain parameters *one at a time* carries a risk that interactions between parameters may not be captured.

A *stochastic cost-effectiveness analysis* is where both costs and effects are determined from data sampled from the same patients in a study. If cost and effect data are sampled and variances are available, then formal statistical methods can be used on observed differences in costs (treatment–control) or effects.

This section examines some of the statistical issues that arise in the conduct of stochastic economic evaluation based on patient-level data. This is an area of methodology that has developed rapidly over the last 10 years, and it is outside the scope of this book to provide a comprehensive guide to all the issues. Rather, the purpose of this section is to summarize the main developments. For more detailed overviews, see Heyse *et al.* (2001), Glick *et al.* (2001), Briggs *et al.* (2002), and Briggs (2003).

8.3.1. The nature of economic data

If the data collected in trials for purposes of economic evaluation were, in terms of their statistical features, very similar to those collected in clinical evaluations, there would be little to write in this section! However, one of the reasons why there has been so much interest in statistical methods for economic evaluation alongside trials is that economic data are not synonymous with clinical data and have required the development of new methods, or the adaptation of existing techniques, to analyse them appropriately. Below some of the characteristics of economic data are described.

1. *Skewed cost data*. Many of the interesting statistical issues in trial-based economic evaluation relate to the analysis of cost data. Cost data are usually right skewed (Briggs and Gray 1999). This is because costs are naturally bounded by zero (they cannot be negative), but they have no logical upper bound. In the context of a trial, it is quite common to have a small proportion of patients with very high costs, perhaps reflecting serious adverse effects of treatment with low prevalence. The cost of this small number of patients has a much bigger effect on mean cost than the median, giving the distribution its characteristic right-skewed shape. This feature of cost data is illustrated in Fig. 8.1 using results from a trial-based economic evaluation of laparoscopic compared to open abdominal hysterectomy (Garry *et al.* 2004; Sculpher *et al.* 2004).

Faced with skewed data, a standard approach in clinical evaluation would be to provide a summary measure of the distribution in the form of the median. In the context of costs, however, this is inappropriate given that the decision-maker needs to be able to link the summary measure of cost per patient to the overall budget impact, and this can only be achieved with the mean. Other ways of dealing with skewed data have been suggested such as data transformations and non-parametric hypothesis tests, but these have limitations (Briggs and Gray 1999). The method of non-parametric bootstrapping is increasingly used to analyse cost data (Briggs and Gray 1998, 1999; Barber and Thompson 1998), but this too has been criticised (O'Hagan and Stevens 2003)

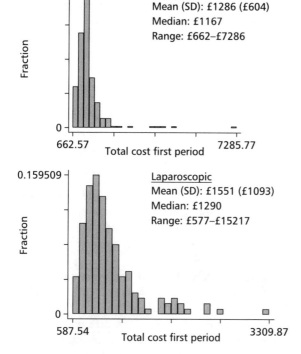

Fig. 8.1 Illustration of right-skewed cost data from a randomized trial comparing laparoscopic and abdominal hysterectomy (Garry *et al.* 2004; Sculpher *et al.* 2004). Costs relate to an initial period of 6 weeks following surgery.

(Section 8.3.2 provides more detail on bootstrapping methods). In addition, some work has been undertaken exploring the use of statistical methods to model the underlying factors that might lead to a patient being an 'outlier' in term of costs, including two-stage regression models (Lipscomb *et al.* 1998; Cooper *et al.* 2003).

Given these methodological uncertainties, the analyst would be well advised to present as much detail about the cost distribution as possible. The development of appropriate methods for the analysis of cost data is an important area for future research.

2. *Missing data*. In all economic studies involving the collection of patient-level data, it is likely that there will be some missing data. This can happen for a variety of reasons including patients failing to respond to questionnaires or being lost to follow-up, or items in CRFs not being completed by clinical or research staff. Missing data on economic measurements can be a particular problem if these items are accorded less priority by clinical and research staff. The problem of missing data also exists in clinical evaluation, but it has some particularly important implications for economic analysis. The estimation of mean cost will typically be based on a number of items of resource use data, each of which is multiplied by a relevant unit cost, and total cost is the aggregation across these items (see Chapter 4). If any one of these resource items is missing for a particular patient, then it is not clear how to estimate that patient's total cost. Various methods are available to address this problem, none of which is specific to the analysis of economic data (Briggs *et al.* 2003). A simple method is to

analyse the costs of those patients for whom complete data are available (this is referred to as *complete case analysis*). However, in studies where there are a lot of resource use data on each patient, a large proportion of patients may have at least one item of missing data. This will mean that complete case analysis will relate to relatively few patients and relevant data will be 'thrown away' resulting in mean costs being estimated with less precision than necessary. Hence it may be the case that, although the proportion of resource use items that is missing is quite small, the proportion of patients with missing total costs is high.

Alternative techniques to 'fill in' the missing data, based on those data that have been collected, are available and have been used in trial-based economic evaluations (Briggs *et al.* 2003). The validity of each method in part rests on the important issue of the extent to which the 'missingness' of the data is random.

3. *Censored cost data*. A specific type of missing data relates to situations where patients have been followed up for differential time periods, which leads to censored data. One example of this is administrative censoring, when patients are recruited into a trial over a period of time (for example, 2 years), but analysis is undertaken at a specific time point based on all available data (for example, 1 year after the last patient is recruited). This means that the extent of follow-up data will vary between patients—in this example, the minimum follow-up period will be 1 year and the maximum 3 years.

A key assumption when analysing censored data is that censoring is 'non-informative'; that is, the patients who are fully followed up (uncensored) are representative of those who are censored. Standard methods exist for the analysis of censored time-to-event data (for example, time until death), typically the Kaplan–Meier estimator (Kahn and Sempos 1989). However, these methods are not appropriate to analyse censored cost data and will lead to biased estimates (Hallstrom and Sullivan, 1998; Etzioni *et al.* 1999). This is because different patients can accumulate costs at different rates over time, so two patients who are censored at the same time, but with different accumulated cost, would ultimately be expected to have different total costs if they had been fully followed up. Hence the assumption of non-informative censoring is no longer tenable. Various methods have been developed in recent years to analyse censored costs appropriately. It is not within the scope of this book to describe these methods in detail, but O'Hagan and Stevens (2004) provide good overviews of the methods and principles and Raikou and McGuire (2004) offer some comparison of methods.

4. *Difficulties with incremental cost-effectiveness ratios*. As described in Chapters 2, 3, and 5, the incremental cost-effectiveness ratio (ICER) is the traditional summary result from a cost-effectiveness or cost–utility analysis. A statistical issue that has been of some interest in the literature since the mid-1990s relates to how to present the statistical uncertainty around the ICER when it is derived from sampled patient-level data on costs and effects (see Section 8.3.2). The development of appropriate methods for this purpose has been hampered by some particular features of the ICER that make it difficult to handle statistically (Briggs 2001). One problem relates to the issue of negative ICERs, and can be described with reference to Box 8.1. The diagram shows a cost-effectiveness plane (see Box 3.1 for an introduction) with two different comparisons of a New Intervention relative to a Standard Intervention. In the top left quadrant, Comparison A shows a situation where the Standard Intervention dominates the New Intervention, with lower costs and higher effects. In the bottom right

Box 8.1 **The problem of negative incremental cost-effectiveness ratios**

Treatment	Costs	Effects	ICER
Comparison A			
New Intervention	80	5	
Standard Intervention	60	7	
Difference	+20	−2	−10
Comparison B			
New Intervention	65	12	
Standard Intervention	85	10	
Difference	−20	+2	−10

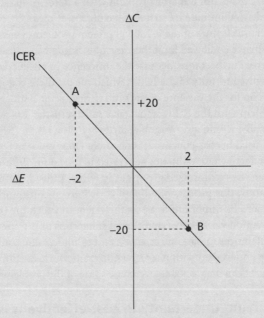

Comparison A (in the top right quadrant) shows that the new intervention is dominated as it has higher costs and lower effects than the standard intervention. For Comparison B, the converse is true with the new intervention dominating the standard intervention. Yet, in these very different situations, the ICER is identical

quadrant, the New Intervention is dominant (Comparison B). Despite these quite different results, the ICER is identical for the two comparisons (−10). This feature of the ICER is not necessarily a problem for a deterministic analysis based on a point estimate of differential cost and effect, because it is clear in which quadrant the comparison is located. However, when the uncertainty around the point estimates is allowed for, the ICER and its uncertainty could span more than one quadrant and the feature of the ICER shown in Box 8.1 can make this uncertainty difficult to present.

A second, and related, problem is that when the comparison is located in the top left and bottom right quadrants of the cost-effectiveness plane where one option is dominant and the ICER is negative, the magnitude of the ICER has no meaning. Consider three different comparisons in the bottom right quadrant:

(1) X results in 1 quality-adjusted life-year (QALY) gained, a saving of £2000, and hence an ICER of –£2000;

(2) Y results in 2 QALYs gained, a saving of £2000, and hence an ICER of –£1000;

(3) Z results in 2 QALYs gained, a saving of £1000, and hence an ICER of –£500.

In terms of ICERs, Z would be preferred to Y, which would be preferred to X. However, in terms of changes in costs and QALYs, Y would clearly be preferred to X and Z as it has the highest combination of QALY gain and cost saving.

Third, if the denominator of the ICER (the difference in effects) is zero, the ratio itself is infinite. This is not a major problem with a deterministic analysis as one treatment is likely to dominate by virtue of having lower mean costs. In a stochastic analysis, however, this feature of the ICER will present problems when the uncertainty in the effect difference is allowed for if there is a non-negligible probability of that difference being zero. Furthermore, because the difference in effects could be negative, this can cause a discontinuity in the ICER, which means there is no mathematically tractable expression for the variance of the ratio (Briggs *et al.* 2002).

A fourth problem with the ICER is that, as a ratio statistic, it is not easy to use as a dependent variable within a regression analysis and, as a result, these methods have not been widely used in cost-effectiveness research. However, it may be important to adjust the cost-effectiveness estimates generated in a trial for differences in patient case mix between the randomized groups at baseline. Indeed, in the context of an observational study, this process of adjusting for known confounding variables is essential. It may also be important to assess the extent to which the cost-effectiveness of a given intervention varies between different subgroups of patients. The process of adjusting for differences in baseline case mix and of undertaking subgroup analysis would ideally be undertaken within a regression framework. Section 8.3.2 describes methods that have been developed to overcome some of the problems with ICERs.

8.3.2. Quantifying uncertainty in cost-effectiveness using patient-level data

It is helpful to distinguish three general approaches to representing uncertainty in cost-effectiveness results: (1) hypothesis testing, (2) estimation, and (3) decision uncertainty. Each of these are dealt with below. It should be noted that these methods have been used to assess uncertainty in cost-effectiveness and cost–utility studies because these are the most popular forms of economic evaluation. They also, however, have relevance to cost–benefit studies.

1. *Hypothesis testing.* When patient-level sample data are available on costs and effects, it is possible to use formal hypothesis testing as a way of reflecting the

uncertainty in cost, effects, and cost-effectiveness (O'Brien *et al.* 1994*b*, *c*). In the analysis of effect data with associated sampling variation, the null hypothesis is usually that there is no difference in outcome between experimental and control therapy, and this is tested against either a one-tailed alternative (usually that the experimental treatment is more effective) or a two-tailed alternative (that the experimental treatment is more or less effective than the control).

A problem with hypothesis-testing as a form of stochastic analysis is that an overemphasis tends to be placed on the statistical significance of results (the size of the *P*-value) in isolation from the magnitude of the effect size. This can be illustrated with reference to Box 2.3. If a formal hypothesis test suggests that there is no statistically significant difference in effects between treatment and control, then it may seem logical to adopt the approach of cost-minimization analysis whereby the less costly treatment is the most cost-effective. However, unless the measure of effect in the cost-effectiveness study is the primary outcome measure, it is very unlikely that the trial would have been 'powered' to find a statistically significant difference in effects. This is likely to be the case, for example, when QALYs are the measure of effect in the study, but the trial was not powered to show a statistical difference in mortality or utility. Therefore, there is likely to be an important risk of rejecting the alternative hypothesis (that treatment is more effective than control) when in fact that hypothesis is correct (that is, a high type II error), and this error will be reflected in the economic evaluation (Briggs and O'Brien 2001).

Even if the trial had been formally powered to test a hypothesis around the effect measure used in the cost-effectiveness study, it may still be inappropriate to conclude that the lack of a statistically significant difference in effectiveness between a new treatment and control is synonymous with there being a difference of zero. The difference between the two sample means remains the best estimate of effect difference rather than zero. The importance of this point can be illustrated using the example of the cost-effectiveness analysis of laparoscopic versus open abdominal hysterectomy introduced above and in Box 8.1 (Garry *et al.* 2004; Sculpher *et al.* 2004). Over the full follow-up period of 1 year (as opposed to the short-term follow-up in Box 8.1), laparoscopic hysterectomy had an additional mean cost of £186 (95% confidence interval (CI), −£26 to £375) and additional mean QALYs of 0.007 (95% CI, −0.008 to 0.023). In neither case, therefore, were these differences statistically significant as the 95% CIs around them both crossed zero. How should a decision-maker react to these results? One option would be to interpret the data as saying that the lack of a statistically significant difference in costs and effects is synonymous with there being zero difference in these endpoints, and hence the options are identical in terms of cost-effectiveness. This is inappropriate as the mean differences remain the best estimates of differential costs and effects.

A second option is to adopt conventional rules of statistical inference and conclude that the data provide no basis, using a threshold *P*-value of 0.05, to reject the null hypotheses that open abdominal hysterectomy is less costly and more effective than the new laparoscopic technique, and that abdominal method should remain the preferred option. However, this assumes that the error probability inherent in the 0.05 *P*-value is appropriate for the decision. It may be the case that the decision-maker is willing to accept a much higher risk of inappropriately rejecting the null hypothesis. A third option is to reject conventional methods of statistical inference and focus on mean differences in costs and effects in which case laparoscopic hysterectomy would be preferred if the ICER (£186/0.007 = £26 571) is considered acceptable by the decision-maker. However, basing the decision on mean costs and effect differences alone would ignore the sampling uncertainty associated with those mean values.

2. *Estimation.* To what extent are these difficulties overcome by using estimation for cost-effectiveness rather than hypothesis testing? This is consistent with clinical evaluation for which statistical guidelines in a number of medical journals have generally recommended that, in preference to reporting only P-values, analyses should report the observed effect size with an associated CI (Gardner and Altman 1989). The advantage of the CI is that it yields information on the *magnitude* of the observed difference (quantitative significance or importance).

Defining a confidence region for cost-effectiveness. Of course, cost-effectiveness incorporates both cost and effect differences. Familiar CIs for the effectiveness of treatment can be defined:

$$(\bar{E}_T - \bar{E}_C) \pm t_{(n_T + n_C - 2, 1 - \frac{\alpha}{2})} \sqrt{\frac{s_{ET}^2}{n_T} + \frac{s_{EC}^2}{n_C}}$$

where s^2_{ET} and s^2_{EC} are the sample estimates of variances. If it is assumed that resource use was measured, patient-specific costs can be estimated from the same trial. Assuming patient i consumes j different types of resources $(j = 1 \dots J)$ in quantity Q_{ij} at unit price P_j, then the costs for individual i can be expressed as

$$C_i = \sum_{j=1}^{j} P_j Q_j$$

Note that the assumption has been made that the prices of resources are known with certainty. This would seem reasonable in that decision-makers in a given locality should know the prices they face. It may be that these prices *vary* between, for example, hospitals, but this is different to their being uncertain. To allow for variability in prices, the analysis could be undertaken as many times as there are different sets of prices.

Summing over i patients $(i = 1 \dots n_T)$ in the treatment group, mean cost per patient can be expressed as

$$\bar{C}_T = \frac{1}{n_T} \sum_{i=1}^{n_T} C_i$$

Therefore, the difference between the mean cost associated with treatment and control can be expressed as a CI. If it is reasonable to assume that the data are normally distributed (which, as discussed above, may be in doubt), this can be expressed as

$$(\bar{C}_T - \bar{C}_C) \pm t_{(n_T + n_C - 2, 1 - \frac{\alpha}{2})} \sqrt{\frac{s_{CT}^2}{n_T} + \frac{s_{CC}^2}{n_C}}$$

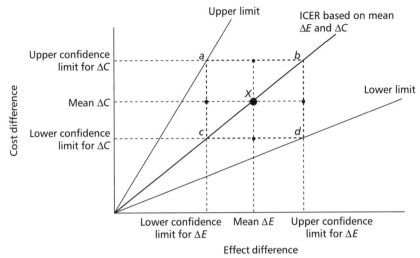

Fig. 8.2 The top right ('north-east') quadrant of the cost-effectiveness plane. This shows mean cost and effect differences (of treatment compared to control) at point X and the associated incremental cost-effectiveness ratio (ICER) represented by the bold line from the origin through that point. The 'confidence box' *abcd* is the combination of confidence intervals in cost and effect differences.

The combination of these simple 95% CIs for cost and effect differences can be portrayed as two-dimensional confidence regions for cost-effectiveness as in Fig. 8.2 (O'Brien *et al.* 1994*b*, *c*). The most simple definition of the confidence region is the 'confidence box' bounded by *abcd*. Rays from the origin passing through points *a* and *d* define a slice of pie based on the upper limits of each CI. The box approach assumes that the difference in costs is independent of (uncorrelated with) the difference in effects which would be unlikely in most situations. It is also the case that, when costs and effects are independent, the confidence box will represent 90% CIs although it is based on 95% intervals on individual costs and effects (Briggs 2001).

In order to reflect the co-variance in cost and effect differences rather than assume independence in these two parts of the ICER, the concept of the confidence ellipse was suggested (O'Brien *et al.* 1994*b*, 1994*c*; van Hout *et al.* 1994). The precise shape of the ellipsoid confidence region will depend upon co-variation between costs and effects (Gold *et al.* 1996). This is illustrated in Figs 8.3 and 8.4, which show situations where there is, respectively, positive and negative correlation between the numerator and denominator of the ICER. The ellipses are derived assuming a joint normal distribution in costs and effects. The rays drawn from the origin as tangents to the ellipses represent approximations to the 95% of the ICER. It is clear from Figs 8.3 and 8.4, however, that the width of the CIs defined by this method are highly dependent on the correlation between costs and effects and would only be the same as that defined by the confidence box by coincidence.

The statistical characteristics of the ICER, which were discussed above, mean that it has not been straightforward to define methods to calculate CIs for this measure of

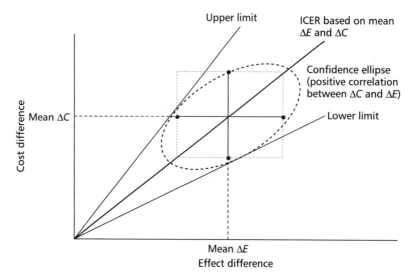

Fig. 8.3 The top right ('north-east') quadrant of the cost-effectiveness plane showing a confidence ellipse when there is positive correlation between costs and effects. ICER: Incremental cost-effectiveness ratio.

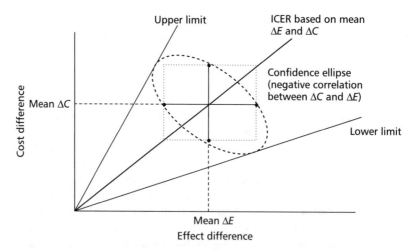

Fig. 8.4 The top right ('north-east') quadrant of the cost-effectiveness plane showing a confidence ellipse when there is negative correlation between costs and effects. ICER: incremental cost-effectiveness ratio.

cost-effectiveness. Several methods have been suggested to overcome these difficulties (see Briggs 2001), but two methods have been used regularly in the applied literature. The first is Fieller's method, which is based on work on ratio statistics undertaken in the 1930s. This was developed as a means of calculating an exact CI for the ICER allowing for the possible skewness in the sampling distribution of the ratio

(Chaudhary and Stearns 1996; Willan and O'Brien 1996). Like the ellipse method, however, the key assumption of Fieller's theorem is that the numerator and denominator of the ICER follow a joint normal distribution. This assumption may be overly strong given the skewness of sampled cost data.

Non-parametric bootstrapping (Efron and Tibshirani 1993) is the second method for deriving CIs for the ICER that has been adopted in applied studies (Chaudhary and Stearns 1996, Briggs *et al.* 1997; Obenchain *et al.* 1997). Rather than making assumptions about the underlying distributions in the ICER, this method re-samples from the original data to build an empirical estimate of the sampling distribution of the ICER. Box 8.2 summarizes the bootstrap method as applied to derivation of CIs for the ICER.

Moving to net benefit. It is clear that there are various statistical issues with the ICER that have complicated efforts to quantify its sampling uncertainty in a trial-based economic evaluation. In the face of these statistical difficulties, the use of net benefit may be one way forward (Willan 2003). The concept of net benefit was introduced in Chapter 5 as a way of moving away from a ratio and placing both costs and effects on a single scale (either net monetary benefit (NMB) or net health benefit). Net monetary benefit is the most widely used version where the difference in effects between two options being evaluated is re-scaled into monetary value using the threshold willingness-to-pay (R_T) for a unit of effect, and the difference in costs between the options is subtracted from this value.

Box 8.2 **Summary of the stages of non-parametric bootstrap methods**

1 Draw a sample from (and of equal size to) the observations of the treatment group by simple random sampling with replacement. Compute $\overline{C}_T^*$ and $\overline{E}_T^*$, the bootstrap replicates of $\overline{C}_T$ and $\overline{E}_T$.

2 Draw a sample from (and of equal size to) the observations of the control group by simple random sampling with replacement. Compute $\overline{C}_C^*$ and $\overline{E}_C^*$, the bootstrap replicates of $\overline{C}_C$ and $\overline{E}_C$.

3 Compute the bootstrap replicate $\hat{R}_b^*$:

$$\hat{R}_b^* = \frac{\overline{C}_T^* - \overline{C}_C^*}{\overline{E}_T^* - \overline{E}_C^*}$$

4 Repeat steps 1–3 a large number of times (say B) and obtain the independent bootstrap replications $\hat{R}_1^*, \hat{R}_2^*, \cdots \hat{R}_B^*$. This is the empirical estimate of the sampling distribution of the ICER.

5 Several methods are then available to calculate CIs from this empirical estimate. For example, a simple approach would be to base a 95% CI on the 2½ and 97½ centiles from the empirical sampling distribution.

For statistical analysis, compared to the ICER, NMB has the advantage of being a linear expression, which means it is more tractable and has a sampling distribution that is easier to work with. The variance of NMB can be easily defined (Briggs *et al.* 2002). The statistical convenience of the net benefit statistic has also allowed consideration of how an appropriate sample size might be determined for trial-based economic evaluation based on standard statistical methods (Willan and Lin 2001).

Given that the value of the threshold willingness-to-pay is not usually known by the analyst (see Chapter 10 for a discussion of this threshold), it is possible to present NMB, and its sampling uncertainty, diagrammatically as a function of the threshold. An example of this is shown in Fig. 8.5 and is similar to that presented, in a deterministic framework, in Chapter 5. The example is taken from the laparoscopic versus abdominal hysterectomy study (Sculpher *et al.* 2004), but using 6-week follow-up data because both CIs for the ICER are undefined for the 1-year follow-up. The bold line on the figure shows mean NMB. Where this line intersects the *x*-axis, NMB is zero and the threshold value on the *x*-axis is equal to the ICER. This line meets the *y*-axis at a value of NMB that is equal to the negative value of the difference in mean cost between the two options. The slope of the NMB line is equal to the difference in effects. The upper and lower 95% CIs in NMB are also shown in the figure as the lighter curves below and above the mean NMB line. Hence, for a given threshold willingness-to-pay value, it is possible to read off the mean NMB as well as the upper and lower 95% CIs. When these CI lines cross the *x*-axis, it is possible to define the 95% CIs for the ICER. In the example shown, the lower 95% CI is defined but this is not the case with the upper 95% CI.

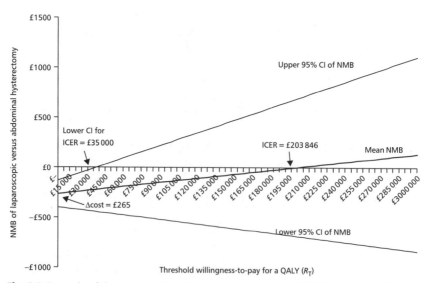

Fig. 8.5 Example of the presentation of net monetary benefit (NMB), together with its sampling uncertainty, as a function of the threshold willingness-to-pay. The example is based on the comparison of laparoscopic and abdominal hysterectomy based on 6-week follow-up (Sculpher *et al.* 2004). CI, confidence interval; ICER, incremental cost-effectiveness ratio; QALY, quality-adjusted life-year.

3. *Decision uncertainty.* Although the use of NMB provides a statistically tractable way of presenting sampling uncertainty in cost-effectiveness measures, it has not been widely used in published applied studies. One method that is increasingly used is the *cost-effectiveness acceptability curve* (CEAC) (van Hout *et al.* 1994). Although the CEAC can be interpreted in terms of standard ('frequentist') statistics, it is usually interpreted using Bayesian statistical methods (Briggs 1999). That is, the CEAC shows the probability that an intervention is more cost-effective than its comparator or, in a study comparing more than two interventions, it shows the probability that a given intervention is the *most* cost-effective given the observed data (Fenwick *et al.* 2001). As for the NMB plot, the CEAC is shown as a function of the threshold willingness-to-pay. In effect, the CEAC can show a decision-maker the probability that, if the intervention is funded or reimbursed, this will be the correct decision.

Figure 8.6 shows how the CEAC is derived from the joint uncertainty in costs and effects, and the corresponding CEAC is shown in Fig. 8.7. The example is based on the analysis of laparoscopic versus open abdominal hysterectomy based on 1-year follow-up (Garry *et al.* 2004; Sculpher *et al.* 2004). The scatter of points on the plane is based on the results of a non-parametric bootstrap analysis. A number of lines is drawn on the figure, each one going through the origin, and these represent alternative values for the threshold willingness-to-pay for an additional QALY. An extreme value would be zero—that is, there is no value attached to an additional QALY—and that is shown by the horizontal line running along the *x*-axis. At the other extreme is a vertical line

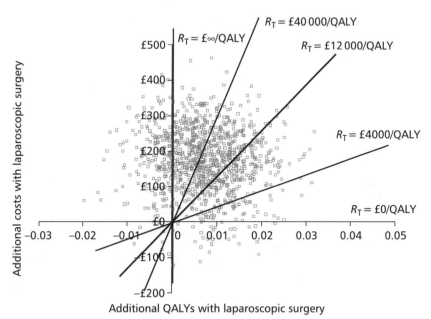

Fig. 8.6 The process of deriving a cost-effectiveness acceptability curve from the joint uncertainty in differential costs and effects on a cost-effectiveness plane. Based on data from a cost-effectiveness analysis of laparoscopic versus abdominal hysterectomy using data from 1-year follow-up (Sculpher *et al.* 2004). QALY, quality-adjusted life-year.

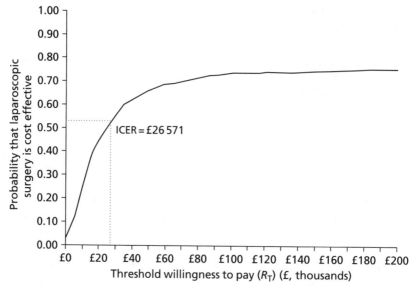

Fig. 8.7 A cost-effectiveness acceptability curve for laparoscopic hysterectomy based on the uncertainty in cost and effect differences shown in Figure 8.6. These results are based on 1-year follow-up. ICER, incremental cost-effectiveness ratio.

running along the y-axis, which corresponds with an infinite threshold willingness-to-pay for an additional QALY. There are then several points between these two extremes: threshold values of £4000, £12 000, and £40 000 are shown.

For a given threshold, all points on the cost-effectiveness plane below the threshold line would be considered cost-effective because laparoscopic surgery is either (1) dominant (that is, in the south-east quadrant); (2) more costly and more effective but with an ICER below the threshold willingness-to-pay (in the north-east quadrant but below the threshold line); or (3) less costly and less effective but abdominal surgery (the comparator) has an ICER above the threshold willingness-to-pay (south-west quadrant but below the threshold line). When a threshold willingness-to-pay of £0 applies (the horizontal threshold), all points on the cost-effectiveness plane below the x-axis (that is, all points where laparoscopic surgery is less costly) would be considered cost-effective. The proportion of points below this threshold would be the corresponding point on the CEAC for a zero threshold. As the threshold increases (pivots around the origin in a counter-clockwise direction), the proportion of points on the plane below the threshold (that is, points that can be defined as cost-effective) changes, and these proportions are shown on the corresponding CEAC. At the extreme, where the threshold willingness-to-pay is infinite (the vertical threshold), the proportion of points to the right of the y-axis (where laparoscopic surgery is more effective) is marked on the CEAC.

Hence Fig. 8.7 shows the CEAC for laparoscopic hysterectomy. As the threshold willingness-to-pay increases, the proportion of bootstrap replicates that are in the cost-effective region of the plane changes, and this can be interpreted as the probability that laparoscopic surgery is more cost-effective. Although it is not shown here, it would be possible also to present the CEAC for abdominal hysterectomy (the comparator). As there were only two options compared in the trial, the vertical sum of the two curves would always sum to 1.

The CEAC also embodies other information about the comparison (Briggs *et al.* 2002). Taking a frequentist perspective, where it cuts the vertical axis is the *P*-value for a (one-sided) hypothesis test for the difference in costs. At the other end, the curve tends towards 1 minus the *P*-value for a (one-sided) hypothesis test for the difference in QALYs. The ICER is also shown on the CEAC. As the ICER is based on mean cost and effect differences, and the 50% point on the CEAC effectively corresponds to the *median* in those differences, the ICER will not necessarily fall at the 50% point (Fenwick *et al.* 2001). The shape of the CEAC will vary depending on the joint uncertainty in cost and effect differences on the cost-effectiveness plane (Fenwick *et al. 2004*).

By showing the decision-maker, who has decided to adopt a particular intervention, the probability (s)he has made the wrong decision, the CEAC represents *the decision uncertainty* in cost-effectiveness analysis. However, it does not indicate the costs of making a wrong decision. This is part of the process of calculating the value of additional information (through extra research), which is described in Chapter 9.

8.3.3. **Explaining variability in cost-effectiveness analysis**

As mentioned in Section 8.3.2, in analysing patient-level data on costs and effects, explaining variability in cost-effectiveness can be very important. Whilst cost-effectiveness analysis was based on deterministic measures of the ICER, formal regression analysis to quantify variability was not possible. One of the implications of moving to stochastic methods in the analysis of patient-level economic data is that regression methods are now feasible. Regression analysis for costs is widely undertaken, although it is complicated by the features of cost data described in Section 8.3.1 (Manning and Mullahy 2001), but this has conventionally not been the case with cost-effectiveness. Hoch *et al.* (2002) made a major contribution to this development by introducing the concept of net benefit regression. When individual patient data on costs and effects exist, as in trial-based studies, NMB can be calculated for each individual (i) in the trial as shown in the equation below where the subscript i indicates that the relevant measure can relate to the individual patient:

$$\text{NMB}_i = (E_i \times R_T) - C_i$$

Using a model regressing this patient-level NMB_i against the treatment arm dummy variable (t_i), Hoch *et al.* (2002) demonstrated the equivalence of a regression-based approach to CEA with a 'standard' stochastic cost-effectiveness analysis. Their regression framework is illustrated in the equation below:

$$\text{NMB}_i = \alpha + \beta t_i + e_i$$

In this formulation, the NMB for the i-th patient in the trial is the patient-level net-benefit defined above and t_i represents a treatment dummy taking the value 0 for 'standard' or comparator therapy and 1 for the new intervention. In the context of a trial, this dummy variable would be defined in terms of the group to which the individual patient is randomized. The coefficients $\alpha + \beta$ are, respectively, the intercept and the slope term obtained from a standard ordinary least-squares (OLS) regression (Seber *et al.* 2003). The term e_i is an error term with constant variance usually assumed to be normally distributed. In terms of the interpretation of the results from the OLS regression, the estimated coefficient α represents the mean NMB in the group receiving the 'standard treatment' in the trial, the sum of the two estimated coefficients $\alpha + \beta$ is the mean net benefit in the new intervention arm, and β is the incremental net benefit between the two arms of the trial. More recent work on regression methods for cost-effectiveness have moved away from using NMB as the dependent variable towards defining two regression equations (one for costs and one for effects) then correlating the error terms (Willan *et al.* 2004). This 'seemingly unrelated regression' approach has the advantage of allowing different co-variates and functional forms for the two equations.

The real value of the framework comes from adding additional co-variates to the single treatment dummy in the simple regression above. These would typically be baseline characteristics of the patient such as age, sex, and a range of clinical characteristics. Regression methods offer three important contributions for cost-effectiveness analysis based on patient-level data. First, they allow baseline differences in patient case mix between the treatment groups in a study to be adjusted for. In the context of a randomized trial, this may provide more precise estimates of cost-effectiveness (for example, narrower CIs) although the random allocation of patients to the arms of the study will ensure unbiased estimates without the need for statistical adjustment. This may be particularly important in the context of QALY calculation (Manca *et al.* in press). In a non-randomized study, the process of adjusting for known differences in case mix is a necessary (but not necessarily sufficient) condition for an *unbiased* estimate. The second contribution of the regression framework is that it facilitates subgroup analysis, that is, a formal means of assessing whether the cost-effectiveness of an intervention systematically varies between patients with different baseline characteristics. The third contribution offered by the framework is to assess whether cost-effectiveness varies according to the location in which the patient was treated (for example, the centre or country in a trial setting). The use of regression methods to explore issues relating to the transferability of economic data from setting to setting is discussed in Chapter 10.

8.4. **Conclusions**

This chapter has indicated that randomized trials have strengths and weaknesses as a vehicle for economic evaluation. It has described the limitations of economic evaluation that is 'piggybacked' on to the design of a typical safety and efficacy trial. An alternative approach was considered where an analyst can mount a specific pragmatic (naturalistic) trial in which randomization is used but protocols for subsequent patient management are more relaxed than is conventional.

Interest in the statistical issues arising from economic evaluations alongside trials is growing rapidly. As studies move toward greater use of sampled data, analysis plans need to be based more on stochastic rather than deterministic methods. Although some of the early work in statistical methods in economic evaluation considered formal hypothesis testing, most work in this area has concentrated on estimation methods. More recently, quantifying the implications of sampling uncertainty for decision uncertainty, typically using the CEAC, has been the major focus.

8.5. **Exercise: economic evaluation alongside clinical trials—a case study in osteoporosis**

Scenario

You have been asked to conduct an economic evaluation of a new drug for treatment of osteoporotic fractures. A large randomized trial is planned and you have the opportunity to build economic and quality-of-life endpoints into this trial.

The drug has a positive effect on rebuilding of bones and is therefore thought to accelerate the healing of fractures. A multicentre clinical trial in hip fracture is to be conducted in the USA and four European countries. The preliminary design of the trial is as follows.

1 The trial will be randomized and double blind, and the new drug will be added from the day of the fracture to standard methods used to treat hip fractures, and compared to placebo. Drug treatment will be for 3 months.

2 The tentative main clinical endpoints are
   - bone building index
   - ability to stand
   - ability to walk 50 metres
   - time to hospital discharge.

3 Sample size calculations, based on the power to detect a clinically important difference in the clinical endpoints, suggest that there will have to be 200 patients in each group.

4 Patients will be assessed at baseline, 1, 3, and 6 months (end of the trial).

5 Because of the potentially toxic nature of the drug, additional monitoring (laboratory tests) will be performed at monthly intervals. In order to preserve blinding, tests will also be performed on the placebo patients.

Tasks

1 Comment critically on the suitability of this trial for the assessment of economic endpoints (give points for and against). If necessary, propose changes to the trial design.

2 Specify the categories of data on resource use you would like to see collected as part of the trial.

3 Discuss whether you would want to collect quality-of-life data in this trial, and if so, would you use a generic or specific quality-of-life scale?

4 Specify any other data that you feel need to be gathered in the five countries to supplement the data being collected as part of the trial.

5 Although the economic data would be collected alongside the clinical trial, do you think that there is any role for modelling in this case? If so, what kind of model would you recommend?

Solutions

1. As we have discussed in this chapter, one of the goals in designing a pragmatic economic trial is to generate evidence on costs and outcomes that are mostly likely to arise in routine practice. There are a number of limitations for this current trial for achieving this goal.

First, this is a placebo-controlled trial which raises the question of the relevance of this comparison. Even though the placebo is adjunctive, are there any other pharmacological or non-pharmacological treatments that would be implemented in the different countries for treatment of hip fractures?

Second, this is a double-blind trial and therefore necessitates additional tests and visits for the placebo group that would not otherwise arise but are there to preserve the blinding. Might it be feasible and desirable to have this as an unblinded trial so that both patients and physicians could be studied in a less artificial environment where they know they were either on or not on the new therapy?

Third, is the trial long enough? Drug treatment will be for 3 months and follow-up will continue to 6 months. It is not clear whether this length of follow-up will be adequate to capture downstream consequences of therapy, such as recurrence of fracture or adverse consequences of medication. One possibility might be to end the complete follow-up at six months but continue a more streamlined follow-up for economic endpoints to 1 year.

Fourth, is it desirable to have this trial conducted in multiple countries? To the extent that practice patterns will vary between the USA and Europe (and even within Europe) it may not be possible to meaningfully pool the economic data. Is it possible to consolidate the trial in one continent or, ideally, in one country to reduce the heterogeneity in the economic data?

2. In addition to hospitalization data that will be collected as part of the main case report form (CRF) for the trial, and depending upon the viewpoint of the economic analysis, it may be desirable to capture the following resource consequences:

- family physician visits
- homemaker/home help costs
- drugs
- nursing home costs
- community nursing costs
- re-hospitalization.

3. A general issue in the collection of quality-of-life data in this trial is whether the period of follow-up (6 months) is going to be sufficiently long to be able to ascertain clinically important changes in these hip fracture patients. In choosing

among general versus disease-specific measures it might be desirable to have both a disease-specific measure that is sensitive to small but clinically important differences but also a more general measure (such as a utility measure) that will afford the study some more general comparability with other disease and treatment areas. A practical concern, however, is whether the measures chosen have been validated and are available in different countries where the study will be conducted. A further concern may be to attempt some measurement of quality-of-life in care-givers for persons with this condition. Before deciding upon any quality-of-life measures to include in the trial it is useful to review what pilot data are available that will give a perspective on whether the measures can detect the kind of changes one can expect to see in the trial.

4. In addition to the resource information being collected as part of the trial, there are at least three categories of information that will be required from each of the participating countries.

(1) Price data to attach to resources measured. These are obvious things such as hospital prices, drug prices, and physician costs in addition to factors such as labour market wage rates if the valuation of productive time is to be measured.

(2) Practice patterns for the management of hip fracture in each of the countries would be useful information to collect. The concern here is that the trial may be an abstraction from routine practice and also that we are seeking to combine information from five different countries where practice patterns may vary. In assessing whether the data are combinable or transferable between countries, some knowledge of variation in practice patterns for the condition will be useful.

(3) Information on reimbursement mechanisms in each of the countries would also be useful in further exploring why variation in management of patients may exist between countries. For example, are physicians paid a fee per item of service to conduct additional tests or procedures or are they reimbursed by salary? Are hospitals reimbursed on the basis of case mix groups such that there is an incentive to reduce length of stay, and so on.

5. There might be a general need for modelling to address two types of questions.

(1) Modelling may be necessary to extrapolate some of the intermediate clinical endpoints to final outcomes. For example, at 6 months we may have knowledge regarding the extent to which bone has been rebuilt, but to what extent does this manifest itself in reduced risk of fracture recurrence in the following year? Hence there may be a need for epidemiologic models that extrapolate bone density and mass to fracture risk.

(2) Modelling may also be necessary to attempt to generalize the findings from this multicountry study to individual countries studied and countries not studied. The general issue here would be to ascertain whether the cost-effectiveness of the therapy was conditional upon the treatment patterns and reimbursement practices in any given country.

References

Anderson, D., O'Brien, B., Levine, M., *et al.* (1993). Efficacy and cost-effectiveness of low molecular weight heparin versus standard heparin in the prevention of deep vein thrombosis following total hip replacement arthroplasty. *Annals of Internal Medicine*, **119**, 1105–12.

Barber, J. A. and Thompson, S. G. (1998). Analysis and interpretation of cost data in randomised controlled trials: review of published studies. *British Medical Journal*, **317**, 1195–200.

Beck, T. M., Ciociola, A. A., Jones, S. E., *et al.* (1993). Efficacy of oral ondansetron in the prevention of emesis in outpatients receiving cyclophosphamide-based chemotherapy. *Annals of Internal Medicine*, **118**, 407–13.

Briggs, A. H. (1999). A Bayesian approach to stochastic cost-effectiveness analysis. *Health Economics*, **8**, 257–62.

Briggs, A. (2001). Handling uncertainty in economic evaluation and presenting the results. In: *Economic evaluation in health care: merging theory with practice* (ed. M. Drummond and A. McGuire), pp. 172–214. Oxford University Press, Oxford.

Briggs, A. (ed.) (2003). *Statistical methods for cost-effectiveness research*. Office of Health Economics, London.

Briggs, A. and Gray, A. (1998). The distribution of health care costs and their statistical analysis for economic evaluation. *Journal of Health Services Research and Policy*, **3**, 233–45.

Briggs, A. H. and Gray, A. M. (1999). Handling uncertainty when performing economic evaluation of healthcare interventions. *Health Technology Assessment*, **3(2)**, 1–134.

Briggs, A. H. and O'Brien, B. J. (2001). The death of cost-minimisation analysis? *Health Economics*, **10**, 179–84.

Briggs, A. H., Wonderling, D. E., and Mooney, C. Z. (1997). Pulling cost-effectiveness analysis up by its bootstraps: a non-parametric approach to confidence interval estimation. *Health Economics*, **6**, 327–40.

Briggs, A. H., O'Brien, B. J., and Blackhouse, G. (2002). Thinking outside the box: recent advances in the analysis and presentation of uncertainty in cost-effectiveness studies. *Annual Review of Public Health*, **23**, 377–401.

Briggs, A. H., Clark, T., Wolstenholme, J., Clarke, P. (2003). Missing . . . presumed at random: cost-analysis of incomplete data. *Health Economics*, **12**, 377–92.

Buxton, M. J. and O'Brien, B. J. (1992). Economic evaluation of ondansetron: preliminary analysis using trial data prior to price setting. *British Journal of Cancer*, **66** (Suppl. XIX), 564–7.

Buxton, M. J., Drummond, M. F., Van Hout, B. A., *et al.* (1997). Modelling in economic evaluation: an unavoidable fact of life. *Health Economics* **6**, 217–27.

Chaudhary, M. A. and Stearns, S. C. (1996). Estimating confidence intervals for cost-effectiveness ratios: an example from a randomized trial. *Statistics in Medicine*, **14**, 1447–58.

Cooper, N. J., Sutton, A. J., Mugford, M., and Abrams, K. R. (2003). Use of Bayesian Markov Chain Monte Carlo methods to model cost data. *Medical Decision Making* **23**, 38–53.

Cubeddu, L. X., Hoffmann, I. S., Fuenmayor, N. T., and Finn, A. L. (1990). Efficacy of ondansetron (GR 38032F) and the role of serotonin in cisplatin-induced nausea and vomiting. *New England Journal of Medicine*, **322**, 810–16.

Drummond, M. F., Bloom, B. S., Carrin, G., *et al.* (1992). Issues in the cross-national assessment of health technology. *International Journal of Technology Assessment in Health Care*, **8**, 671–82.

Efron, B. and Tibshirani, R. (1993). *An introduction to the bootstrap*. Chapman and Hall, New York.

Etzioni, R. D., Feuer, E. J., Sullivan, S. D., Lin, D., Hu, C., and Ramsey, S. D. (1999). On the use of survival analysis techniques to estimate medical care costs. *Journal of Health Economics*, 18, 365–80.

Fenwick, E., Claxton, K., and Sculpher, M. (2001). Representing uncertainty: the role of cost-effectiveness acceptability curves. *Health Economics*, 10, 779–89.

Fenwick, E., O'Brien B. J., and Briggs, A. (2004). Cost-effectiveness acceptability curves—facts, fallacies and frequently asked questions. *Health Economics*, 13, 405–15.

Freemantle, N. and Drummond, M. F. (1997). Should clinical trials with concurrent economic analyses be blinded? *Journal of the American Medical Association*, 277, 63–4.

Gardner, M. J. and Altman, D. G. (1989). *Statistics with confidence—confidence intervals and statistical guidelines*. British Medical Association, London.

Garry, R., Fountain, J., Brown, J., *et al.* (2004). EVALUATE hysterectomy trial: a multicentre randomised trial comparing abdominal, vaginal and laparoscopic methods of hysterectomy. *Health Technology Assessment*, 8(26), 1–154.

Glick, H., Polsky, D., and Schulman, K. (2001). Trial-based economic evaluations: an overview of design and analysis. In: *Economic evaluation in health care: merging theory with practice* (ed. M. F. Drummond and A. McGuire), pp. 113–140. Oxford University Press, Oxford.

Gold, M. R., Siegel, J. E., Russell, L. B., and Weinstein, M. C. (1996). *Cost-effectiveness in health and medicine*. Oxford University Press, Oxford.

Hallstrom, A. P. and Sullivan, S. D. (1998). On estimating costs for economic evaluation in failure time studies. *Medical Care* 36, 433–6.

Heart Protection Study Collaborative Group (2002). MRC/BHF Heart Protection Study of cholesterol lowering with simvastatin in 20536 high-risk individuals: a randomised placebo-controlled trial. *Lancet* 360, 7–22.

Heyse, J., Cook, J., and Carides, G. (2001). Statistical considerations in analysing health care resource utilisation and cost data. In: *Economic evaluation in health care: merging theory with practice* (ed. M. F. Drummond and A. McGuire), pp. 215–35. Oxford University Press, Oxford.

Hoch, J. S., Briggs, A. H., and Willan, A. (2002). Something old, something new, something borrowed, something BLUE: a framework for the marriage of health econometrics and cost-effectiveness analysis. *Health Economics*, 11, 415–30.

Hughes, D. A., Bagust, A., Haycox, A., and Walley, T. (2001). The impact of non-compliance on the cost-effectiveness of pharmaceuticals: a review of the literature. *Health Economics*, 10, 601–15.

Johannesson, M., Jönsson, B., Kjekshus, J., *et al.* (1997). Cost effectiveness of simvastatin treatment to lower cholesterol levels in patients with coronary heart disease. *New England Journal of Medicine*, 336, 332–6.

Kahn, H. A. and Sempos, C. T. (1989). *Statistical methods in epidemiology*. Oxford University Press, New York.

Lipid Research Clinics Programme (1984). The Lipid Research Clinics coronary primary prevention trial results: I Reductions in the incidence of coronary heart disease. *Journal of the American Medical Association*, 251, 351–64.

Lipscomb, J., Ancukiewicz, M., Parmigiani, G., Hasselblad, V., Samsa, G., and Matchar, D. B. (1998). Predicting the cost of illness: a comparison of alternative models applied to stroke. *Medical Decision Making* 18 (Suppl.), S39–56.

Manca, A., Hawkins, N., and Sculpher, M. (in press). Estimating mean QALYs in trial-based cost-effectiveness analysis: the importance of controlling for baseline utility. *Health Economics*.

Manning, W. G. and Mullahy, J. (2001). Estimating log models: to transform or not to transform? *Journal of Health Economics* **20**: 461–94.

Mauskopf, J., Schulman, K., Bell, L., and Glick, H. (1996). A strategy for collecting pharmacoeconomic data during phase II/III clinical trials. *PharmacoEconomics*, **9**, 264–77.

Morris, S., McGuire, A., Caro, J., and Pettitt, D. (1997). Strategies for the management of hypercholesterolaemia: a systematic review of the cost-effectiveness literature. *Journal of Health Services Research and Policy*, **2**, 231–50.

Obenchain, R. L., Melfi, C. A., Croghan, T. W., and Buesching, D. P. (1997). Bootstrap analyses of cost effectiveness in antidepressant pharmacotherapy. *PharmacoEconomics* **11**, 464–72.

O'Brien, B. J. (1991). *Cholesterol and coronary heart disease: consensus or controversy?* Office of Health Economics, London.

O'Brien, B. J., Anderson, D., and Goeree, R. (1994*a*). Cost-effectiveness of enoxaparin versus warfarin prophylaxis against deep vein thrombosis after total hip replacement. *Canadian Medical Association Journal*, **150**, 1083–172.

O'Brien, B. J. and Drummond, M. F. (1994*b*). Statistical versus quantitative importance in the socio-economic evaluation of medicines. *PharmacoEconomics*, **5**, 389–98.

O'Brien, B. J., Drummond, M. F., Labelle, R. J., and Willan, A. (1994*c*). In search of power and significance: issues in the decision and analysis of stochastic cost-effectiveness studies in health care. *Medical Care*, **32**, 150–63.

O'Hagan, A. and Stevens, J. W. (2003). Assessing and comparing costs: How robust are the bootstrap and methods based on asymptotic normality? *Health Economics*, **12**, 33–49.

O'Hagan, A. and Stevens, J. W. (2004). On estimators of medical costs with censored data. *Journal of Health Economics*, **23**, 615–25.

Oster, G., Borok, G. M., Menzin, J., *et al.* (1995). A randomised trial to assess effectiveness and cost in clinical practice: rationale and design of the Cholesterol Reduction Intervention Study (CRIS). *Controlled Clinical Trials*, **16**, 3–16.

Oster, G., Borok, G. M., Menzin, J., *et al.* (1996). Cholesterol-reduction intervention study (CRIS): a randomized trial to assess effectiveness and costs in clinical practice. *Archives of Internal Medicine*, **156**, 731–9.

Paiment, G. D., Wessinger, S. J., and Harris, W. H. (1987). Survey of prophylaxis against venous thromboembolism in adults undergoing hip surgery. *Clinical Orthopedics*, **223**, 188–93.

Raikou, M. and McGuire, A. (2004). Estimating medical care costs under conditions of censoring. *Journal of Health Economics*, **23**, 443–70.

Rusthoven, J., O'Brien, B. J., and Rocchi, A. (1992). Ondansetron versus metoclopramide in the prevention of chemotherapy-induced emesis and nausea: a meta-analysis. *International Journal of Oncology*, **1**, 443–50.

Scandinavian Simvastatin Survival Study Group (1994). Randomised trial of cholesterol lowering in 4444 patients with coronary heart disease: the Scandinavian Simvastatin Survival Study (4S). *Lancet*, **344**, 1383–9.

Schulman KA, Buxton MJ, Glick H., *et al.* (1996). Results of the economic evaluation of the FIRST study: a multinational prospective evaluation. *International Journal of Technology Assessment in Health Care*, **12**(4), 698–713.

Schwartz, D. and Lellouch, J. (1967). Explanatory and pragmatic attitudes in therapeutic trials. *Journal of Chronic Disease*, **20**, 637–48.

Sculpher, M. J., Manca, A., Abbott, J., Fountain, J., Mason, S., and Garry, R. (2004). Cost-effectiveness analysis of laparoscopic-assisted hysterectomy in comparison with standard hysterectomy: results from a randomised trial. *British Medical Journal*, **328**, 134–40.

Seber, G. A. F., Lee, A. J., Seber, G. A. F., and Lee, A. J. (2003). *Linear regression analysis* (2nd edn). Wiley, Chichester.

Thompson, M. S., Read, J. L., Hutchings, H. C., and Harris, E. D. (1989). The cost-effectiveness of auranofin: results of a randomized clinical trial. *Journal of Rheumatology*, 15, 35–42.

van Hout, B. A., Al, M. J., Gordon, G. S., and Rutten, F. F. H. (1994). Costs, effects and c/e-ratios alongside a clinical trial. *Health Economics*, 3, 309–19.

Walt, R. P., Hunt, R. H., Misiewicz, J. J., *et al.* (1984). Comparison of ranitidine and cimetidine maintenance treatment of duodenal ulcer. *Scandinavian Journal of Gastroenterology*, 19, 1045–7.

Willan, A. (2003). Analysing cost-effectiveness trials: net benefits. In: *Statistical methods for cost-effectiveness research: a guide to current issues and future developments* (ed. A. Briggs), pp. 8–23. Office for Health Economics, London.

Willan, A. and O'Brien, B. J. (1996). Confidence intervals for cost-effectiveness ratios: An application of Fieller's theorem. *Health Economics*, 5, 297–305.

Willan, A. R. and Lin, D.Y. (2001). Incremental net benefit in randomized clinical trials. *Statistics in Medicine*, 20(11), 1563–74.

Willan, A. R., Briggs, A. H., and Hoch, J. S. (2004). Regression methods for covariate adjustment and subgroup analysis for non-censored cost-effectiveness data. *Health Economics*, 13, 461–75.

Wilby, J., Kainth, K., Hawkins, *et al.* (in press). A rapid and systematic review of the clinical effectiveness, tolerability and cost effectiveness of newer drugs for epilepsy in adults. *Health Technology Assessment*.

Chapter 9

Economic evaluation using decision analytic modelling·

9.1. **Some basics**

The ultimate purpose of economic evaluation is to inform different types of decision-makers about the efficient allocation of health care resources. In recent years, economic evaluation has been increasingly undertaken for specific decision-makers, who formally require economic evidence (Hjelmgren *et al.* 2001). For example, a number of health care systems now use economic evaluation to help them decide whether new health technologies (particularly pharmaceuticals) represent sufficient value for money to be funded. The role of economic evaluation in decision-making is discussed in more detail in Chapter 10, but the greater use of these methods to inform particular decisions in specific jurisdictions has had implications for economic evaluation (Claxton *et al.* 2002). In particular, it has indicated that relying on a randomized trial as a single vehicle for economic evaluation, in which data on resource use and effectiveness are collected simultaneously, has a number of limitations. As a result, economic evaluation for decision-making will usually need to draw on evidence from a range of sources. These could include economic data collected alongside randomized trials, but are also likely to include clinical, cost, and health-related quality of life data from other types of study such as cohort studies and surveys. Decision analytic models provide a means of bringing this evidence together.

Decision analytic modelling has its theoretical foundations in statistical decision theory (Raiffa and Schlaifer 1959; Raiffa 1968), and shares common theoretical origins with expected utility theory (discussed in Chapter 6). It also has a close association with Bayesian statistics where statistical analysis is closely related to decision-making (Spiegelhalter *et al.* 2003). Decision analysis has been widely used outside health care, such as in business and engineering. It has an established basis as a framework for *clinical* decision-making—that is, decision-making relating to individual patients when costs are not necessarily a primary consideration, and several good texts exist introducing decision analysis in health care generally (Weinstein and Fineberg 1980; Sox *et al.* 1988; Hunink *et al.* 2001). This chapter introduces the use of these methods in economic evaluation in particular.

Decision analytical modelling provides a framework for decision-making under conditions of uncertainty. As a set of methods, it can satisfy five important objectives for any economic evaluation.

1 *Structure*. It can provide a structure that appropriately reflects the possible prognoses that individuals of interest may experience, and how the treatments

and programmes being evaluated may impact on these prognoses. The structure will have to reflect the variability between apparently similar individuals in their prognoses and in the effect of interventions. The individuals will often be patients with a particular condition, but may be healthy or asymptomatic in the context, for example, of a screening or preventative programme.

2 *Evidence*. It offers an analytic framework within which evidence relevant to the study question can be brought to bear. This is achieved partly through the structure of the model, but also in the estimates of the input parameters of the model.

3 *Evaluation*. It provides a means of translating the relevant evidence into estimates of the cost and effects of the alternative options being compared. Using appropriate decision rules for the relevant study types (that is, cost-effectiveness, cost–utility, or cost–benefit analysis), the option that the analysis identifies as the best or 'optimal' can be identified based on the available evidence.

4 *Uncertainty and variability*. It facilitates an assessment of the various types of uncertainty relating to the evaluation. As outlined in Chapter 3, this includes uncertainty relating to model structure and input parameters. Models also provide flexibility to characterize heterogeneity across different subgroups of individuals.

5 *Future research*. Through the assessment of uncertainty, it can identify likely priorities for future research, which can generate further evidence to re-assess the question in the future.

9.2. **The role of decision analytic models for economic evaluation**

In considering the role of decision models in economic evaluation, it is useful to contrast two different activities in health care evaluation—measurement and decision analysis—which are summarized in Box 9.1. In part, economic evaluation is concerned with the process of measurement through the collection of data relating to effectiveness, resource use, unit costs, and utilities, often alongside randomized trials. Ultimately, though, economic evaluation is concerned with informing appropriate decisions in health care about resource allocation under conditions of uncertainty. This will require the appropriate synthesis of all relevant evidence. Being clear about these different roles for economic evaluation emphasizes that decision models and randomized trials are not competing alternatives. Rather, randomized trials are focused on different types of measurement, whilst decision models are concerned with informing specific decisions.

This section considers the features of economic evaluation for decision-making that frequently necessitate the use of decision analytic models rather than reliance on a single data source such as a randomized controlled trial. There are several different requirements for an economic evaluation that are relevant, and these are detailed below.

Box 9.1 **Contrasting activities in economic evaluation: measurement versus decision analysis**

Health care evaluation in general, and economic evaluation in particular, involves two important but separate activities: measurement and decision analysis. Both are important in establishing the most economically appropriate form of management or intervention, but they have distinct roles. The process of measurement has the following features.

1 A focus on estimating and testing hypotheses relating to particular parameters and relationships between parameters (for example, event rates, relative treatment effects, resource use, and quality of life effects).

2 A concentration on relatively few parameters.

3 A primary interest in randomized trials as a vehicle for measurement, particularly of relative treatment effects.

4 A focus on uncertainty in parameters.

The activity of decision analysis can be characterized as:

1 The primacy of identifying an appropriate course of action from amongst alternatives for a specific recipient group.

2 The process of informing decisions based on currently available evidence.

3 Identification of a preferred option based on the expected values of the alternatives rather than on individual parameters.

4 An explicit acceptance that decisions will always be taken under conditions of uncertainty.

9.2.1. **The need for comparison of all relevant options**

As described in Chapters 2 and 3, economic evaluation is about comparing the value for money of alternative courses of action (or options) for particular recipient groups. It is possible that decision-makers will be misled by a study that fails to compare all the relevant options, which might include more than one option that is currently used as well as the new option(s) available. However, as discussed in Chapter 8, in randomized trials it is rarely the practice to compare all relevant options and a subset are typically studied. In some studies, moreover, the comparator is not an active intervention at all, but a placebo. To compare all relevant options, it is likely that effectiveness data will have to be taken from several trials. For example, in a model of the cost-effectiveness of glycoprotein IIb/IIIa antagonists in acute coronary syndrome, 18 trials randomizing nearly 50 000 patients were used to generate the evidence on effectiveness (Palmer *et al.* in press). Meta-analysis will be necessary to synthesize this type of evidence, but the decision model will provide the framework to combine it with other types of evidence.

9.2.2. **The need to reflect all appropriate evidence**

To offer a decision-maker guidance on the economically optimal course of action for a given patient group, it is important that all appropriate evidence is brought to bear. This is consistent with the axioms of evidence-based medicine, where appropriate evidence is systematically and comprehensibly used to make clinical decisions (Sackett *et al.* 1996). For economic evaluation, however, it is not just effectiveness evidence that is required. In addition, evidence relating to resource use, unit costs, and, for cost–utility analysis, data on health-related quality of life and preferences, are required. This array of evidence is rarely collected in trials and, if it is, it is unlikely to be the only source. Again, the decision model is used to combine all sources of evidence.

9.2.3. **The need to link intermediate to final endpoints**

Chapter 5 described the situation that exists in some cost-effectiveness studies where available trial evidence compares interventions in terms of intermediate endpoints rather than final outcomes. This is frequently the case, for example, in cost–utility analysis when the trials have measured one or a series of clinical endpoints, which may or may not include mortality, but the economic evaluation requires that these are linked to health-related quality of life and hence to utilities and quality-adjusted life-years (QALYs). Box 9.2 provides examples of economic evaluation studies where a decision model has been used to link one or more intermediate endpoints with final outcomes.

9.2.4. **The need to extrapolate over the appropriate time horizon of the evaluation**

In Chapter 3, the issue of the appropriate time horizon for an economic evaluation was discussed. In principle, this should be the period over which the costs and/or effects of the alternative options being compared might differ. Often the appropriate time horizon will be the patient's lifetime. For example, in the case of the treatment of chronic disease where the initiation of an intervention in a middle-aged patient may have cost and effect implications on the remainder of their life. Except in rare cases where palliative treatments are being compared (for example, for advanced cancer), randomized trials will not follow all patients up for the remainder of their lives. An important role of decision models, then, is to bridge the gap between what has been observed in trials and what would be expected to happen, in terms of costs and effects, over a long-term time horizon.

It is frequently necessary to extrapolate when the options being compared differ in terms of mortality and this difference is to be expressed in terms of life-years or QALYs gained. This is illustrated in Fig. 9.1 in the form of the survival curves of two interventions (treatment and control) being compared in a randomized trial. These show the proportion of patients surviving until particular points of follow-up (measured in months). Figure 9.1(a) relates to the maximum follow-up during the

Box 9.2 **Examples of studies where decision models have been used to extrapolate between intermediate endpoints and measures of health gain**

Study	Intermediate endpoints	Method of extrapolation
(Glick et al. 1992.) A general model to establish the cost effectiveness of a range of possible cholesterol-lowering interventions as a form of primary prevention of coronary heart disease (CHD)	Assumed treatment effects for cholesterol-lowering therapies in terms of percentage reduction in cholesterol level	A Markov-type model with the following states: alive and free of CHD, alive with CHD, dead from CHD, and dead from non-CHD causes. The probability of getting CHD was estimated using risk equations from the Framingham Heart Study. This risk is conditional on factors including age, gender, cholesterol level, systolic blood pressure, and smoking status. Changes in this risk would change the proportion of patients experiencing CHD and hence life expectancy and life-term costs. A therapy that reduced cholesterol levels—one of the risk factors in the equation—could then be evaluated in terms of patients' long-term costs and life expectancy
(Neumann et al. 1999.) A model to assess the cost-effectiveness of donepezil in mild to moderate Alzheimer's disease (AD)	Treatment effect from trial between baseline and 24 weeks in terms of transition between Clinical Dementia Rating (CDR) scale 2 (moderate) and CDR 0.5 or 1 (mild)	Markov model with states defined in terms of mild, moderate, and severe disease (in terms of CDR); also a dead state. Baseline disease progression between states was taken from a longitudinal cohort study. Utilities were estimated for each Markov state using the Health Utilities Index-2 (see Chapter 6) in a cross-sectional survey of caregivers of AD patients. The treatment effect was applied to the baseline transitions, with several alternative durations. After coming off the drug, patients return to baseline progression rates
(Kobelt et al. 2003.) A model to assess the cost-effectiveness of infliximab in rheumatoid arthritis	Treatment effect in terms of change in Health Assessment Questionnaire (HAQ)-score, which is focused on functional disability—over a period of 54 weeks	A Markov model was developed with seven states—six relating to HAQ levels (functional disability) and one for death. Utility estimates for each HAQ state were estimated using the EQ-5D. The trial data were used to show short-term movements between the HAQ states on infliximab and for its comparator. Data from epidemiological cohort studies were used to estimate longer-term transitions between states

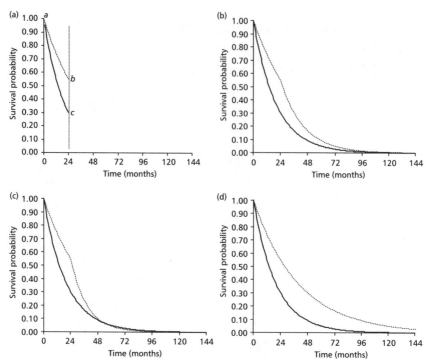

Fig. 9.1 Series of charts showing alternative extrapolation assumptions relating to survival data observed in a trial over a 24-month follow-up. —, control; ..... treatment. (a) The curves as observed in the trial, with a 50% reduction in mortality with treatment compared with control. (b) The survival curves extrapolated over 144 months with the assumption of a 'one-time' benefit to patients. (c) Extrapolation with a rebound effect. (d) Illustration of the assumption of a continuous treatment effect.

trial of 24 months. It indicates that, in terms of mortality, treatment is more effective than control as it reduces the mortality rate by 50%. If the time horizon of the study is taken to be the same as the maximum follow-up in the trial, the measure of life-years gained from surgery is equivalent to the area between the two curves over 2 years (area *abc* in Fig. 9.1(a)). The assumption with a 2-year time horizon is that the patients who remain alive at the end of trial follow-up receive a maximum benefit of 2 years additional life expectancy—this effectively assumes that they die at the end of the trial! This assumption is often called 'stop and drop'. In reality, the additional patients living at the end of the trial having received the treatment will live for a longer time period and this 'within-trial' measure of life-years gained will inevitably be an underestimate.

The use of modelling to extrapolate beyond the trial follow-up period involves predicting what the survival curves will look like beyond what has been observed.

This does not necessarily require a decision model; for example, survival regression can be used when patient-level data are available (Collett 1994). However, when working with summary data from the literature (which will usually be the case when data from several sources are being employed), a decision model is usually the vehicle for extrapolation. A key question with extrapolation relates to the appropriate assumption about the shape of the survival curves after follow-up. For interventions that take place only during the trial period, a popular assumption is that the more effective treatment during the trial confers a 'one-time' benefit to patients. As illustrated in Fig. 9.1(b), this means that beyond the period of the trial the rate of death per period of time, conditional on surviving until the end of the trial, is the same for patients originally allocated to treatment and to control. In other words, beyond the 24-month period, the 50% reduction in the rate of mortality in the trial is assumed to end and both groups become identical in terms of the mortality rate. The area between the two survival curves represents the gain in mean survival duration with treatment. This is effectively the approach to extrapolation undertaken by Mark *et al.* in the base-case cost-effectiveness analysis of alternative thrombolytic therapies for acute myocardial infarction considered in Chapter 3 (Mark *et al.* 1995). That study used a separate source of data (a registry of patients who had experienced acute myocardial infarction and survived the first year) to provide 15-year estimates of risk of mortality; beyond 15 years these risks were based on general population data.

This assumption of a one-time benefit has been used in several studies, particularly in the cardiac field. However, it might be inappropriate. It might be more appropriate to assume that the survival curves converge more rapidly after the trial follow-up period. That is, the conditional rate of death beyond trial follow-up becomes higher with treatment compared to control. Here is it assumed that, beyond the trial follow-up period, the mortality rate increases by 40% in the treatment arm compared to control. This could happen, for example, if the more effective intervention delays the death of a high-risk subgroup of patients who, once treatment is ended (at the end of trial follow-up), die at a faster rate than those patients surviving in the other arm. This scenario is sometimes known as a 'rebound effect'. It can be seen that the area between the survival curves (the gain in mean survival duration with treatment) is less than when a 'one-time' benefit is assumed.

At the other extreme, it may be reasonable to assume that the treatment confers a continuous benefit beyond trial follow-up, and this is shown in Fig. 9.1(d). That is, the curves continue to diverge in the longer term and the 50% reduction in mortality of treatment continues and patients randomized to that option continue to die at a slower rate. It can be seen that the area between the curves assuming a continuous benefit is larger than in Figs 9.1(b) and 9.1(c). This may be a more appropriate assumption when treatment is still ongoing at the end of trial follow-up when, of course, costs are extrapolated as well as benefits. The issue of the most reasonable assumption can be informed by the shape of the survival curves within the trial. For example, if they are ceasing to diverge in the latter period of follow-up, an assumption of continued divergence in the extrapolation is likely to be unwarranted. External non-trial data may also hold some clues. It is also important, however, to identify an appropriate assumption on the basis of what is known about the biology of the intervention—for example, in the case of a pharmaceutical, the length of time it remains active in the patient's body.

The choice of assumption made regarding extrapolation may have major implications on study results. For example, in an early cost-effectiveness study of therapy for patients with HIV, Schulman *et al.* (1991) estimated the incremental cost per life-year gained under two alternative assumptions about the effect of zidovudine on the development of AIDS and hence on mortality: a one-time effect and a continuous effect. The incremental cost per life-year gained of therapy ranged from $6553 to $70 526 under those two scenarios. This shows that it is important to run alternative scenarios regarding plausible extrapolation assumptions. The judgements about plausibility are usually based on our knowledge about the epidemiology of the disease and the effects of other treatments that have been evaluated in the past.

Another example is a model to evaluate the cost-effectiveness of new pharmaceuticals for multiple sclerosis (Chilcott *et al.* 2003). It was assumed that, once patients come off the new treatment, disease progression, in terms of the Kurtzke Expanded Disability Status Scale, continued as it would have under conventional therapy, which is equivalent to the one-time benefit scenario described above. The authors intended that this assumption was optimistic to the new therapies, which were found to have an incremental cost per QALY gained ranging from £42 000 to £98 000. They recognized that if a rebound effect was assumed, these ratios would be markedly higher.

9.2.5. The need to make results applicable to the decision-making context

Another situation where there may be a gap between the available evidence, particularly from randomized trials, and the requirements for a decision, relates to situations where the decision problem being addressed is inconsistent with the nature of the available trial evidence. One example of this was considered in Chapter 5 (Box 5.1) relating to the cost-effectiveness of strategies for the long-term management of duodenal ulcer. Here a model was used to adjust for the fact that the measure of efficacy was based on endoscopic measurements of recurrence, which would not be carried out in routine practice in patients without symptoms. Another example of the use of decision models to relate available evidence to a particular decision context is the adjustment of effectiveness evidence that is generated in one location and making it relevant to an economic evaluation in another jurisdiction. This use of models to 'transfer' results between settings is discussed more fully in Chapter 10.

A third example concerns the use of decision models to focus an economic evaluation on one or more specific subgroups of patients, based on available clinical evidence that may relate to a mix of patients. In decision models, the methods used to estimate cost-effectiveness for specific subgroups often divides the absolute benefit of a treatment upon which cost-effectiveness is based (for example, the absolute reduction in an event such as the rate of myocardial infarction following an intervention) into two elements: baseline effects and relative effects. Baseline effects are the measure of events in the comparator group. The relative treatment effect is a ratio (for example, an odds ratio, relative risk, or hazard ratio) representing the effectiveness of the newer therapy relative to the control group, which is typically the main focus when the clinical results of a randomized trial are reported (Kahn and Sempos 1989). Often the clinical report of a trial will indicate that there is no evidence of differences between subgroups (defined in terms of one more patient characteristics collected at the start of the trial) in terms of relative treatment effect. However, cost-effectiveness is driven by *absolute* benefit, and there may still be important variation between subgroups in baseline event rates. Indeed, this assumption of constant relative effects being applied to subgroup-specific baseline event rates is common in cost-effectiveness models. Its use will mean that, all other things being equal, a subgroup with a higher baseline risk of an undesirable clinical event will be more cost-effective to treat with an intervention that confers a proportional risk reduction than a subgroup with a lower baseline risk.

An example of a modelling study using this assumption compared lifetime costs and QALYs of two alternative hip prostheses used in primary hip replacement (Briggs *et al.* 2004). The effectiveness of the two prostheses, in terms of their failure rate over time, was taken from a large registry developed in Sweden. Reflecting the registry data, the model allowed the baseline failure rate (that for the 'usual care' prosthesis) to vary by the patient's age and sex. The relative reduction in failure rate with the newer prosthesis was, however, assumed constant over those subgroups. It is also important to note that the 'background' mortality rate (that is, the population rate from all causes) is known to vary by age and sex. As death from reasons unrelated to hip replacement was also included in the model (a 'competing risk'), this increases the differences between age and sex subgroups in terms of the cost-effectiveness of the newer prosthesis. Using the top and bottom right quadrants of the cost-effectiveness plane (see Chapter 3), Fig. 9.2 shows how the cost-effectiveness of the newer prosthesis varied by age and sex. The top line relates to incremental costs and effects of the newer prosthesis relative to the old for females, with various points on that line representing patient age. The lower line shows the similar relationship for males. It can be seen that, for both males and females, the newer prosthesis is more cost-effective for the younger age groups: the newer device is dominant for men aged 70 or younger and for women aged 60 or younger. This is because the lifetime risk of failure with the older prosthesis is higher in younger patients because they impose greater wear and tear on their hips due to their greater activity, and because they would be expected to live longer. Therefore, a constant relative reduction in the failure rate with the newer prosthesis will confer a greater absolute benefit in these younger age groups. In addition to variation in the

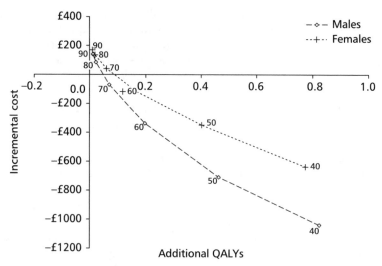

Fig. 9.2 Results of a cost-effectiveness study by Briggs *et al.* showing how the cost-effectiveness of a newer prosthesis varies by patient subgroup defined in terms of age and sex. QALY, quality-adjusted life-year. From Briggs *et al.* (2004).

cost-effectiveness of the newer prosthesis by age, it is also less cost-effective in women (that is, the line in Fig. 9.2 is higher). Again, this is because men have a higher baseline event rate with the existing prosthesis as their activity levels place greater stress on the hip.

Other studies have made both the baseline event rate and the relative treatment effect specific to the subgroup of interest. For example, in their cost–utility analysis of glycoprotein IIb/IIIa antagonists (GPAs) in acute coronary syndrome (ACS), Palmer *et al.* (in press) considered the cost-effectiveness of different ways of using the drug in all patients with ACS, and in those at high risk of future cardiac events. The baseline event rate in the high-risk group was taken from an observational study of ACS, and the relative treatment effect of GPAs in that subgroup was taken from a meta-analysis of trials. As for all sub-group analyses, there should always be a plausible clinical explanation of subgroup effects, rather than crude data mining. Furthermore, the uncertainty associated with subgroup analysis should also be fully assessed (see Section 9.4.6).

9.3. **Key elements of decision analytic modelling**

There are some key elements to decision analysis that are common to all models. These are probabilities and expected values. Different model types such as decision trees could also be added to this list, but these are discussed more fully in Section 9.4.

9.3.1. **Probabilities**

Probabilities are used widely in quantitative methods in many fields, and have an important role in clinical decision-making (Weinstein and Fineberg 1980). A common way of thinking about probability is as the measured frequency of an event in a given sample or population. For example, if 200 patients are treated with a particular medicine and 10 have an adverse event, the proportion of 0.05 can be taken as an estimate of the probability of a patient experiencing an adverse event with that therapy in the future. Although the next patient to be treated will either experience the adverse event or not, when the decision is being taken regarding whether to administer the therapy the uncertain outcome for the individual can be expressed in terms of a probability estimated from the experiences of other patients.

This concept of probability as a number indicating whether an event will or will not take place is a feature of Bayesian statistics, and is not shared with classical or 'Frequentist' statistical methods that are widely used in the analysis of randomized trials (O'Hagan and Luce 2003). This emphasizes the common origins of decision analysis and Bayesian statistics. This concept of probability can be generalized to represent a strength of belief which, for a given individual, is based on their previous knowledge and experience. This view of probability is important in decision analysis as, in many analyses, the likelihood of particular events may not have been informed by formal studies such as trials, and estimates from relevant experts may need to be elicited. This use of expert opinion in decision analysis may be considered a weakness of the methods. However, another perspective is that decisions about the use of health care interventions have to be taken regardless of the strength of the evidence available. The spirit of decision analysis is that these decisions should be taken on an analytical basis based on explicit methods and assumptions. Because, in the absence of formal evidence, the decision will still have to be taken on the basis of assumptions and judgements, decision analysis provides an analytical framework within which this can be done explicitly.

Some specific probability principles are also important in decision analysis, and these are summarized in Box 9.3.

Box 9.3 **Probability concepts**

Joint probability	The probability of two events occurring concomitantly. In terms of notation, the joint probability of events A and B: $P[A \text{ and } B]$. When the events are independent $P[A \text{ and } B] = P[A] \times P[B]$
Conditional probability	The probability of an event A given that an event B is known to have occurred. The notation is $P[A|B]$. Joint and conditional probabilities are related in the following equation: $P[A \text{ and } B] = P[A|B] \times P[B]$
Independence	Events A and B are independent if $P[A]$ is the same as $P[A|B]$.

9.3.2. **Expected values**

A key concept in decision analysis is the expected value. This is illustrated in Fig. 9.3, which compares two alternative interventions, medical and surgical. For each intervention, a given patient can follow one of three possible pathways where these are defined in terms of a bad, intermediate, or good outcome. Prior to treatment, it is unknown which pathway a specific patient will follow, but probabilities are used to express the likelihood of each occuring. These are likely to differ by therapy. For the alternative therapies, each pathway has a cost and an outcome expressed in terms of QALYs; there is also a cost of the intervention itself which is incurred whatever pathway the patient follows. For each of the therapies, an expected cost and expected outcome can be calculated. The expected cost is the cost of the intervention plus the therapy-specific sum of the costs of the three pathways weighted by the probability of a patient following each pathway with that treatment. The same idea is applied to calculate expected outcome. On that basis, it is clear that surgery has both a higher expected cost and higher expected QALYs. Using the methods of incremental analysis introduced in Chapter 3, the incremental cost per additional QALY generated by surgery can be calculated.

The concept of expected value is clearly analogous to the mean value of an endpoint when sample data are available. In a trial-based cost–utility analysis, for example, the mean costs and QALYs across patients in each of the randomized groups are used as

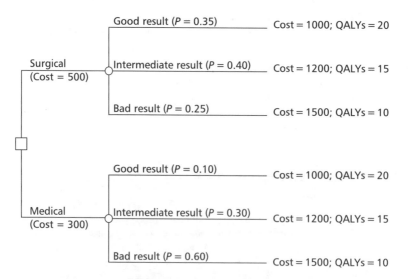

Expected cost of surgery: $500 + (0.35 \times 1000) + (0.40 \times 1200) + (0.25 \times 1500) = 1705$
Expected QALYs of surgery: $(0.35 \times 20) + (0.40 \times 15) + (0.25 \times 10) = 15.5$
Expected cost of medicine: $300 + (0.10 \times 1000) + (0.30 \times 1200) + (0.60 \times 1500) = 1660$
Expected QALYs of medicine: $(0.10 \times 20) + (0.30 \times 15) + (0.60 \times 10) = 12.5$

Incremental cost per QALY gained of surgery: $(1705 - 1660)/(15.5 - 12.5) = 15$

Fig. 9.3 Simple decision tree showing example of the calculation of expected values. QALY, quality-adjusted life-year.

the basis of the incremental analysis. As for mean values in trial-based studies, the expected value from a decision model represents the best estimate of the endpoints of interest for decision-making. As decision analysis shares common theoretical origins with the expected utility theory described in Chapter 6, the expected values calculated in decision models should strictly be von Neumann–Morgenstern utilities. Given that expected utility theory is a normative framework for decision-making under conditions of uncertainty, the expected utilities from decision models would provide a clear indication of the preferred option from those being compared. However, decision analysis is widely used for situations when outcomes other than von Neumann–Morgenstern utilities are used. The expected value should still provide the key input for decision-making as long as the outcomes have been chosen appropriately, as discussed in earlier chapters.

9.4. The stages in the development of a decision analytic model

The development of a decision analytic model for economic evaluation involves a number of stages. This section considers each of the stages to provide a fuller understanding of the role of decision modelling in this field.

9.4.1. Defining the decision problem

One of the key stages in the development of the model is the specification of the question being addressed, sometimes called the decision problem. This process closely mirrors the specification of the study question for economic evaluation in general as discussed in Chapter 3. In particular, there is a need to define the recipient group (patients or others) and the relevant options being compared. It is important to emphasize that, in defining these options, this may include more than specific interventions. It may include, for instance, starting and stopping rules for treatments—for example, when to start and stop medical therapy for a particular chronic condition. For some evaluations, the options will represent *clinical treatment strategies or pathways*, such as the sequence of therapies that might be used for the treatment of a condition characterized by treatment failure with some therapies. An example of such a study is a decision model looking at the cost-effectiveness of alternative therapies for epilepsy where assumptions were made about which therapies patients were placed on if they failed on initial treatment (Wilby *et al.* 2003).

9.4.2. Defining the boundaries of the model

All models are simplifications of reality so, in developing an analysis, decisions have to be taken about what to include. In part, this relates to general issues in economic evaluation such as the choice of perspective, the appropriate measure of effect/benefit, and the time horizon (see Chapter 3). However, it is sometimes important to consider how far a model should go to cover all the possible implications of an intervention or programme. For example, in considering the cost-effectiveness of antibiotic treatment for a given condition, the issue of the cost and health effects of antibiotic resistance could be an issue for decision-making, but relatively few cost-effectiveness models have considered this aspect of therapy—that is, they have drawn the boundaries of the model to exclude it from consideration. Another example is a decision model that was developed to assess the cost-effectiveness of routine ante-natal HIV testing (Ades *et al.* 1999). Ades *et al.* assessed the impact of different screening strategies on the extent to which a woman's HIV status was known during pregnancy. Through the use of interventions, this knowledge could have three beneficial health effects: (1) on the woman through earlier use of antiretroviral therapy; (2) on the child through the use of interventions to reduce the mother-to-child (vertical) transmission rate; and (3) on the child through the earlier use of antiretroviral therapy and prophylaxis if the child is born with HIV. The broader health benefit relating to reductions in infections to others through changes in sexual behaviour (horizontal transmission) was not, however, considered in the model, thus defining the study boundary. Decisions about the boundaries in decision models will partly be based on the availability of data and complexity of the modelling task, but they should mainly be driven by the extent to which extending the boundaries (adding complexity) is considered likely to impact on the cost-effectiveness of the options being compared.

9.4.3. **Structuring a decision model**

A key stage in the development of a decision model is the process of deciding on a structure. Formally, this involves a series of decisions concerning how the input parameters in the model are to be related and, in particular, choices about how to characterize the clinical events of interest (for example, episodes of a disease, disease progression, case identification). Each economic evaluation brings with it different structural issues, but a few common ones are given below.

1 Do the events of interest occur just once (for example, death) or can it happen several times over the relevant time horizon (for example, a non-fatal myocardial infarction)?

2 Is there a series of competing event risks that need to be considered (for example, the risk of a heart attack but also of death)?

3 As discussed in Section 9.2.4, when extrapolating events over time, what is the durability of the effectiveness of a particular intervention?

4 Do the probabilities of events change as time elapses or are they constant with respect to time?

5 Are all important events included and has double-counting of events been avoided?

6 For the management of a chronic disease, does the structure of the model allow for the costs and effects of subsequent therapies to be included?

The way in which an analyst handles these issues can essentially be defined as a series of mathematical relationships between parameters. Indeed some studies present the structure of their decision models in terms of a series of equations

(Spiegelhalter and Best 2003). Most decision models used in economic evaluation, however, present the structure of their model schematically. Two model structures predominate in the economic evaluation literature, decision trees and Markov models.

1. *The decision tree.* The decision tree is probably the most common structure for decision models in economic evaluation. It represents individuals' possible prognoses, following some sort of intervention, by a series of pathways. A simple example was considered in Fig. 9.2 to illustrate expected values. Decision trees were also used in Chapter 5 to illustrate how this type of model structure was used in a cost-effectiveness analysis of different interventions for the prevention of pulmonary embolism. Another clinical example is used here to illustrate the use of decision models in more detail—the comparison of two antiemetic prophylactic therapies for patients undergoing chemotherapy for cancer. The example is based on a published study comparing ondansetron and metoclopramide which was undertaken prior to a price having been determined for ondansetron (Buxton and O'Brien 1992). The study considered the acquisition cost of the therapies, the cost of the adverse events and of their treatment, and the cost of treatment failure (that is, an episode of emesis). Effects were in terms of the probability of a patient being successfully treated, which was defined as the absence of emesis and adverse events. The decision tree is shown in Fig. 9.4, and this can be used to describe a series of general features with this sort of model structure.

Decision nodes. The square box at the start of the decision tree is a decision node and represents the decision being addressed in the model: which of ondansetron and metoclopramide is the more cost-effective in preventing episodes of emesis without adverse events?

Chance nodes. Coming out of the decision node is the range of possible pathways that characterize the effects of the alternative therapies. The pathways are built up through a series of branches representing particular events. Here the events are significant emesis, significant adverse events, the treatment of adverse events, and the resolution of adverse events. Given that, *ex ante*, it is not known whether a patient will experience a given event and follow a particular branch, the circular nodes (chance nodes) define points of uncertainty in the tree.

Branch probabilities. The branches issuing from a chance node represent the possible events patients may experience at that point in the tree. The likelihood of the event is represented in terms of branch probabilities. For both treatments, the first chance node relates to whether or not a patient experiences an episode of emesis, and the probability of emesis and its complement (that is, 1—the probability of that event) are shown on the respective branches. Moving from left to right, chance nodes show subsequent uncertain events. The probabilities of these subsequent events are conditional probabilities because they only relate to those patients who have experienced particular previous events. For example, for those patients who have experienced an episode of emesis on metoclopramide, the conditional probability of significant adverse events is 0.34; and the probability of treatment conditional on such an event is 0.6. It can be seen that, although the possible events are the same

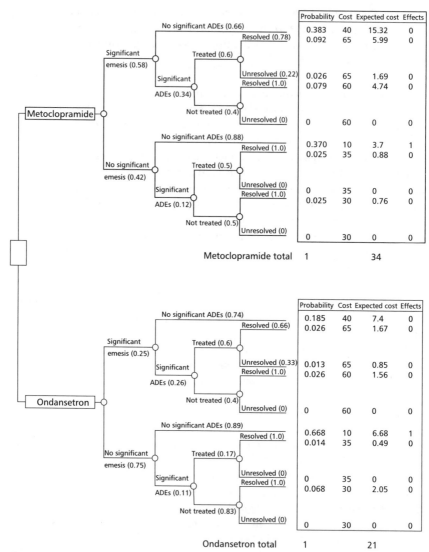

Fig. 9.4 Example of a decision tree taken from Buxton and O'Brien (1992). ADE, adverse drug events. Other inputs into the model: price of both treatments, £10; cost of an episode of emesis, £30; cost of side-effects, £20; cost of treating side-effects, £5.

for the two therapies, the probabilities in the two parts of the tree are not the same. Specifically, the efficacy of ondansetron was considered higher than that of metoclopramide, so there is a lower probability of emesis. Ondansetron was also considered less toxic, as the probabilities of adverse events (whether or not the drug had been efficacious) are lower than those for metoclopramide. There are also differences between the two therapies in the probabilities of an adverse event being treated and of it resolving.

Pathways. The combination of the different branches in the tree determines a series of pathways along which patients can pass in the tree. For both treatments, there are 10 possible pathways. The top pathway for each treatment is significant emesis and no adverse events; the second pathway is significant emesis and a significant adverse event that is treated and resolves, and so on. The final pathway for each treatment is no significant emesis and an adverse event that is not treated and that does not resolve. These pathways are mutually exclusive (a given patient can only follow one of the pathways) and exhaustive (a given patient must follow one of the pathways).

Pathway probabilities. To the right of the decision tree in Fig. 9.4 is a series of columns of numbers. The first is the probability of a given patient passing along each of the pathways. These probabilities are calculated by multiplying the initial branch probability by subsequent conditional probabilities. So the probability of the first pathway with ondansetron is the product of the probability of significant emesis (0.25) and the probability of no significant adverse events conditional on significant emesis (0.74), which equals 0.185. As the pathways are mutually exclusive, the probabilities for a given treatment must sum to 1.

Pathway costs. Each pathway in the tree also has costs associated with it. These represent the sum of the costs of each of the events a patient experiences in that pathway. For the first pathway for example, the relevant costs are the cost of the drug itself (£10) and the cost of significant emesis (£30), totalling £40. The second pathway cost is the sum of the drug cost (£10), significant emesis (£30), and significant adverse events (£20) which are treated (£5), equalling £65. The same principle is applied to the other pathways in the tree. It can be seen that the pathway costs are the same for metoclopramide and ondansetron as it is assumed that the two products have the same acquisition price and event costs.

Expected values. The expected cost for the two therapies can be calculated by weighting each pathway cost by its respective probability, and then summing across all the pathways. This can be seen in the expected cost column of Fig. 9.3. Adding down this column generates an expected cost for metoclopramide and ondansetron of £34 and £21, respectively. This decision model is used as a basis for a cost-effectiveness analysis using the probability of successful treatment as the relevant measure of effect (no emesis and no adverse events). In terms of expected values, this is equivalent to giving the pathway of no emesis and no adverse events the value 1 and all other pathways the value 0. Assuming equal prices for the products, this version of the model indicates that ondansetron is dominant, as it has a lower expected cost than metoclopramide and a higher expected effect. The original paper considered a number of sensitivity analyses involving alternative assumptions about the prices for the products. Another way of working out the expected costs and effectiveness for a given option in a decision tree is by 'rolling back' the tree. It will give exactly the same answer as the approach outlined above, but involves working from the right-hand side of the tree towards the left, calculating expected values at each chance node. Box 9.4 shows how the decision tree for the alternative antiemetics is rolled back to estimate expected costs for metoclopramide.

Limitations of the decision tree. The decision tree is widely used in economic evaluation, but has important limitations. The first is that events are implicitly taken

Box 9.4 **The process of 'rolling back' a decision tree to calculate expected values**

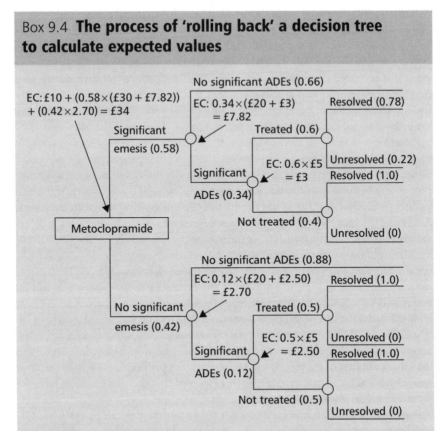

EC, expected costs, ADE, adverse drug events. The example shows the calculation of expected cost for metoclopramide in the decision tree shown in Fig. 9.4.

as occurring over an instantaneous discrete period. In the antiemetic case study discussed above, for example, costs and effects over an undefined treatment period were considered. In other words, time is not explicitly defined in a decision tree unless the analyst does so in determining the different branches. As there is no explicit time variable in a decision tree, those elements of an economic evaluation that are time dependent can be difficult to implement. This is true of discounting, where the time at which costs and outcomes are accrued is very important. It also applies to the process of adjusting survival duration for health-related quality of life in cost–utility analysis where it is necessary to know when a change in health status occurs.

The second, and related, limitation of decision trees is that they can get very complex when they are used to model complicated long-term prognoses, particularly related to chronic diseases. For example, to model the future prognosis of a woman with early-stage breast cancer, a decision tree would have to characterize a whole series of competing risks that a woman would have to face including adverse treatment effects, cancer recurrence (of various types), remission from cancer, and death. Given the chronic nature of the disease, once an event is experienced in one time period (for example, cancer recurrence), a series of new risks may present themselves for future time periods. In principle, these recurring events could be structured using a decision tree where a set of chance nodes and branches could be used to characterize events in a particular time period, and the same or similar ones could be used for subsequent time periods. However, for a long-term chronic disease, where a patient is at risk of events for many years, the tree could become very 'bushy', with many mutually exclusive pathways. A model of this type would probably be very time consuming to programme and analyse.

2. *The Markov model.* The limitations of the decision tree are the main reasons why another model structure—Markov models—are also widely used in economic evaluation to handle particular decision problems (Sonnenberg and Beck 1993; Briggs and Sculpher 1998). Whereas decision trees characterize possible prognoses in terms of alternative branches, Markov models are based on a series of 'states' that a patient can occupy at a given point in time. Time elapses explicitly with a Markov model, with the probability of a patient occupying a given state assessed over a series of discrete time periods, called cycles. The length of these cycles will depend on the disease and interventions being evaluated, but might be a month or a year. Each state in the model has a cost associated with it and, for cost–utility analysis, a utility value. The time duration during which the average patient occupies the various states in the model will, when weighted by the relevant cost or utility, be used to calculate expected costs and outcomes. The speed with which patients move between the states in the model is determined by a set of transition probabilities.

These concepts are described in more detail using an example from the published literature, which evaluated the cost-effectiveness of two antiretroviral therapies (zidovudine monotherapy versus zidovudine plus lamivudine combination therapy) for patients with HIV infection (Chancellor *et al.* 1997).

Markov states. Figure 9.5 shows a schematic of the Markov model used in the HIV example. The model is structured in terms of four Markov states. Two of these are related to a patient's CD4 count, which indicates the strength of their immune system. State A represents the healthiest patients with relatively high CD4 counts, and State B includes patients with lower CD4 counts. State C includes patients who have progressed to AIDS, and the patient moves to State D when they die. The arrows in the model show how patients can progress through the model over the cycles, which were taken to be 1 year. If a patient starts in State A in the first cycle, various transitions are possible in the second cycle: the patient can (1) remain in State A; (2) move to State B as their CD4 count drops; (3) move to State C if they suffer an AIDS-defining illness; or (4) move to State D if they die. Once a patient has moved to State B, in the next cycle they can remain in this state, or progress to State C or to State D. In this model, it is not possible for a patient's health to improve, so they cannot, for example, move from State B to State A. Once in State C, in the next cycle they can remain in that state or die, but not move back to States A or B. State D (death) is an absorbing state from which, sadly, there is no escape!

Transition probabilities. Figure 9.5 shows the transition probabilities that define the speed at which patients move between the Markov states, and the cycle length is 1 year.

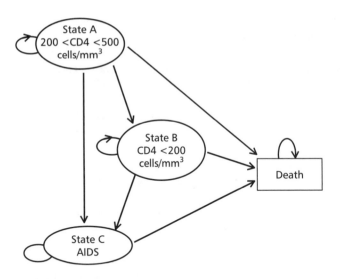

Transition probabilities—monotherapy

	Transition to			
Transition from	State A	State B	State C	State D
State A	0.721	0.202	0.067	0.01
State B	0	0.581	0.407	0.012
State C	0	0	0.75	0.25
State D	0	0	0	1

Transition probabilities—combination therapy

	Transition to			
Transition from	State A State B		State C	State D
State A	0.858 0.103		0.034	0.005
	(1−sum) (0.202×RR)		(0.067×RR)	(0.01×RR)
State B	0 0.787		0.207	0.006
	(1−sum)		(0.407×RR)	(0.012×RR)
State C	0 0		0.873	0.127
			(1−sum)	(0.25×RR)
State D	0 0		0	1

Fig. 9.5 Markov diagram for a cost-effectiveness model in HIV taken from Chancellor *et al.* (1997). Below the diagram are the transition probabilities used for the two interventions that were evaluated. RR is the relative risk of combination therapy compared to monotherapy in terms of disease progression.

Two sets of probabilities are shown—one for monotherapy (the comparator therapy), and one for combination therapy (the new therapy). The two matrices show the state the patient starts the cycle in, and the probabilities associated with the various transitions during that cycle. For example, if a patient is in State A on monotherapy, there is a probability of 0.721 that they will remain in that state in the next cycle, of 0.202 that they will progress to State B, of 0.067 that they will progress to State C, and of 0.01 that they will die. The zeros in the matrix represent situations where backwards transitions are not permitted. It can be seen that, because a patient always has to be in one of the states, the sum of the probabilities across the lines must always equal 1. These 'baseline' probabilities, relating to what was then current practice, were taken from a longitudinal cohort study, which is a common source for these parameters. Appropriate analytical methods are required to translate longitudinal data into transition probabilities over discrete cycles. This will often require survival analysis (Kuntz and Weinstein 2001), and there will always need to be an awareness of the distinction between rates and probabilities (Miller and Homan 1994). This is essential when probabilities identified in the literature relate to different time periods than the cycle length in the Markov model.

The second matrix shows the transition probabilities for combination therapy. Based on the relative risk from a meta-analysis of 0.509, the authors assumed that the new therapy would reduce each transition probability to a worse state by about 50%. To ensure that the line of probabilities continued to sum to 1, this required the probabilities of remaining in a state to be increased to compensate.

In this model the transition probabilities are the same for every cycle in the model. This implies, for example, that a patient with AIDS is at the same risk of death over the next year regardless of factors such as their age or the duration of time they have had AIDS. Markov models with fixed transition probabilities with respect to time are known as Markov chains.

Costs and outcomes. In the Markov model, costs are typically implemented each cycle according to the state a patient occupies. For the two therapies being evaluated in the HIV example, the cost of being in a given state is the same, and the only difference is in the acquisition price of the therapies. Hence, as for the decision tree example above, the only elements of the Markov model that differ between the two therapies are the acquisition cost of the therapies themselves and the probabilities that determine how a patient moves through the model. On the outcome side, the HIV model was a cost-effectiveness analysis in which expected survival duration (life-years) was the measure of effectiveness, and this was evaluated over a life-time time horizon.

Expected values. The process of calculating expected costs and effectiveness with a Markov model is very similar to that in a decision tree. Instead of summing pathway costs and effects and weighting by their probabilities as with the decision tree (or rolling back the tree), the costs and values of each Markov state are weighted by the time a patient spends in that state. This is made up of two stages. In the first, the probability of a patient being in a given state for each cycle is calculated. There are several ways in which this can be calculated, but this is usually done in a spreadsheet or similar software using an approach method known as the cohort method, which produces a 'Markov trace' showing the proportion of the cohort in each state over time.

This is illustrated in Fig. 9.6 with respect to the monotherapy intervention in the HIV example, using 20 annual cycles. It is assumed that 1000 patients begin in the cohort, but the number is irrelevant as only the proportions of the cohort in particular states at a given time-point matter. One patient or one million patients could be used as the starting cohort, and the answer will be the same. For each cycle, the proportion of the cohort in each state is calculated on the basis of the proportions in the various

Cycle	State A	State B	State C	State D	Total
0	1000	0	0	0	1000
	1000×0.721	1000×0.202	1000×0.067	1000×0.01	
1	721	202	67	10	1000
2	520	263	181	36	1000
3	375	258	277	90	1000
4	270	226	338	166	1000
5	195	186	363	256	1000
6	140	147	361	351	1000
7	101	114	340	445	1000
8	73	87	308	532	1000
9	53	65	271	611	1000
10	38	48	234	680	1000
11	27	36	197	739	1000
12	20	26	164	789	1000
13	14	19	135	831	1000
14	10	14	110	865	1000
15	7	10	89	893	1000
16	5	7	72	916	1000
17	4	5	57	934	1000
18	3	4	45	948	1000
19	2	3	36	959	1000
20	1	2	28	968	1000

Fig. 9.6 The results of the Markov trace for the monotherapy group in the HIV example. The trace assumes a starting cohort of 1000 beginning in State A.

states in the last cycle and the transition probabilities. Figure 9.6 shows the calculations for the first cycle. In a spreadsheet, once the equations have been determined for the first cycle, it is normally a case of simply copying down the formulas for subsequent cycles. As more and more cycles are added, the proportion of the cohort in the absorbing state (here death) increases, and all but a very small proportion should have died once a cycle number that is consistent with the relevant life expectancy has been reached.

Once the proportion of patients (or, in other words, the probability of a given patient being) in each state for each cycle has been calculated, the second stage involves working out expected costs and effects. On the cost side, this involves calculating an expected cost per cycle by adding the cost of each cycle weighted by the proportion of the cohort in each state. The overall expected cost then simply involves summing the expected cost of each cycle. Implementing discounting is straightforward, with the standard formula (see Chapter 4) used to adjust the expected cost of every individual cycle. Expected outcomes are calculated on a similar basis. In the case of survival duration, this simply involves weighting the proportion of patients in each state per cycle by 1 if they are alive, and by 0 if the are dead. Adding up across the cycles (with or without discounting as necessary) will provide the expected number of life-years experienced by the cohort. In the case of QALYs, this is slightly different because the proportion of the cohort in each state is weighted by the utility value associated with that state, and then summed across the cycles.

A cohort simulation is undertaken for each option being evaluated. In the case of the HIV model, a cohort simulation was undertaken separately with the two sets of transition probabilities shown in Fig. 9.5. On this basis, combination therapy was found to be more costly and more effective, with an incremental cost per life-year gained of £6276.

3. *Other approaches to structuring decision models.* This chapter has considered two popular model structures used in economic evaluation. The Markov model is used in situations when the decision tree would become too unwieldy, typically when events can recur over a long time horizon. In some situations, a decision analysis may involve the combination of both a decision tree and a Markov. This was the case in evaluation of glycoprotein IIb/IIIa antagonists by Palmer *et al.* (in press), for example. A short-term decision tree was used to establish the proportion of patients with each therapy experiencing myocardial infarction or death over an initial 6-month period; a Markov model was used to calculate long-term expected costs and quality-adjusted survival duration conditional on which events had been experienced in the short-term model.

The Markov model may be unsuitable to model some prognoses. The HIV example described above, for example, assumed that transition probabilities did not vary over time. However, in some situations, this assumption may be difficult to sustain because of evidence suggesting that the probability increases or decreases with time. Some forms of 'time dependency' in transition probabilities can be handled quite easily in Markov models. This is the case, for instance, when the transition probability changes as the age of the patient increases. This can be implemented simply by having a different transition probability for each cycle in the cohort simulation. Similarly, it is not difficult to implement transition probabilities that change as a function of the time a patient has been in a state, as long as all patients start in that state, and none return to it once they have left it.

In other situations, it is less straightforward to implement time dependency in transition probabilities because of the key assumption underlying Markov models. This 'Markov assumption' is often described as the memoryless feature of these models. It holds that the probability of a given transition in the model is independent of the nature or timing of earlier transitions. This can be illustrated using the HIV model shown in Fig. 9.5. In this model, patients can enter the AIDS state (State C) from either State A or State B. However, once a patient has entered the AIDS state, the model cannot 'remember' where the patient came from; that is, it cannot distinguish the origin of the patients in the state at a given time point and treats them as homogenous. This assumption might be difficult to justify if evidence suggests, for example, that mortality risk is higher in patients who have experienced AIDS-defining events having previously had lower CD4 counts. If the memoryless feature represents an oversimplification of the epidemiological evidence, then it is always possible to add additional states to the Markov model. In the example above, two AIDS states could be used: one containing patients who moved there from State A and the other including patients who arrived from State B. These two AIDS states could then differ with respect to the risk of mortality and, if necessary, in terms of the cost per cycle of occupying that state.

Giving a Markov model additional 'memory' by adding states can, however, become unwieldy if numerous additional states have to be added. In this situation, one option for the analyst is to move to a different modelling approach. The decision tree and Markov model are usually analysed as *cohort models*. As shown above, this involves calculating the proportion of a homogeneous cohort that would move along particular pathways or occupy specific Markov states. Using these proportions to weight the costs and outcomes associated with pathways or Markov states, this provides the route to calculating overall expected costs and outcomes for each of the options being compared. An alternative approach to decision modelling is to move away from the cohort model towards modelling individual patients moving through models. These '*micro simulation*' or '*individual sampling*' models literally track the process of individual patients through particular states, and allow them to accumulate costs and benefit over time. They have the potential to offer greater flexibility than cohort models as the future prognosis of a given patient can vary according to their 'history'. In the case of the HIV example, the use of a micro simulation would mean that a patient who experiences an AIDS event with a CD4 count of 400 could have a different risk of future events than a patient who experienced such an event with a CD4 count of 200. Given the focus of economic evaluation on expected values, such a model has to simulate the costs and outcomes of a large number of patients and work out the average over those simulations. More detail about the use of micro simulation models in economic evaluation can be found elsewhere (Davies 1985; Barton *et al.* 2004), as can examples of their use (Paltiel *et al.* 1998; Karnon 2003).

Structuring decision models using micro simulations does have some limitations, however. The opportunity to incorporate patient history with such models may allow greater structural flexibility, but it will often require additional evidence to populate such models. This is because parameters representing possible future prognoses for a given patient need to be conditional on history, thus increasing the number of parameters to be estimated. A second limitation is that the simulation requirements of these models can be time consuming even with modern computers. This is particularly the case when probabilistic sensitivity analysis (PSA) is undertaken to quantify parameter uncertainty (see Section 9.4.5).

Identifying an appropriate structure is an extremely important stage of the decision-modelling process. It is not possible to provide definitive guidelines for the selection of a particular model structure, as these have to depend on the overall objective of the economic evaluation as well as the nature of the disease process and impacts of the interventions. It has to be emphasized that all models are a simplification of reality, and the ultimate objective in selecting an appropriate structure for a decision model is to make the model no more complex than it has to be to address the policy questions appropriately.

9.4.4. Identifying and synthesizing evidence

Once the appropriate structure of the model as been established it is necessary to identify available data with which to populate the model. As described in Chapter 5 and Section 9.2.2, the principles of evidence-based medicine and policy require that evidence is not identified selectively. This means that the evidence going into decision models needs to be identified systematically. There are well-known methods for the identification and quality assessment of effectiveness data (Centre for Reviews and Dissemination 2001). As yet, relatively little work has been done on systematic review methods for other types of parameters in decision models such as baseline event rates, resource use, unit costs, and utilities. Further methods research in this area is needed as the design hierarchy relating to relative effectiveness (see Chapter 5) is not directly relevant to many of the other parameters used in economic evaluation. For example, an estimate of the mean utility associated with a patient who experiences a myocardial infarction need not necessarily come from a randomized trial because it is not a parameter that directly relates to the comparison of alternative interventions, so selection bias is not an issue.

Given that a specific parameter in a decision model may have a number of sources of evidence informing it, evidence synthesis is an important prerequisite to decision modelling. For effectiveness parameters (particularly relative treatment effects such as a an odds ratio or relative risk) there is an extensive literature on the methods of meta-analysis (Sutton *et al.* 2000). The needs of policy relevant decision analysis do, however, pose some difficult questions for the methods of evidence synthesis, even relating to effectiveness parameters. These methods challenges relate to issues such as how to use observational data in estimating treatment effects (Prevost *et al.* 2000), how to generate indirect effectiveness estimates when the interventions of interest have not been directly compared in 'head-to-head' trials (Hasselblad 1998), and how to estimate treatment effects when different follow-up periods have been used (Nam *et al.* 2003). The methods of evidence synthesis for clinical parameters are becoming increasingly sophisticated (Sutton and Abrams 2001), and these will have benefits for economic evaluation using decision models. Indeed, there are now examples of economic studies where the synthesis of clinical data and the decision analysis have been undertaken as one comprehensive statistical model (Cooper *et al.* 2004).

The literature on methods to synthesize evidence for the estimation of parameters other than those relating to treatment effects is limited, and this represents an important area of future research.

9.4.5. **Dealing with uncertainty**

The different types of uncertainty that exist in decision analytic models was summarized in Chapter 3 (Box 3.3), following earlier classifications (Gold *et al.* 1996; Briggs 2001). Each of these types of uncertainty is important, and it is crucial to assess their implications for the model's results. The issues relating to methodological uncertainty, generalizability/transferability and 'process' uncertainty are largely general to economic evaluation and are not specific to decision modelling. There are particular features of parameter and structural uncertainty, however, which are specific to decision modelling, and these are considered in more detail below.

1. *Parameter uncertainty.* Chapter 8 discussed the development of statistical methods to reflect the sampling uncertainty inherent in economic evaluation studies

undertaken using patient-level data (for example, randomized trials). The need for these methods reflects the fact that any measurements made on the basis of sampled data are estimated imprecisely. For example, the mean cost measured in a sample of patients is estimated with uncertainty as represented in terms, for example, of the standard error of the mean. In decision analytic models, this imprecision is reflected in the input parameters that go into the model because usually these will be estimated from sampled data. This applies to parameters such as event probabilities, costs, utilities, and treatment effects. It is important to emphasize that, for economic evaluation, the ultimate purpose of a model is to estimate expected (or mean) costs and effectiveness. In the cohort models that are typically used in this area, therefore, the input parameters will represent the mean value for a particular population or subgroup, but these are estimated with uncertainty from sampled data.

In order to handle this *parameter uncertainty* in decision models, there needs to be an assessment of how it impacts on the results of the analysis. Until recently this was undertaken using standard sensitivity analysis, which involves varying individual input parameters across a range and assessing how this changes the model's results. As mentioned in Chapter 3, this form of sensitivity analysis has several drawbacks. First, with standard sensitivity analysis it is only practical to vary a small number of parameters simultaneously. In most cases only one parameter is varied at a time (one-way sensitivity analysis), but it is possible to vary two or perhaps three at the same time. However, most models include many more input parameters than this, each of which is usually estimated with uncertainty. To assess the implications of uncertainty in all these parameters, standard sensitivity analysis has to be undertaken sequentially, taking individual parameters (or small groups) one at a time. Not only is this tedious and often difficult to communicate to decision-makers but it is partial and fails to provide a complete picture of the joint parameter uncertainty. A second drawback relates to situations when input parameters in the model are correlated. This can occur, for example, when more than one parameter is estimated from some form of regression analysis. A third drawback is that there is no suitable summary measure of the implications of the uncertainty. It is only possible to show decision-makers the range of results associated with varying a particular input parameter rather than indicating the likelihood of particular results.

In the face of the limitations of standard sensitivity analyses, another form of sensitivity analysis is being increasingly used to handle parameter uncertainty. Probabilistic sensitivity analysis has been discussed for some years (Doubilet *et al.* 1985; Critchfield *et al.* 1986), but not until more recent advances in computer power have these methods been routinely applied. Probabilistic sensitivity analysis (PSA) has a number of elements, as described below.

1. *Characterize uncertainty in input parameters.* In standard sensitivity analysis, this takes the form of the definition of a 'best estimate' plus a range. With PSA, inputs are defined in as probability distributions to reflect their full uncertainty. Although a large number of distributions are available to use for this purpose, relatively few types of input parameters are used in most models, and the nature of these data is such that only a relatively small number of alternative distributions are available (Briggs et al. 2002). For example, most models include a number of

probability parameters, and the uncertainty in these parameters would be characterized as a beta distribution because this is bounded between 0 and 1. Selection from a similarly small subset of distributions would be made to characterize uncertainty in mean costs, mean utilities, and a relative treatment effect. When two or more parameters are correlated, multivariate distributions would be appropriate.

2. *Propagate the uncertainty through the model.* The second stage of PSA is to assess the implications for the results of the study of the uncertainty in all of the input parameters simultaneously. This process of *propagating* parameter uncertainty through the model would normally be undertaken using simulation techniques. A popular method is Monte Carlo simulation where the model is evaluated (that is, expected values are calculated) a large number of times, with each simulation involving a random draw from each of the input parameter distributions. The end result of the process is a large number (for example, 10 000) of sets of expected costs and effects that reflect the combined parameter uncertainty in the model. As mentioned in Section 9.4.3, in some situations micro simulation models may be used to provide more structural flexibility over cohort models. These models use simulation methods to calculate expected costs assuming a fixed (that is, certain) set of input parameter. To undertake PSA with such models, therefore, requires a second level of simulations for different values of uncertain input parameters. This can represent a major computational task, but short-cuts are available (Stevenson *et al.* 2004).

3. *Present the implications of parameter uncertainty.* The third step is to present the results of the PSA in an appropriate format. Once the simulation process has been undertaken, the situation is comparable to one where sample data are available (for example, from a trial) and provides estimates of mean overall cost and effect by intervention. Hence the methods discussed in Chapter 8 can be used to summarize the overall parameter uncertainty in the model. These include confidence intervals around an incremental ratio or incremental net benefit. Increasingly, cost-effectiveness acceptability curves (see Chapter 8) are being used to provide a full picture of parameter uncertainty, perhaps complemented by a scatter-plot of the simulations on the cost-effectiveness plane.

2. *Structural uncertainty.* Briggs refers to two forms of modelling uncertainty, structural and process (Briggs 2001). With respect to the former, decision modelling seeks to be of value for decision-making by simplifying the often highly complex process underlying the possible prognoses a patient can experience and the way interventions interact with these. As discussed in Section 9.4.3, any process of simplification will require assumptions, and these are embodied within the judgements made about the appropriate structure of the model. The extent to which a particular structural assumption has an important impact on the results should, as far as possible, be assessed as part of the analysis. In principle, this could be done using the methods of PSA. This would require the model to incorporate 'competing' structural assumptions, with weights placed on each to represent their relative plausibility. This has also been referred to as 'model averaging' (Hoeting *et al.* 1999), but there are few, if any, examples in the economic evaluation literature. To the extent

that this form of uncertainty is formally considered at all, it is usually achieved using standard sensitivity analysis. This represents 'standard' sensitivity in as much as the model is re-run with an alternative structural assumption to that in the base-case (or primary) analysis, but these methods have also been referred to as scenario analysis. An example of addressing structural uncertainty in this way is the model of combination therapy in HIV described in Section 9.4.3 (Chancellor *et al.* 1997). As part of their sensitivity analysis the authors explored the implications of the structural assumption that the duration of the treatment effect of combination therapy would be 2 years by varying this, in alternative scenarios, between 1 year and a continuous effect.

In some situations, a series of structural assumptions is so engrained in the model that assessing the implications and varying these using sensitivity analysis are not straightforward. This is the case, for example, in comparing the cost and effectiveness estimates based on a micro simulation model with those of a cohort model, which would, in effect, require two models to be developed. Karnon undertook such an analysis in the context of a cost-effectiveness analysis of tamoxifen plus chemotherapy versus chemotherapy alone in breast cancer (Karnon 2003). He compared his results based on a discrete event simulation and on a Markov model, and found these to be very similar. He concluded that, given the additional data needed to populate a micro simulation model, the Markov model was probably preferable in the circumstances. Inevitably the results of any decision analytic model are conditional on its input parameters and structural assumptions. It will rarely be possible to subject every structural feature of a model to sensitivity analysis, and there will always be a need, on an iterative basis, for the decision-maker and the analyst to identify what is considered to be the most appropriate structure of a model given the nature of the decision problem and the available evidence. There remains an important research agenda regarding an appropriate process to identify a 'preferred' model structure and to assess structural uncertainty.

9.4.6. Dealing with variability

As discussed in Chapters 3 and 8, it is important to draw a distinction in economic evaluation between uncertainty and variability. The former refers to situations where a model input is not known precisely and can, in principle at least, be characterized as a random variable. Variability is concerned with situations where input parameters might vary systematically between recipients or locations. As discussed in Chapter 8, to the extent to which the results (and potential conclusions) of an analysis might vary according to the characteristics and/or location of recipients, the appropriate way to deal with this heterogeneity is to run the model, and to present its results, separately for each relevant subgroup of recipient. As mentioned in Section 9.2.5, the decision model provides a flexible framework to assess the implications of different assumptions about the nature of the heterogeneity; for example, whether it relates to baseline events with the relative treatment effects being generalizable or whether both the baseline and relative effectiveness varies by subgroup. Of course, there will always remain uncertainty in estimates of input parameters that are specific to particular subgroups, so there will be a need to deal with parameter uncertainty appropriately for each subgroup. Indeed, given that the process of estimating subgroup-specific input parameters usually involves reducing sample size, it is even more important to assess the implications of parameter uncertainty fully.

9.4.7. Using models to assess the value of additional research

As discussed in Section 9.2, the role of economic evaluation is ultimately to improve decision-making regarding resource allocation. The value of decision modelling, in particular, is to bring to bear available evidence within an appropriately structured framework as an input into clearly defined decision problems. Typically, a decision problem will be defined in terms of whether resources should be made available for a particular intervention for a specific population. To inform this question, a decision model will provide an estimate of *expected* costs and effects for each intervention being evaluated, *based on currently available data*, from which the preferred option can be identified.

The various forms of uncertainty discussed in Section 9.4.5 generate a distribution around overall expected costs and effects. This results in what has been termed 'decision uncertainty'—that is, the probability that a given decision about a preferred intervention is the correct one. This can be calculated formally using stochastic analysis based on patient-level data or PSA, and is the focus of the cost-effectiveness acceptability curve introduced in Chapter 8. To the extent that there are different mean results for altern-ative scenarios relating to structural assumptions, measures of decision uncertainty should be presented for each of these. The same applies when different results are pre-sented for alternative patient subgroups. The extent to which decision uncertainty should impact on the choice of preferred option is controversial (see Chapter 10). However, there is no doubt that decision uncertainty is important to consider in addressing another decision: whether or not to undertake or require additional research.

There are examples of the use of decision models to inform research priorities without formally quantifying the decision uncertainty associated with identifying a preferred option based on currently available evidence (Detsky 1989; Drummond *et al.* 1992; Townsend and Buxton 1997). However, the use of PSA in decision models extends these methods by providing the opportunity to use value of information methods that have a firm foundation in statistical decision theory (Schlaiffer 1958) and have been applied in other areas of evaluation (Thompson and Evans 1997). In the context of health care evaluation, Claxton has set out the methods required to estimate the expected value of perfect information (EVPI) (Claxton and Posnett 1996; Claxton 1999). These can be summarized in a number of steps.

1 Expected costs and effects of the alternative options being compared from a PSA would be used to identify the preferred option from those being compared based on existing evidence. In the context of cost–utility/cost-effectiveness analysis, for example (see Chapter 3), an option would be preferred if it dominates its comparators or has an incremental cost per additional QALY that is less than the decision-maker's threshold willingness-to-pay (see Chapter 10 for further discussion of this threshold).

2 As shown in cost-effectiveness acceptability curves, the decision uncertainty quantified through PSA will indicate the probability that this decision is the correct one or, alternatively, the probability that in choosing this option the decision-maker is making an error.

3 The results of PSA can also be used to quantify the cost of making a wrong decision, both in terms of forgone health gain to patients and in terms of wasted resources. Combining this cost with the probability of making a wrong decision represents the expected cost of uncertainty, which can be considered synonymous with the EVPI because, if research could remove all uncertainty, its value would be the cost of that uncertainty. Because of the public good features of information (when it is made available to for one patient, it is available for all), the *population* EVPI relates to all patients who could potentially benefit from additional research over a period of time.

Therefore, EVPI represents a notional maximum value of further research against which the cost of undertaking a particular study can be compared. The overall measure of EVPI represents the expected cost of uncertainty relating to all input parameters in a decision model. It is also possible quantify the EVPI relating to individual parameters within a model that reflects the extent to which the uncertainty associated with a particular parameter is contributing to the cost of uncertainty (Ades *et al.* 2003).

An important implication of value of information methods is that the question of how much research is efficient to undertake is an empirical question as the value of research will vary between different technologies. Furthermore, the value of information about individual parameters will have implications for the different types of research that should be undertaken. For example, if there is a high EVPI for a relative treatment effect, then this would suggest a randomized trial may be necessary. However, if a cost or utility parameter has a high EVPI, then a non-experimental design may be acceptable. Value of information for a given technology is also likely to vary for different patient subgroups.

There have now been a number of applications of these methods in applied economic evaluations (Fenwick *et al.* 2000; Claxton *et al.* 2001). They have also been used in a pilot study to inform priority setting in research as part of the UK's National Health Service Health Technology Assessment Programme (Claxton *et al.* 2004). Figure 9.7 summarizes the results of one of these analyses relating to a cost–utility analysis of the use of prophylactic low-dose antibiotics in children with recurrent urinary tract infections (Claxton *et al.* 2004).

A *necessary* condition for the economic efficiency of additional research is that its cost is less than its EVPI (that is, less than its maximum value). However, this is not a *sufficient* condition for such research to be funded as decisions need to be taken about the optimal design of the research. Value of information methods can be extended to address the issue of design. Methods to quantify the EVSI can be used, for example, to balance the marginal cost of adding additional patients to a randomized trial with the consequent marginal reduction in the cost of uncertainty (Claxton 1999; Ades *et al.* 2003). These methods can also be used to identify the optimal allocation of patients to each arm of a trial, appropriate endpoints and stopping rules

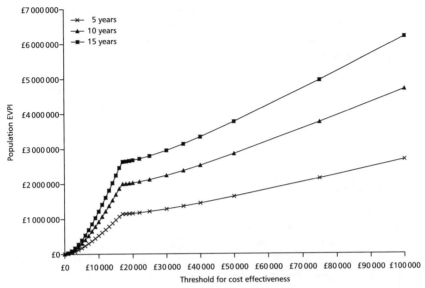

Fig. 9.7 An example of the use of expected value of perfect information (EVPI) analysis. The example relates to a model of the cost-effectiveness of prophylactic low-dose antibiotics in children with recurrent urinary tract infections (Claxton *et al.* 2004). This graph shows population EVPI for girls with vesico-ureteral reflux under three alternative assumptions about the length of time the research is likely to be useful.

(Claxton and Thompson 2001). The use of EVSI methods to inform research design has huge potential, but the general application of these methods represents a major computational burden as they are based on multiple levels of simulation. There is an important research programme around ways to increase computational efficiency in this area.

9.5. **Critical appraisal of decision analytic models**

Although decision analytic modelling can provide a valuable framework for economic evaluation, its results are always conditional on data and structural assumptions. In other words, there are good and bad decision models. As for any other form of evaluation, it is crucial that decision models are subject to careful critical review, and their results should not be used blindly in decision modelling. There are a number of examples in the literature of papers that have discussed the characteristics of 'a good model' (Eddy 1985; Halpern *et al.* 1998; Akehurst *et al.* 2000; International Society for Pharmacoeconomics and Outcomes Research 2000; McCabe and Dixon 2000; Sculpher *et al.* 2000; Weinstein *et al.* 2001).

Recently methods guidelines in decision modelling were reviewed to compare and contrast their recommendations for good practice (Philips *et al.* 2004). There was a fair amount of consistency between the papers in their guidelines, but some areas of conflict. One example of this was the extent to which the availability of data should constrain the structure of a model as opposed to structure being determined based on a theoretical understanding of a condition and the effect of a treatment. The authors argued that, in principle, structure should not be influenced by the extent or quality of the data available to populate a model but, in practice, this will not always be possible and more detailed guidance would be of value for analysts. Philips *et al.* went on to synthesize the available guidelines and, based on this, came up with a checklist to apply to specific decision models used in economic evaluation. It should be emphasized that this checklist relates to models and is not a substitute for those that relate to economic evaluation in general, including the one introduced in Chapter 3. This modelling checklist is reproduced in the Annex 9.1.

9.6. **Conclusions**

Decision modelling is increasingly seen as an important vehicle for economic evaluation, particularly where there is a specific resource-allocation decision to be taken. The value of a formal analytic framework for decision-making is that it offers a means of synthesizing available evidence from a range of sources rather than relying on a *single study*, provides a way of relating the available evidence to the specific decision problem being posed, provides a framework within which the limitations of randomized trials *as a vehicle for economic evaluation* can be addressed, helps decision-makers identify optimal interventions under conditions of uncertainty, and can contribute to the process of setting research priorities.

This chapter has provided an introduction to these methods, and further reading is available for the those who are interested (Kuntz and Weinstein 2001). There remain important methods questions to address in decision modelling. These include how to develop efficient methods to identify evidence relating to all parameters in decision models and not just those relating to treatment effects, how to synthesize all available evidence in models and reflect the uncertainty and correlation in these data, and how to deal with uncertainty in the structure of decision models and reflect this in the value of information analysis. Whilst decision modelling has the potential to provide a powerful input for decision-making, there are good and bad applications of these methods, and critical appraisal is essential.

9.7. **Exercise: developing a decision analytic model**

Background

Imagine that you have been asked to advise local decision-makers on the cost-effectiveness of ante-natal HIV testing (that is, testing pregnant women for the HIV virus). You undertake a literature search to identify published economic evaluations—but find nothing to help you in your analysis. You quickly realize that you will have to undertake a decision analysis of your own using data from available sources.

The data

From a literature search you identify publications that provide you with the following information.

1 If a woman has HIV and her infection is not known during pregnancy, the probability that she will transmit the infection to her child is 26%.

2 If a woman's infection is known during pregnancy, however, it is possible to use risk-reduction interventions such as caesarean section, antiretroviral therapy and bottle feeding. These interventions cost £800 more than a normal delivery and reduce the probability of vertical transmission to 7%, but only 95% of infected women accept them.

3 Discussion with midwifery staff indicates that offering the test to women could be achieved at negligible additional cost, but your pathology laboratories suggest that each blood test will cost £10; they also indicate that the tests are 100% accurate (that is, there are no false negatives or false positives).

4 A published paper suggests that the prevalence of previously undetected HIV in the ante-natal population in your area is 5%.

Assumptions

Discussions with professional staff indicate that the following assumptions can be justified.

1 No woman will select to terminate on discovering she has HIV infection.

2 All women who are tested positive will be offered risk-reduction interventions.

The task

Your task is the following.

1 To structure a decision tree characterizing the decision regarding whether or not to offer ante-natal HIV testing.

2 To calculate the expected cost per true positive case detected.

3 What are likely to be the key sensitivity analyses to undertake?

4 What are the weaknesses of the analysis?

Solutions

1 The decision tree is shown in Fig. 9.8.

2 Expected cost of testing = $(810 \times 0.0033) + (810 \times 0.0441) + (10 \times 0.0007)$
$+ (10 \times 0.0019) + (10 \times 0.95) = 47.92$.

Probability of vertical transmission with testing $= 0.0033 + 0.0007 = 0.004$.

Expected cost of no testing $= 0$.

Probability of vertical transmission $= 0.013$.

Additional expected cost per HIV-infected child avoided:

- additional cost $= 47.92$
- reduced vertical transmission $= 0.013 - 0.004 = 0.009$
- additional cost per HIV-infected birth avoided $= 47.92/0.009 = £5324$.

3 The following sensitivity analyses would be warranted.

Due to parameter uncertainty

- Probabilities of transmission
- probability of acceptance of interventions
- prevalence.

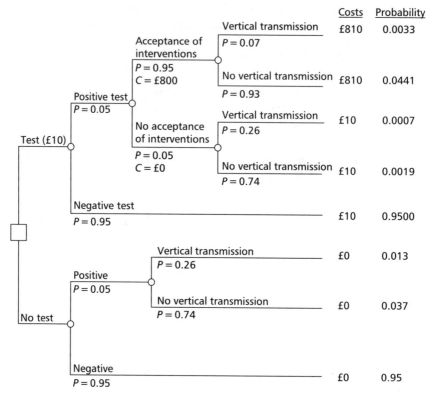

Fig. 9.8 Decision tree for antenatal HIV testing from the exercise.

Due to variability

- Costs
- probability of acceptance of interventions
- prevalence.

Due to structural uncertainty

- Accuracy of test (need to re-structure tree)
- termination rate: in this model, termination may increase or decrease costs; there would be a difficulty in how this is dealt with on the outcomes side
- uptake of test will not affect cost-effectiveness.

4 Weaknesses of the analysis:

(1) in reality, the relevant options to compare would be more likely to be universal testing versus high-risk group testing versus on-demand testing, rather than testing versus not;

(2) a full PBA would ideally be undertaken for to assess parameter uncertainty;

(3) the scope of analysis is limited:
- should have a longer term model to include an assessment of the costs and (quality-adjusted) life-years conditional on HIV transmission;
- should be a consideration of lifetime costs and outcomes;
- should consider effect of testing on the women themselves in terms of the costs and outcomes of earlier treatment than would be expected without testing;
- possible effects on horizontal transmission might be considered in a wider scope.

References

Ades, A. E., Sculpher, M. J., Gibb, D. M., Gupta, R., and Ratcliffe, J. (1999). Cost effectiveness analysis of antenatal HIV screening in United Kingdom. *British Medical Journal*, **319**, 1230–4.

Ades, A. E., Lu, G., and Claxton, K. (2003). Expected value of sample information in medical decision modelling. *Medical Decision Making*, **24**, 207–27.

Akehurst, R., Anderson, P., Brazier, J., *et al.* (2000). Decision analytic modelling in the economic evaluation of health technologies—a consensus statement. *PharamacoEconomics*, **17**, 443–4.

Barton, P., Bryan, S., and Robinson, S. (2004). Modelling in the economic evaluation of health care: selecting the appropriate approach. *Journal of Health Services Research and Policy*, **9**, 110–18.

Briggs, A. H. (2001). Handling uncertainty in economic evaluation and handling results. In: *Economic evaluation in health care: merging theory with practice* (ed. M. F. Drummond and A. McGuire). Oxford University Press, Oxford.

Briggs, A. and Sculpher, M. J. (1998). An introduction to Markov modelling for economic evaluation. *Pharmacoeconomics*, **13**, 397–409.

Briggs, A. H., Goeree, R., Blackhouse, G., and O'Brien, B. J. (2002). Probabilistic analysis of cost-effectiveness models: choosing between treatment strategies for gastroesophageal reflux disease. *Medical Decision Making*, **22**, 290–308.

Briggs, A., Sculpher, M., Dawson, J., FitzPatrick, R., Murray, D., and Malchau, H. (2004). The use of probabilistic decision models in technology assessment: the case of hip replacement. *Applied Health Economics and Policy*, **3**, 79–89.

Buxton, M. J. and O'Brien, B. J. (1992). Economic evaluation of ondansetron: preliminary analysis using clinical trial data prior to price setting. *British Journal of Cancer*, **66**, S64–7.

Centre for Reviews and Dissemination (2001). *Undertaking systematic reviews of research on effectiveness: CRD's guidance for carrying out or commissioning reviews*, Report 4. York: CRD.

Chancellor, J. V., Hill, A. M., Sabin, C. A., Simpson, K. N., and Youle, M. (1997). Modelling the cost effectiveness of lamivudine/zidovudine combination therapy in HIV infection. *PharmacoEconomics*, **12**, 1–13.

Chilcott, J., McCabe, C., Tappenden, P., *et al.* (2003). Modelling the cost effectiveness of interferon beta and glatiramer acete in the management of multiple sclerosis. *British Medical Journal*, **326**, 522.

Claxton, K. (1999). The irrelevance of inference: a decision-making approach to the stochastic evaluation of health care technologies. *Journal of Health Economics*, **18**, 342–64.

Claxton, K. and Posnett, J. (1996). An economic approach to clinical trial design and research priority-setting. *Health Economics*, **5**, 513–24.

Claxton, K. and Thompson, K. (2001). A dynamic programming approach to efficient clinical trial design. *Journal of Health Economics*, **20**, 797–822.

Claxton, K., Neumann, P. J., Araki, S. S., and Weinstein, M. C. (2001). The value of information: an application to a policy model of Alzheimer's disease. *International Journal of Technology Assessment in Health Care*, **17**, 38–55.

Claxton, K., Sculpher, M., and Drummond, M. (2002). A rational framework for decision making by the National Institute for Clinical Excellence. *Lancet*, **360**, 711–15.

Claxton, K., Ginnelly, L., Sculpher, M., Philips, Z., and Palmer, S. (2004). A pilot study on the use of decision theory and value of information analysis as part of the National Health Service Health Technology Assessment Programme. *Health Technology Assessment*, **8(31)**, 1–103.

Collett, D. (1994). *Modelling survival data in medical research*. Chapman and Hall/CRC, London.

Cooper, N. J., Sutton, A. J., Abrams, K. R., Turner, D., and Wailoo, A. (2004). Comprehensive decision analytical modelling in economic evaluation: a Bayesian approach. *Health Economics*, **13**, 203–26.

Critchfield, G. C., Willard, K. E., and Connelly, D. P. (1986). Probabilistic analysis of decision trees using Monte Carlo simulation. *Medical Decision Making*, **6**, 85–92.

Davies, R. (1985). An assessment of models of a health system. *Journal of the Operational Research Society*, **36**, 679–87.

Detsky, A. S. (1989). Are clinical trials a cost-effective investment? *Journal of the American Medical Association*, **262**, 1795–1800.

Doubilet, P., Begg, C. B., Weinstein, M. C., Braun, P., and McNeil, B. J. (1985). Probabilistic sensitivity analysis using Monte Carlo simulation. *Medical Decision Making*, **5**, 157–77.

Drummond, M. F., Davies, L. M., and Ferris, F. L. (1992). Assessing the costs and benefits of medical research: the diabetic retinopathy study. *Social Science and Medicine*, **34**, 973–81.

Eddy, D. M. (1985). Technology assessment: the role of mathematical modeling. In: *Assessing medical technologies* (ed. F. Mosteller), pp. 144–153. National Academy Press, Washington DC.

Fenwick, E., Claxton, K., Sculpher, M., and Briggs, A. (2000). *Improving the efficiency and relevance of health technology assessment: The role of decision analytic modelling*, Centre for Health Economics Discussion Paper 179. York: CHE.

Glick, H., Heyse, J. F., Thompson, D., *et al.* (1992). A model for evaluating the cost-effectiveness of cholesterol-lowering treatment. *International Journal of Technology Assessment in Health Care*, **8**, 719–734.

Gold, M. R., Siegel, J. E., Russell, L. B., and Weinstein, M. C. (1996). *Cost-effectiveness in health and medicine*. Oxford University Press, New York.

Halpern, M. T., McKenna, M., and Hutton, J. (1998). Modeling in economic evaluation: an unavoidable fact of life. *Health Economics*, **7**, 741–2.

Hasselblad, V. (1998). Meta-analysis of multi-treatment studies. *Medical Decision Making*, **18**, 37–43.

Hjelmgren, J., Berggren, F., and Andersson, F. (2001). Health economic guidelines—similarities, differences and some implications. *Value in Health*, **4**, 225–50.

Hoeting, J. A., Madigan, D., Raftery, A. E., and Volinsky, C. T. (1999). Bayesian model averaging: a tutorial. *Statistical Science*, **14**, 382–417.

Hunink, M., Glaziou, P., Siegel, J., *et al.* (2001). *Decision making in health and medicine. Integrating evidence and values*. Cambridge University Press, Cambridge.

International Society for Pharmacoeconomics and Outcomes Research (2000). *A report of the ISPOR Health Science Committee—Task Force on Good Research Practices—modelling studies.* http://www.ispor.org/workpaper/healthscience/TFModeling.pdf.

Kahn, H. A. and Sempos, C. T. (1989). *Statistical methods in epidemiology.* Oxford University Press, New York.

Karnon, J. (2003). Alternative decision modelling techniques for evaluation of health care technologies: Markov processes verses discrete event simulation. *Health Economics*, **12**, 837–48.

Kobelt, G., Jonsson, B., Young, A., and Eberhardt, K. (2003). The cost-effectiveness of infliximab (Remicade) in the treatment of rheumatoid arthritis in Sweden and the United Kingdom based on the ATTRACT study. *Rheumatology*, **42**, 326–35.

Kuntz, K. and Weinstein, M. (2001). Modelling in economic evaluation. In: *Economic evaluation in health care: merging theory with practice* (ed. M. F. Drummond and A. E. McGuire). Oxford University Press, Oxford.

Mark, D. B., Hlatky, M. A., Califf, R. M., *et al.* (1995). Cost effectiveness of thrombolytic therapy with tissue plasminogen activator as compared with streptokinase for acute myocardial infarction. *New England Journal of Medicine*, **332**, 1418–24.

McCabe, C. and Dixon, S. (2000). Testing the validity of cost-effectiveness models. *PharmacoEconomics*, **17**, 501–13.

Miller, D. K. and Homan, S. M. (1994). Determining transition probabilities: confusion and suggestions. *Medical Decision Making*, **14**, 52–8.

Nam, I.-S., Mengerson, K., and Garthwaite, P. (2003). Multivariate meta-analysis. *Statistics in Medicine*, **22**, 2309–33.

Neumann, P. J., Hermann, R. C., and Kuntz, K. M. (1999). Cost-effectiveness of donepezil in the treatment of mild or moderate Alzheimer's disease. *Neurology*, **52**, 1138–45.

O'Hagan, A. and Luce, B. (2003). *A primer on Bayesian statistics in health economics and outcomes research.* Medtap International, Bethesda, Maryland.

Palmer, S., Sculpher, M., Philips, Z., *et al.* (in press). Management of non-ST-elevation acute coronary syndromes: how cost-effective are glycoprotein IIb/IIIa antagonists in the UK National Health Service? *International Journal of Cardiology.*

Paltiel, A. D., Scharfstein, J. A., Seage III, G. R., Losina, E., Goldie, S. J., and Weinstein, M. C. (1998). A Monte Carlo simulation of advanced HIV disease. *Medical Decision Making*, **18 (Suppl.)**, S93–105.

Philips, Z., Ginnelly, L., Sculpher, M., *et al.* (2004). A review of guidelines for good practice in decision-analytic modelling in health technology assessment. *Health Technology Assessment*, **8(36)**, 1–158.

Prevost, T. C., Abrams, K., and Jones, D. (2000). Hierarchical models in generalised synthesis of evidence: an example based on studies of breast cancer. *Statistics in Medicine*, **19**, 3359–76.

Raiffa, H. (1968). Decision analysis: introductory lectures on choices under uncertainty. Addison-Wesley, Reading, Massachusetts.

Raiffa, H. and Schlaifer, R. (1959). *Probability and statistics for business decisions.* McGraw-Hill, New York.

Sackett, D. L., Rosenberg, W. M. C., Gray, J. A. M., Haynes, R. B., and Richardson, W. S. (1996). Evidence-based medicine: what it is and what it isn't. *British Medical Journal*, **312**, 71–2.

Schlaiffer, R. (1958). *Probability and statistics for business decisions.* McGraw-Hill, New York.

Sculpher, M., Fenwick, E., and Claxton, K. (2000). Assessing quality in decision analytic cost-effectiveness models. A suggested framework and example of application. *PharmacoEconomics*, **17**, 461–77.

Sonnenberg, F. A. and Beck, J. R. (1993). Markov models in medical decision making. *Medical Decision Making*, **13**, 322–38.

Sox, H. C., Blatt, M. A., Higgins, M. C., and Marton, K. I. (1988). *Medical decision making*. Butterworths, Stoneham, Massachusetts.

Spiegelhalter, D. J. and Best, N. G. (2003). Bayesian approaches to multiple sources of evidence and uncertainty in complex cost-effectiveness modelling. *Statistics in Medicine*, **22**, 3687–709.

Spiegelhalter, D. J., Abrams, K. R., and Myles, J. P. (2003). *Bayesian approaches to clinical trials and health-care evaluation*. Wiley, Chichester.

Stevenson, M. D., Oakley, J., and Chilcott, J. B. (2004). Gaussian process modelling in conjunction with individual patient simulation modelling: a case study describing the calculation of cost-effectiveness ratios for the treatment of established osteoporosis. *Medical Decision Making*, **24**, 89–100.

Sutton, A. J. and Abrams, K. R. (2001). Bayesian methods in meta-analysis and evidence synthesis. *Statistical Methods in Medical Research*, **10**, 277–303.

Sutton, A. J., Abrams, K. R., Jones, D. R., Sheldon, T. A., and Song, T. A. (2000). *Methods for meta-analysis in medical research*. Wiley, Chichester.

Thompson, K. M. and Evans, J. S. (1997). The value of improved national exposure information for perchloroethylene (perc): a case study for dry cleaners. *Risk Analysis*, **17**, 253–71.

Townsend, J. and Buxton, M. (1997). Cost effectiveness scenario analysis for a proposed trial of hormone replacement therapy. *Health Policy*, **39**, 181–94.

Weinstein, M. C. and Fineberg, H. V. (1980). *Clinical decision analysis*. Saunders, Philadelphia.

Weinstein, M. C., Toy, E. L., Sandberg, E. A., *et al.* (2001). Modeling for health care and other policy decisions: uses, roles, and validity. *Value in Health*, **4**, 348–61.

Wilby, J., Kainth, K., Hawkins, N., *et al.* (2003). *A rapid and systematic review of the clinical effectiveness, tolerability and cost effectiveness of newer drugs for epilepsy in adults*, www.nice.org.uk. National Institute for Clinical Excellence, London.

Annex 9.1. A suggested checklist for assessing quality in decision analytic models (from Philips et al. 2004)

Dimension of quality		Attributes of good practice	Questions for critical appraisal
Structure			
S1	Statement of decision problem/objective	There should be a clear statement of the decision problem prompting the analysis.	Is there a clear statement of the decision problem?
		The objective of the evaluation and of the model should be defined.	Is the objective of the evaluation and model specified and consistent with the stated decision problem?
		The primary decision-maker should be stated clearly.	Is the primary decision-maker specified?
S2	Statement of scope/perspective	The perspective of the model (relevant costs and consequences) should be stated clearly, and the model inputs should be consistent with the stated perspective and overall objective of the model.	Is the perspective of the model stated clearly?
			Are the model inputs consistent with the stated perspective?
		The scope of the decision model should be specified and justified.	Has the scope of the model been stated and justified?
		The outcomes of the model should reflect the perspective and scope of the model and should be consistent with the objective of the evaluation.	Are the outcomes of the model consistent with the perspective, scope, and overall objective of the model?

Annex 9.1. (Continued)

Dimension of quality	Attributes of good practice	Questions for critical appraisal
S3 Rationale for structure	The structure of the model should be consistent with a coherent theory of the health condition under evaluation and the treatment pathways (disease states or branches) should be chosen to reflect the underlying biological process of the disease in question and the impact of the intervention. The structure should not be dictated by current patterns of service provision. All sources of evidence used to develop and inform the structure of the model (that is, the theory of disease) should be described. The structure should be consistent with this evidence.	Is the structure of the model consistent with a coherent theory of the health condition under evaluation? Are the sources of data used to develop the structure of the model specified? Are the causal relationships described by the model structure justified appropriately?
S4 Structural assumptions	All structural assumptions should be transparent and justified. They should be reasonable in the light of the needs and purposes of the decision-maker.	Are the structural assumptions transparent and justified? Are the structural assumptions reasonable given the overall objective, perspective, and scope of the model?
S5 Strategies/comparators	There should be a clear definition of the options under evaluation. All feasible and practical options relating to the stated decision problem should be evaluated.	Is there a clear definition of the options under evaluation? Have all feasible and practical options been evaluated?

S6	Model type	Options should not be constrained by the immediate concerns of the decision-maker, or data availability, nor limited to current clinical practice.	Is there justification for the exclusion of feasible options?
		The appropriate model type will be dictated by the stated decision problem and the choices made regarding the causal relationships within the model.	Is the chosen model type appropriate given the decision problem and specified causal relationships within the model?
S7	Time horizon	A model's time horizon should extend far enough into the future in order for it to reflect important differences between options.	Is the time horizon of the model sufficient to reflect all important differences between options?
		It is important to distinguish between the time horizon of the model, the duration of treatment and the duration of treatment effect.	Are the time horizon of the model, the duration of treatment, and the duration of treatment effect described and justified?
S8	Disease states/pathways	Disease states/pathways should reflect the underlying biological process of the disease in question and the impact of interventions.	Do the disease states (state transition model) or the pathways (decision tree model) reflect the underlying biological process of the disease in question and the impact of interventions?
S9	Cycle length	For discrete time models, the cycle length should be dictated by the natural history of disease. It should be the minimum interval over which the pathology or symptoms are expected to alter.	Is the cycle length defined and justified in terms of the natural history of disease?

Annex 9.1. (*Continued*)

Dimension of quality		Attributes of good practice	Questions for critical appraisal
Data			
D1	Data identification	Methods for identifying data should be transparent and it should be clear that the data identified are appropriate given the objectives of the model. There should be justification of any choices that have been made about which specific data inputs are included in a model. It should be clear that particular attention has been paid to identifying data for those parameters to which the results of the model are particularly sensitive. Where expert opinion has been used to estimate particular parameters, sources and methods of elicitation should be described.	Are the data identification methods transparent and appropriate given the objectives of the model? Where choices have been made between data sources, are these justified appropriately? Has particular attention been paid to identifying data for the important parameters in the model? Has the quality of the data been assessed appropriately? Where expert opinion has been used, are the methods described and justified?
D2	Data modelling	All data modelling methodology should be described and based on justifiable statistical and epidemiological methods. Specific issues to consider include those below.	Is the data modelling methodology based on justifiable statistical and epidemiological techniques?
D2a	Baseline data	Baseline probabilities may be based on natural history data derived from epidemiological/observational studies or relate to the control group of an experimental study.	Is the choice of baseline data described and a justified? Are transition probabilities calculated appropriately?

		Rates and interval probabilities should be transformed into transition probabilities appropriately. If there is evidence that time is an important factor in the calculation of transition probabilities in state transition models, this should be incorporated. If a half-cycle correction has not been used on all transitions in state transition model (costs and outcomes), this should be justified.	Has a half-cycle correction been applied to both cost and outcome? If not, has this omission been justified?
D2b	Treatment effects	Relative treatment effects derived from trial data should be synthesized using recognized meta-analytic techniques. The methods and assumptions that are used to extrapolate short-term results to final outcomes should be documented and justified. This should include justification of the choice of survival function (for example, exponential or Weibull forms). Alternative assumptions should be explored through sensitivity analysis. Assumptions regarding the continuing effect of treatment once treatment is complete should be documented and justified. If evidence regarding the long-term effect of treatment is lacking, alternative assumptions should be explored through sensitivity analysis.	If relative treatment effects have been derived from trial data, have they been synthesized using appropriate techniques? Have the methods and assumptions used to extrapolate short-term results to final outcomes been documented and justified? Have alternative assumptions been explored through sensitivity analysis? Have assumptions regarding the continuing effect of treatment once treatment is complete been documented and justified? Have alternative assumptions been explored through sensitivity analysis?

Annex 9.1. (*Continued*)

Dimension of quality		Attributes of good practice	Questions for critical appraisal
D2c	Costs	Costing and discounting methods should accord with standard guidelines for economic evaluation.	Are the costs incorporated into the model justified? Has the source for all costs been described? Have discount rates been described and justified given the target decision-maker?
D2d	Quality of life weights (utilities)	Utilities incorporated into the model should be appropriate for the specified decision problem.	Are the utilities incorporated into the model appropriate? Is the source for the utility weights referenced? Are the methods of derivation for the utility weights justified?
D3	Data incorporation	All data incorporated into the model should be described and the sources of all data should be given and reported in sufficient detail to allow the reader to be aware of the type of data that have been incorporated. Where data are not mutually consistent in the model, the choices and assumptions that have been made should be explicit and justified.	Have all data incorporated into the model been described and referenced in sufficient detail? Has the use of mutually inconsistent data been justified (that is, are assumptions and choices appropriate)? Is the process of data incorporation transparent?

		The process of data incorporation should be transparent. It should be clear whether data are incorporated as a point estimate or as a distribution. If data have been incorporated as distributions as part of probabilistic analysis, the choice of distribution and its parameters should be described and justified.	If data have been incorporated as distributions, has the choice of distribution for each parameter been described and justified? If data have been incorporated as distributions, is it clear that second-order uncertainty is reflected?
D4	Assessment of uncertainty	In assessing uncertainty, modellers should distinguish between the four principal types of uncertainty.	Have the four principal types of uncertainty been addressed? If not, has the omission of particular forms of uncertainty been justified?
D4a	Methodological	Methodological uncertainty relates to whether particular analytic steps taken in the analysis are the most appropriate.	Have methodological uncertainties been addressed by running alternative versions of the model with different methodological assumptions?
D4b	Structural	There should be evidence that structural uncertainties have been evaluated using sensitivity analysis.	Is there evidence that structural uncertainties have been addressed via sensitivity analysis?
D4c	Heterogeneity	It is important to distinguish between uncertainty resulting from the process of sampling from a population and variability due to heterogeneity (that is, systematic differences between patient subgroups).	Has heterogeneity been dealt with by running the model separately for different subgroups?

Annex 9.1. (Continued)

Dimension of quality		Attributes of good practice	Questions for critical appraisal
D4d	Parameter	Where data have been incorporated into the model as point estimates, the ranges used for sensitivity analysis should be stated and justified. Probabilistic analysis is the most appropriate method of handling parameter uncertainty because it facilitates assessment of the joint effect of uncertainty over all parameters (see data incorporation).	Are the methods of assessment of parameter uncertainty appropriate? If data are incorporated as point estimates, are the ranges used for sensitivity analysis stated clearly and justified?
Consistency			
C1	Internal consistency	There should be evidence that the internal consistency of the model has been evaluated in terms of its mathematical logic.	Is there evidence that the mathematical logic of the model has been tested thoroughly before use?
C2	External consistency	The results of a model should be explicable. Results should either make intuitive sense or counter-intuitive results should be fully explained. All relevant available data should be incorporated into a model. Data should not be withheld for purposes of assessing external consistency. The results of a model should be compared with those of previous models and any differences should be explained.	Are any counter-intuitive results from the model explained and justified? If the model has been calibrated against independent data, have any differences been explained and justified? Have the results of the model been compared with those of previous models and any differences in results explained?

Chapter 10

Presentation and use of economic evaluation results

10.1. Introduction

The implicit or explicit objective of economic evaluation is to improve decisions about the allocation of health care resources. Therefore, in this penultimate chapter we discuss issues relating to the presentation and use of economic evaluation results.

In Chapter 3 we pointed out that, in order to assess the usefulness of economic evaluation results, readers (users) of studies needed to answer the following questions.

1 Are the methods employed in the study appropriate and are the results valid?

2 If the results are valid, would they apply to my setting?

The problems and prospects for using economic evaluation in health care decision-making have been widely debated in recent years, following the attempts to use it in priority setting in the State of Oregon's plan to revise its Medicaid programme (Eddy 1991), the inclusion of a formal requirement for economic analysis in the process for reimbursement of pharmaceuticals in Australia (Commonwealth of Australia 1995) and several provinces of Canada (Ontario Ministry of Health 1994; Anis and Gagnon 2000), and the use of economic modelling in technology appraisals undertaken by the National Institute for Clinical Excellence (NICE) in England and Wales (National Institute for Clinical Excellence 2004).

It is not the purpose here to provide a detailed policy commentary on these developments, because the formal position *vis-à-vis* economic evaluation is likely to change over time. (Indeed the list of applications listed above is not exhaustive.) Rather, the intention is to draw out the *methodological lessons* from the use of economic evaluation in decision-making, particularly as these relate to the conduct and reporting of studies.

The next two sections of the chapter deal with aspects of *validity*. First, the various proposed reporting frameworks for economic evaluation are reviewed, with an emphasis on the methods for ensuring transparency in the reporting of results. Then the interpretation of cost-effectiveness evidence, including the practice of comparing economic evaluation results in cost-effectiveness rankings or 'league tables' is discussed and the major pitfalls identified.

The following two sections of the chapter deal with aspects of *applicability* of economic evaluation. First, the issue of transferring results from one setting to another is discussed, along with some examples. Then the problems and prospects for using economic evaluation are explored, based on the experience gained so far.

The chapter ends with a reminder about the limitations of economic evaluation in health care decision-making.

10.2. Reporting formats for economic evaluation

10.2.1. Why insist on a common reporting format?

Several of the published methodological guidelines for economic evaluation include a suggested reporting format. There are a number of reasons why a common reporting format for economic evaluations would be desirable. First, it may increase the transparency of studies; that is, it would be easier to assess precisely what the analyst had done and, hence, whether the methods were appropriate. Second, it might facilitate comparisons between studies; that is, if all analysts reported their results in a similar fashion, the user could be more confident that differences (say) in cost-effectiveness ratios reflect the characteristics of the interventions or programmes being evaluated, rather than differences in study methodology. Third, it might improve the general quality of evaluations undertaken, because the requirements of the reporting format would lead analysts to address important methodological considerations.

Some of the arguments for a common reporting format are not clear cut. For example, as we shall discuss later in Section 10.3, comparisons between the results of studies, especially in 'league tables', can be problematical. Also, it might be argued that, far from stimulating methodological improvements, a common reporting format might stifle them if analysts interpreted this as a maximum, rather than a minimum, standard that had to be achieved.

The transparency argument is probably the strongest one in favor of a common reporting framework and this was one objectives of the Public Health Services Panel on Cost-effectiveness in Health and Medicine (Gold *et al.* 1996) and the prime motivation for the recommendations of the *British Medical Journal* (*BMJ*) Working Party on Economic Evaluation (1996). The Public Health Services Panel recommended that reports of economic evaluations should always include the panel's chosen 'reference case', in order to enable study results to be compared. (The concept of the 'reference case' was discussed in Chapter 3.) The *BMJ* Working Party acknowledged that there are still many methodological debates in economic evaluation and that it may therefore be difficult to develop standards in all areas. However, it would be possible to standardize the reporting, thereby increasing the transparency of studies. Therefore, it specified reporting guidelines that would be used by peer reviewers of articles submitted to the *BMJ*.

10.2.2. The 10-point checklist as a reporting framework

The 10-point checklist introduced in Chapter 3 is primarily intended as a structure for the critical appraisal of published papers. However, the same questions can serve as a guide to analysts seeking to improve the quality of their study report. If the report is written in a way that would enable the reader to answer all the checklist questions, the analyst would be a long way towards satisfying the basic requirements of transparency.

10.2.3. **Similarities and dissimilarities of existing reporting formats**

The proposals of the *BMJ* Working Party on Economic Evaluation and the checklist in Chapter 3 represent but two of a growing number of suggested reporting formats for economic evaluation. There are a number of different motivations for the various proposals. Some, like the reporting formats suggested by the Commonwealth of Australia (1995), the Ontario Ministry of Health (1994), the Canadian Coordinating Office for Health Technology Assessment (1997), and the National Institute for Clinical Excellence (2004), are linked to a formal requirement for the provision of economic data prior to the reimbursement (public subsidy) of pharmaceuticals. Others, such as that suggested by the US Public Health Service Panel on Cost-effectiveness in Health and Medicine (Gold *et al.* 1996), are more concerned with the maintenance of methodological standards in published work and the interpretation of economic evaluation results by decision-makers. Yet others, such as the proposals of the Task Force on Principles of Economic Analysis of Health Care Technology (1995), also stress the importance of procedural issues, including the contractual relationship between analyst and research sponsor.

The precise content of the various proposals, especially the level of detail, reflects their different objectives (Drummond 1994*a*). Several reviews comparing and contrasting the different suggestions have already been published (Jacobs *et al.* 1995; Hjelmgren *et al.* 2001; Drummond *et al.* 2003) and others will follow as additional recommendations are made in the future. However, two general points have already emerged.

First, although there are differences among the various proposals, there are a number of recommendations common to many of the existing reporting formats. These include the provision for details on

(1) the background (importance) of the question (problem);

(2) the viewpoint for the analysis;

(3) the reasons for selecting a particular form of analysis;

(4) the (patient) population to which the analysis applies;

(5) the comparators being assessed;

(6) the source of the medical evidence and its quality;

(7) the range of costs considered and their measurement (in physical and money terms);

(8) the measure of benefit in the economic study (for example, life-years gained, quality-adjusted life-years (QALYs) gained);

(9) the methods for adjusting for timing of costs and benefits;

(10) the methods for dealing with uncertainty;

(11) the incremental analysis of costs and benefits;

(12) the overall results of the study and its limitations.

This list should come as no surprise to readers of this and other texts on economic evaluation of health care programmes. It signifies that there is now a fair amount of agreement on the need to report major elements of study methodology. Obviously, there is not complete agreement on how each of these methodological issues should be dealt with. However, in a review of 25 published guidelines for economic evaluation, Hjelmgren *et al.* (2001) found that the guidelines were in agreement for about 75% of methodological aspects. The main areas of disagreement were in the choice of perspective, the range of costs and benefits to be included, and their monetary valuation. They note that such differences are to be expected, given differences in countries' health systems and the different purposes of guidelines. In particular, those guidelines that have been developed in conjunction with formal requirements for the use of economic data in reimbursement decisions for health technologies are, by their very nature, more prescriptive.

The second general point to emerge is that full reporting on all relevant aspects of economic evaluation methodology would require considerable space, certainly more than is typically available in mainstream medical journals. One possible solution is to produce a separate technical report that would be made available to interested parties (Gold *et al.* 1996). Another possibility is that detailed analyses of published studies could be provided by structured databases of economic evaluations, which already exist in the UK (Centre for Reviews and Dissemination 2004; Office of Health Economics 2004), the USA (Harvard School of Public Health 2004), France (Collège des Économists de la Santé 2004), and the European Union (Nixon *et al.* 2004). However, the reality is that most users of economic evaluations will be consulting the journal publication, so analysts should ensure that this is as informative as possible, using the 10-point checklist or another reporting format as a template.

10.3. **Interpreting cost-effectiveness evidence**

The vast majority of published economic evaluations are either cost-effectiveness analyses (CEAs) or cost–utility analyses (CUAs). In part, this reflects the published guidelines for economic evaluation discussed above, most of which favor CEA/CUA over cost–benefit analysis (CBA). However, as mentioned in Chapter 7, in the absence of full measurement and valuation of all the costs and consequences of the alternatives being compared (that is, in a CBA), the results of economic evaluations can only be interpreted by reference to an external standard. This can be a comparison with the results from other, independent, programmes, a comparison with a cost-effectiveness threshold reflecting the value for money of existing programmes, or a comparison with the programme to be excluded at the margin (that is, the opportunity cost of the budget constraint).

10.3.1. **Motivations behind the 'league table' approach**

In the 1980s and 1990s it became fashionable to make comparisons between health care interventions in terms of their relative cost-effectiveness, in cost per life-year or cost per QALY gained. The first published ranking or 'league table' for the UK was that derived by Williams (1985). League tables of interventions in North America have been published by Torrance and Zipursky (1984) and Schulman et al. (1991). An example of a league table is given in Table 10.1. In the more recent literature, it is less common to see league tables presented. However, authors still commonly state that the treatment being evaluated has a cost-effectiveness ratio 'which compares favourably with that of other health care interventions', or is below some arbitrary threshold (for example, $50 000 per QALY). (See the study by Mark et al. (1995), which was the subject of a critical appraisal in Chapter 3.)

Table 10.1 League table of costs and quality-adjusted life-years for selected health care interventions

	Cost/QALY (£ August 1990)
Cholesterol testing and diet therapy only (all adults, aged 40–69 years)	220
Neurosurgical intervention for head injury	240
General practitioner advice to stop smoking	270
Neurosurgical intervention for subarachnoid haemorrhage	490
Antihypertensive therapy to prevent stroke (ages 45–64 years)	940
Pacemaker implantation	1100
Hip replacement	1180
Valve replacement for aortic stenosis	1140
Cholesterol testing and treatment	1480
Coronary artery bypass graft (left main vessel disease, severe angina)	2090
Kidney transplant	4710
Breast cancer screening	5780
Heart transplantation	7840
Cholesterol testing and treatment (incrementally) of all adults aged 25–39 years	14 150
Home haemodialysis	17 260
CABG (one-vessel disease, moderate angina)	18 830
Continuous ambulatory peritoneal dialysis	19 870
Hospital haemodialysis	21 970
Erythropoietin treatment for anaemia in dialysis patients (assuming a 10% reduction in mortality)	54 380
Neurosurgical intervention for malignant intracranial tumours	107 780
Erythropoietin treatment for anaemia in dialysis patients (assuming no increase in survival)	126 290

From Maynard (1991).

There are two, quite distinct, motivations behind the league table approach. First, analysts undertaking an evaluation of a particular health treatment or programme often seek, quite appropriately, to place their findings in a broader context. For example, Schulman *et al.* (1991) compared their estimates of the cost per life-year gained from early treatment of asymptomatic people with HIV infection with a broader range of interventions, including treatment for elevated cholesterol, mammography, and renal dialysis. Second, some analysts seek to inform decisions about the allocation of health care resources between alternative programmes. For example, Williams (1985) calculated the cost per QALY of a range of health care interventions and divided them into 'strong candidates for expansion' and 'less strong candidates for expansion', although in part his analysis was designed to illustrate what could be achieved by using available data and to argue for further refinements. Also, in Canada, Laupacis *et al.* (1992) argued that the adoption and utilization of new health technologies could be classified into five grades of recommendation based on their incremental cost per QALY, although they acknowledged that many other issues apart from cost-effectiveness, such as ethical and political considerations, affect the implementation of a new technology.

Most of the criticisms of league tables are directed at the second of these two potential motivations (Laupacis *et al.* 1993; Naylor *et al.* 1993). However, in reality most analysts quoting league tables have either not been clear about their motivation, or have had the first, more limited, objective in mind. Nevertheless, the concerns need to be addressed.

10.3.2. Methodological considerations in the construction and use of league tables

For the information in league tables to be of any use to decision-makers, we need to be confident that the methodology of the source studies (contained in the table) is sound and that it is relatively homogenous among the various studies.

Drummond *et al.* (1993) explored these issues with particular reference to the league table shown in Table 10.1. They found that there was considerable variation in methodology among the source studies generating the 21 estimates of cost per QALY in the table. They argued that in interpreting the league table a number of methodological features are particularly important. These are (1) the discount rate, (2) the method for estimating health state preferences, (3) the range of costs and consequences considered, and (4) the choice of comparison programme. The methodological issues surrounding the choice of discount rate, the inclusion/exclusion of costs and consequences, and the estimation of health state preferences have been discussed elsewhere in this book. However, the fourth issue, the choice of comparison programme, is probably the most important in the interpretation of league tables and is discussed in Box 10.1.

Another problem with the presentation of league tables is that they rarely include measures of uncertainty of the cost-effectiveness estimates (Mauskopf *et al.* 2003). As part of the World Health Organization project on generalized CEA (Tan-Torres Edejer *et al.* 2003), Hutubessy *et al.* (2003) proposed the concept of stochastic league tables to be used in the budgetary context. The proposed approach may also consider different budget levels to inform about a 'budget expansion path'.

Box 10.1 **Is the programme cost-effective? It all depends on what we compare it to**

Suppose our interest is in programme A_2. This could be because it is a new screening programme proposed by public health specialists or a new drug suggested for reimbursement. Compared with 'doing nothing', A_2 costs an additional $100 000 and generates 11 extra QALYs, with an incremental cost-effectiveness ratio of $9100 per QALY. This might be the figure included in a league table for comparison with other interventions. (The cost per QALY ratio between two points is given by the slope of the line and is indicated on the graph.)

However, suppose current practice is to have programme A_1. This costs $50 000 yet generates only one QALY. If we chose to compare A_2 with A_1 we would obtain a more attractive incremental cost-effectiveness ratio of $5000 per QALY. But A_1 is a dominated programme (see Chapter 5) and should not feature in the relevant set of alternatives. Therefore the incremental analysis of A_2 over A_1 would be misleading.

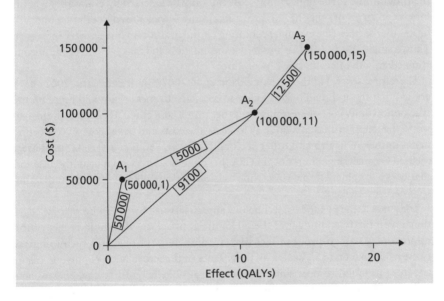

An alternative approach for presenting the uncertainty in the cost-effectiveness estimates is to report the variance of the ratio estimate as well as the mean value. Alternative programmes can then be compared in two dimensions, expected return and variance of the expected return. A risk-neutral decision-maker would rank treatments based only on the mean values of the ratios, whereas a risk-averse decision-maker would take into account the variance of the ratios (O'Brien and Sculpher 2000). The estimate of uncertainty is also useful in assessing the value of obtaining further information (see Section 9.4.7). Section 10.3.4 discusses in more detail issues related to the role of uncertainty in decisions about cost-effectiveness.

10.3.3. **The notion of a cost-effectiveness threshold**

One of the implications of making comparisons of the cost-effectiveness of different interventions is that there is some threshold ratio above which a programme would be deemed *not* cost-effective. The objections to the specification of a cost-effectiveness threshold are numerous and have already been touched on at various points in this book.

First, the outcome measure used in most cost-effectiveness league tables (that is, the QALY) may not capture all the relevant benefits of health care programmes (see the discussion in Chapter 2). Second, most cost-effectiveness league tables include studies from a range of settings and economic data may not be transferable from one setting to another. (This issue is discussed in Section 10.5.) Third, the adoption of a threshold implies a 'shadow price' for a QALY. (This issue was raised in Section 5.5.) Whereas it might be argued that the shadow price represents society's willingness-to-pay (WTP) for a QALY, Gafni and Birch (1993) argue that it is unlikely that the shadow price would be independent of the size of the health programme being considered. That is, the programme's true opportunity cost can only be assessed by examining what is forgone in terms of other health care programmes (given a fixed health care budget), or in other sectors (for example, education) if the health care budget were increased. Thus, a single cost per QALY threshold is meaningless and may be a recipe for unconstrained growth of health care expenditures.

Therefore, several authors (Donaldson *et al.* 2002; Birch and Gafni 2002) have argued that there should be less focus on cost-effectiveness ratios and more on the true opportunity cost of adopting the programme concerned. Of course, in the real world the decision-maker is unlikely to know the costs and benefits of all competing programmes in health and other sectors. However, Sendi *et al.* (2002) propose a method for analysing uncertainty in CEA that directly addresses opportunity costs and that uses a graphical framework (the 'decision-making plane') for communicating with decision-makers.

The guide to the methods of technology appraisal issued by NICE also acknowledges that 'given the fixed budget of the NHS, the appropriate threshold is that of the opportunity cost of programmes displaced by new, more costly, technologies'. However, it goes on to argue that, in the absence of the information required to calculate this threshold, 'comparisons of the most plausible incremental cost-effectiveness ratio (ICER) of a particular technology compared with other programmes that are currently funded are possible and are a legitimate reference (for the Committee). Such comparisons are helpful when the technology has an ICER that is lower than programmes that are widely regarded as cost-effective, substantially higher than other currently funded programmes, or higher than programmes previously rejected as not cost-effective (by the Committee)' (National Institute for Clinical Excellence 2004, p. 33).

A further complication was introduced by O'Brien *et al.* (2002) who, in a review of published studies, found that individuals' willingness-to-accept (WTA) monetary compensation to forgo a programme was consistently greater than their stated WTP for the same benefit. They questioned whether, given that WTA is greater than WTP based on individual preferences, societal preferences used to determine cost-effectiveness thresholds reflect this disparity.

Of course, one way forward would be to estimate society's WTP for a QALY empirically. An analytic approach for this was proposed by Reed Johnson *et al.* (1997), but was limited by the relatively small number of morbidity-valuation studies available at the time. It is likely that more attempts to estimate society's WTP for a QALY will be made in the near future. If successful, they offer the possibility of reconciling the CUA and CBA literature.

10.3.4. The role of uncertainty in decision-making

One of the main areas of methods development in economic evaluation over the last decade relates to the quantification of uncertainty in economic evaluation. This includes advances in statistical analysis of patient-level data (for example, from randomized trials) to quantify the implications of sampling variability on the precision of an estimate of, for example, cost-effectiveness. It also relates to quantification of parameter uncertainty in economic studies based on decision analytic models, where probabilistic sensitivity analysis offers more rigor than standard one-way or multiway sensitivity analysis. The typical economic analysis therefore presents more information on the uncertainty in its results than was the case 10 years ago. But how should this information feed into decision-making?

Like so much in the field of policy evaluations, there are different answers to this question which, in part, reflect alternative disciplinary perspectives. In clinical evaluation, particularly in the context of randomized trials undertaken with the purpose of supporting licence applications for new pharmaceuticals, the traditional rules of statistical inference usually predominate. That is, a new medicine is subject to stringent statistical tests whereby the null hypothesis that it is no more efficacious than its comparator is only rejected if the trial data are consistent with the comparator being more efficacious with a probability of less than 0.05 (Pocock 1983).

There has long been the view in public policy analysis, however, that decisions about resource allocation should be based on the *expected* (that is, mean) measure of value (for example, a cost-effectiveness ratio) (Arrow and Lind 1970). This is based on the idea that, when the risks of investment are spread over the entire population, then that falling on any one individual is too small to have any influence on the decision. In the context of resource allocation in health care, Claxton has argued that, if the health system's objective is to maximize health gain from available resources, the decision about whether an intervention should be funded (reimbursed) should be based on expected cost-effectiveness alone (Claxton 1999). In other words, the use of traditional rules of statistical inference based on P-values is not only arbitrary, but would be expected to lead to reductions in health gain and/or higher costs compared to basing decisions on expected cost-effectiveness. Claxton emphasizes that 'the irrelevance of inference' does not imply that uncertainty in cost-effectiveness is irrelevant to decision-making. Rather, quantification of decision uncertainty is important as a key input into decisions about future research priorities. Chapter 9 has discussed the role of value of information analysis which provides a way of quantifying, in monetary terms, the value of various types of research, and this is based on the cost of uncertainty based on currently available evidence (Claxton and Posnett 1996).

What effect has this methodological tension had on the practice of economic evaluation? As discussed in Chapter 8 in the context of the analysis of patient-level data, there has been an interest in estimation rather than hypothesis testing, including reporting confidence intervals around incremental cost-effectiveness ratios and measures of net benefit. However, there has also been a move away from the fixed error probabilities, which are as much part of standard confidence intervals as hypothesis tests, towards the more flexible cost-effectiveness acceptability curve (CEAC) (van Hout et al. 1994; Fenwick et al. 2001). By showing the probability that a given therapy is the more or most cost-effective, the CEAC presents the error probability, which varies according to the value associated with an extra unit of outcome. The decision-making authority then has the ultimate decision about whether to base its decision on expected values or to use some sort of threshold error probability. If it is the latter, then the CEAC offers flexibility regarding which is selected. The quantification of uncertainty in economic evaluation, and its use in decision-making, is likely to continue to be an area of methodological interest in the future.

10.4. Transfering economic evaluation results from setting to setting

In the discussion of league tables we mentioned that the studies being compared often come from a range of settings. In interpreting economic evaluation results, decision-makers need to form a view on whether the results apply in their own setting. Some scientific data are clearly transferable. For example, the clinical effect of a patient taking a given medicine is likely to be similar in the USA and Canada. However, the same may not be true of the same operation performed by different surgeons. Also, in some cases the clinical endpoints may not be totally independent of the health care setting. For example, the Evaluation of 7E3 for the Prevention of Ischemic Complications (EPIC) trial of a new drug in cardiology (EPIC Investigators 1994) used a combined endpoint of death, non-fatal myocardial infarction, unplanned surgical revascularization, unplanned repeat percutaneous transluminal coronary angioplasty, unplanned insertion of an intra-aortic balloon pump for refractory ischaemia, and unplanned implantation of a coronary stent. Because of these issues, the applicability of economic evaluation results from one setting to another has been widely debated and is an issue both within countries and between countries (Drummond and Pang 2001; Sculpher et al. 2004).

With the growing international literature on economic evaluation and the rapid international spread of new health technologies, there is a need to undertake, or at least interpret, economic evaluations on the international level. For example, health care decision-makers, especially in those countries having limited resources for health technology assessment, may wish to re-interpret in their own setting the results of an economic evaluation that was done elsewhere. Also, controlled clinical trials are often mounted on an international basis in order to recruit sufficient numbers of patients or to satisfy the needs of different national medical and regulatory agencies that like to see evidence of efficacy in their own patient population. Increasingly, these trials may incorporate the gathering of economic data.

However, the gathering of economic data poses different challenges and the results of studies may not be transferable from one setting to another. Indeed, one of the countries to require economic data in support of submissions for government reimbursement of pharmaceuticals has pointed out that the data need to be relevant to local circumstances (Commonwealth of Australia 1995). The suggestion is that demonstrating the cost-effectiveness of a new medicine in (say) the USA may not of itself prove that the same product would be good value for money in Australia. A recent review of economic evaluations of pharmaceuticals in western Europe showed that there are variations in cost-effectiveness estimates between countries and that these variations are not systematic (Barbieri *et al.* in press).

There are a number of reasons to suppose why economic data may not be easily transferable. These include differences in the availability of alternative treatments, in clinical practice patterns, in relative prices, and in the incentives to health care professionals and institutions. The next section discusses in more depth the differences between countries or locations likely to affect cost-effectiveness.

10.4.1. Factors likely to affect cost-effectiveness

1. *Basic demography and epidemiology of disease.* Countries differ in respect of the age structure of their population and the incidence of various diseases. In some cases this will affect the cost-effectiveness of health care programmes, particularly those delivered on a population basis. For example, programmes of immunization or screening and treatment of disease are likely to be more cost-effective in populations where the incidence of the disease in question is high. Different age structures between countries are likely to lead to different levels of incidence in various countries and hence the size of the overall economic burden. The cost-effectiveness of treatment is also likely to vary by patient characteristics, including age, lifestyle, and medical history. Therefore, when discussing the cost-effectiveness of health care treatments and programmes, it is important to specify the patient population to which any statements apply.

2. *Availability of health care resources and variations in clinical practice.* Countries differ in respect of the range of treatments and health care facilities available to their populations. In the case of treatment for ulcer, the availability of surgery could vary from place to place. In some countries with national health care systems, such as Sweden and the UK, rationing takes place, with waiting lists for hospital admission. The availability of important diagnostic facilities, such as endoscopy, could also vary from one location to another. In turn, the availability of resources may affect the way medicine is practised. For example, if there are long waiting times for endoscopy, a clinician may try a therapeutic dose of a drug for a patient experiencing ulcer-type pain without waiting to confirm the diagnosis. Another difference between countries, more directly related to drug therapy, is the range of licensed products and availability of generics.

Although clinical practice is partly constrained by the available alternatives, it is known that practice varies among clinicians in the same geographical area facing essentially the same range of treatment options (McPherson *et al.* 1982). To the extent that clinical practice varies systematically between countries, this is likely to affect the relative cost-effectiveness of therapies.

3. *Incentives to health care professionals and institutions.* In some health care systems the level of remuneration of health care professionals and institutions is largely independent of the level of service delivered. For example, hospitals are given a global budget and physicians are paid by salary. In other systems physicians are paid by fee per item of service and hospitals reimbursed by the number of cases in each category treated.

It has often been suggested that physicians operating under a fee-for-service system are more likely to generate extra demand for their services, whereas those paid by salary or capitation are more likely to deter demand. This may affect the number of physician visits and diagnostic tests performed for a given patient suffering from (say) ulcer-type pain.

In the case of hospital treatment for ulcer, the method of reimbursement could affect which services are delivered on an out-patient basis and also the length of stay for in-patients. A hospital being paid a fixed amount for treating a given case has more incentives to free the bed for the next patient than a hospital being funded through a global budget.

4. *Relative prices or costs.* It is well known that absolute price levels vary between countries. However, from the point of view of cost-effectiveness assessments, the critical issue is whether the *relative* prices of health care resources differ. Most obviously, if the relative prices of the main drugs for a given condition differ between countries, then their relative cost-effectiveness will differ.

Perhaps less obvious is the fact that the relative cost-effectiveness of drugs will differ if the relative prices of *other* health care resources differ between countries. For example, a drug with greater efficacy, a better side-effect profile, or more convenient route of administration, will appear better value for money in a country where the costs of investigations, hospitalizations, surgery, and physician visits are relatively higher, because consumption of these items is likely to be reduced. For example, Hull *et al.* (1981) found that the relative price of venography (a diagnostic test for deep-vein thrombosis (DVT)) differed between the USA and Canada. This affected the relative cost-effectiveness of alternative diagnostic strategies for DVT in the two countries and would also affect the estimates of the value for money of drugs to prevent DVT.

It should also be remembered from Chapter 4 that the prices of health care resources do not always reflect costs, although it is often a tacit assumption of economic evaluations that they do. Therefore, in arguing that savings in other health care resources, such as surgical time, justify a more expensive but more efficacious drug, some consideration should be given to whether the prices of those resources really reflect their true opportunity costs.

5. *Population values.* The results of CBA and CUAs depend on how the outcomes of treatments or interventions are valued by the general population. The values placed

on health states could conceivably vary from place to place and the guidance for conducting economic evaluations issued by the National Institute for Clinical Excellence (2004) requires that 'health states should be measured in patients using a generic and validated classification system for which reliable UK population preference values, elicited using a choice-base method such as the time trade-off or standard gamble (but not rating scale), are available'.

There has been some exploration of the extent to which health state preference values vary by geographical location, although more research is required. However, as discussed in Chapter 6, the research to date on health 'utilities' suggests that the mean values for different health states do not vary greatly (Johnson *et al.* 2000; Le Gales *et al.* 2000).

10.4.2. Ways of adapting results from setting to setting

An analyst seeking to adapt economic evaluation results from one setting to another could be faced with one of three situations. First, only clinical data may have been collected in the clinical trials and there is a need to produce economic evaluations for more than one country or setting. Here the appropriate option is likely to be to undertake a modelling study, where the clinical data are combined with cost (and possibly quality of life) data from a number of sources (for example, routinely available statistics, free-standing cost studies, and so on).

Second, economic data (for example, quantities of resource use) may have been collected alongside a clinical trial undertaken in one country, but economic evaluations are required for other settings. Here, a modelling study using only the clinical data could be undertaken, as above. Alternatively, the resource use data could be adapted in some way in order to make them relevant to another setting.

Third, economic data may have been collected alongside a multinational clinical trial and economic evaluations are required for all the countries enrolling patients in the trial. Here the analyst has a number of options for analysing the resource use data. They could be pooled, as is common for the clinical data, and priced separately for each country. Another option is that the resource use data for patients from each country could be allowed to vary in the analysis and then priced for each country as above. In this case the analysts would also have the option of calculating cost-effectiveness ratios for each country using the pooled clinical results or using the individual clinical results for each country. Another option would be to estimate cost-effectiveness for each country but for this to be based on a combination of data from the country of interest and those from other countries.

The alternative situations present analytical challenges and there are currently very few examples in the published literature. However, some studies are discussed below.

1. *Using modelling to adapt results from one setting to another.* An example here is the study by Drummond *et al.* (1992) of misoprostol, a drug for prophylaxis of gastric ulcers in patients on long-term non-steroidal anti-inflammatory drug (NSAID) use experiencing abdominal pain. A clinical trial, undertaken in the USA (Graham *et al.* 1988), had shown that patients with osteoarthritis (OA) given misoprostol (400 µg daily) for 3 months, had a lower rate of endoscopically determined lesions

than those receiving placebo (5.6% versus 21.7%). With the higher dose, of 800 μg daily, the rate of lesions fell to 1.7%.

Apart from conferring clinical benefits, a lower rate of gastric lesions is likely to generate economic benefits. Namely, if fewer patients have lesions it is likely that fewer will require diagnostic work-up for suspected ulcer and fewer will require treatment in ambulatory care or in hospital. Therefore, an economic evaluation could assess whether these potential savings in resources justify the costs of adding misoprostol.

Drummond *et al.* wanted to conduct economic evaluations in Belgium, France, the UK, and the USA. However, whereas the clinical data might be considered applicable in all countries, other factors might differ. These could include the compliance with therapy, the method of diagnostic work-up, the nature and extent of ambulatory care for ulcer, the rate of hospitalization for ulcer, the level of surgical intervention, and the length of hospital stay. In addition, it was known that the prices of resources, including the acquisition cost of misoprostol, differed from place to place. Whereas the drug price was broadly similar in the three European countries studied, it was around 40% higher in the USA.

In order to model the expected cost of adding 3 months' prophylaxis, Drummond *et al.* devised a decision tree (see Box 10.2). This provided a framework for combining the clinical data from the trial with other data obtained by additional study. For example, the nature of diagnostic work-up and ambulatory care was ascertained by asking expert panels of physicians in the four countries. Hospital admission rates for ulcer were determined from epidemiological surveys, whereas surgical rates and length of hospital stay were obtained from routine hospital statistics. The method of obtaining the relevant financial data varied from country to country. In some countries data on fees and charges were available; in others free-standing costing studies were carried out.

The results (see Table 10.2) showed that indeed there was some variation between countries. It is particularly interesting to note that in the USA, where the acquisition cost of misoprostol is highest, the overall economic results are the most favourable. At the high dose the expected cost of adding 3 months prophylaxis is the lowest in the four countries and at the lower dose there is a net saving. This is because of the relatively higher cost of *other* resources in the US health care system, especially surgery. However, it should be remembered that the savings in this case represent the value of resources that could potentially be freed for other uses.

A more recent, and more sophisticated, example of using modelling to adapt results from one setting to another is the study by Palmer *et al.* (2005) on the cost-effectiveness of glycoprotein 11b/111a antagonists (GPAs) in the management of non-ST-elevation acute coronary syndromes (ACS), which was also referred to in Chapter 9. Although a considerable number of clinical trials of GPAs had been conducted, these had been undertaken largely or wholly outside the UK. Therefore, in building a model to assess the cost-effectiveness of GPAs, the authors had to consider (1) whether the use of GPAs in trials reflected their use in routine UK practice, (2) whether the baseline event rates in the trials were relevant to UK practice, and (3) whether the relative risk reductions estimated from the trials were related to baseline risks.

Box 10.2 **Using a decision tree to adapt data from setting to setting**

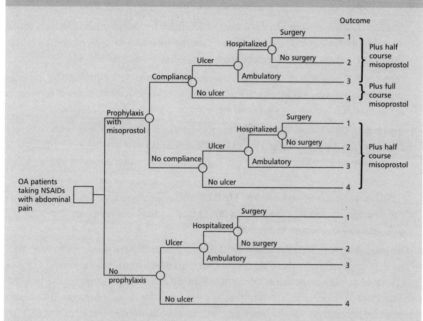

From Drummond *et al.* (1992).

In the decision tree above prophylaxis is compared with no prophylaxis. With no prophylaxis it was assumed that the ulcer rate approximated to that in the placebo group in the clinical trial, although an adjustment was made for the fact that around 40% of lesions discovered endoscopically will be 'silent' (that is, not bothersome to the patient). Thus, these will not require costs in diagnostic work-up or therapy. In the treatment arm the non-compliers were also assigned the trial placebo ulcer rate. The difference in expected cost is driven by the clinical data, but the calculation in both arms requires data that was not gathered in the trial.

Table 10.2 Expected costs (savings) per patient for 3 months' prophylaxis ($)*

	Belgium	France	UK	USA
High dose	32	61	55	22
Low dose	5	15	3	(40)

*Ulcers 0.3 cm or larger, silent ulcer rate of 40%.

2. *Does the use of glycoprotein 11b/111a antagonists in trials reflect their use in routine National Health Service practice?* The evidence base contained two types of GPA trial: those comparing the drugs with standard practice (that is, management without GPAs) in all patients with non-ST elevation ACS regardless of whether percutaneous

coronary intervention (PCI) was subsequently undertaken (medical management); and those looking at GPAs as an adjunct to PCI. However, it was possible to identify four strategies relating to how these drugs were being used in clinical practice in the UK, as outlined below:

Strategy 1. Glycoprotein 11b/111a antagonist as part of initial medical management. This involves patients with ACS receiving an infusion of GPA as soon as their 'high risk' nature has been established.

Strategy 2. Glycoprotein 11b/111a antagonist in patients with planned percutaneous coronary interventions. Glycoprotein 11b/111a antagonist is started once a decision to undertake PCI (or angiography with a view to proceeding to PCI) has been made.

Strategy 3. Glycoprotein 11b/111a antagonist as adjunct to percutaneous coronary intervention. Glycoprotein 11b/111a antagonist is used at the time of PCI or is started up to 1 hour before the procedure in those patients undergoing such a procedure.

Strategy 4. No use of glycoprotein 11b/111a antagonist. With this strategy, patients are assumed to receive standard therapies (for example, heparin, aspirin, nitrates, and analgesia), without the use of GPA.

The model was, therefore, structured directly to compare these four strategies. Given that none of the trials directly compared all of these strategies, however, it was necessary to re-structure the effectiveness data to reflect the nature of the indirect clinical comparison that was needed to populate the decision model. This was achieved by separating out the baseline event rates measured in the standard therapy control groups in the trials from the treatment effect observed in the GPA arms relative to the control group. The relative treatment effects were pooled across the various groups of trials. The relative treatment effect for Strategy 1 was based on seven medical management trials randomizing a total of 30 280 patients; the relative risk reduction for Strategy 2 was taken from a single trial of 1265 patients; and the treatment effect of Strategy 3 was based on 10 trials randomizing a total of 15 951 patients. In principle, the baseline event rates of interest (that is, rates of death, myocardial infarction, and revascularization) could have been taken from pooled control group data from trials. This could have been taken as representing event rates in Strategy 4 (no use of GPAs). For reasons described below, however, baseline event rates were actually taken from another source.

3. *Are baseline event rates in the trials relevant to UK practice?* Given that the trials were undertaken largely outside the UK, the baseline event rates in patients not having GPAs in the UK may be quite different to those patients randomized to the control groups in the trials. This could reflect differences in the epidemiology of the disease or, more probably, differences in overall management of patients with ischaemic heart disease in the UK. Traditionally, the principal difference in the management of ischaemic heart disease in the UK, compared to that in other developed countries, is that fewer patients are considered for PCI. This is important for two reasons. Firstly, early use of PCI in ACS patients has been shown to reduce rates of death and myocardial infarction in recent randomized trials, hence lower rates of PCI

in the UK may have the effect of generating higher baseline event rates than seen in the GPA trials. Second, the limited availability of 'acute' PCI (that is, percutaneous procedures undertaken in non-ST elevation patients shortly after presentation) in the National Health Service may cause clinicians to select ACS patients for acute PCI in a different way than clinicians in the GPA trials.

Therefore, in developing the decision model, baseline event rate data that were specific to UK practice were sought. These data were taken from the Prospective Registry of Acute Ischaemic Syndromes in the UK (PRAIS-UK) (Collinson *et al.* 2001). This is an observational cohort registry of 1046 patients admitted to 56 UK hospitals with ACS in 1999. Patients were followed up for 6 months after their index hospital admission and the hospitals included in PRAIS-UK served 24% of the UK population. For the purposes of the study, patients who received GPA in PRAIS-UK ($n = 13$, 1%) were excluded from the analysis. The parameter estimates from PRAIS-UK relating to patients who received a PCI during the acute phase of their ACS were based on a relatively small number of patients ($n = 53$). For this reason, an audit of unstable angina patients undergoing acute PCI at a large UK cardiac centre (Leeds) was undertaken to supplement data from PRAIS-UK ($n = 231$).

4. *Are the relative risk reductions estimated from the trials related to baseline risks?* One way of adapting the clinical results from international trials to the UK setting is by separating out the baseline event rates associated with standard management (without GPAs), estimating those parameters from UK-specific data, and applying the pooled relative treatment effects, for Strategies 1–3 relative to Strategy 4, from the trials. This approach effectively assumes that baseline risks are not transferable internationally, but relative risk reductions are. It may be, however, that the relative treatment effect is itself related to baseline risk—for example, the higher the baseline risk, the lower the treatment effect—in which case the assumed independence between the two components of clinical effectiveness would not be sustainable.

In order to investigate whether the log relative risk in the individual trials varied with log baseline risk (that is, the log event rate in the control group), a random effects meta-regression model was used.

In effect, this form of meta-regression works by fitting a regression line between the event rates measured in the control groups of the trials and those of the experimental (that is, GPA) groups, with the number of points from which the estimate is made being the number of available trials. This function characterizes the relationship between the baseline risks and the relative risks, and this can either be positive or negative. This can then be used in the decision model to adjust the relative risk estimates according to the baseline risk employed in the model. In the context of the GPA trial, the value of this approach relates to the potentially different baseline risk in patients presenting with non-ST elevation ACS in the UK compared to those randomized into the international trials. Once the function has been estimated in the meta-regression, the pooled relative risk estimates from the trials could be adjusted according to the point on the regression line that accords with the UK baseline risk.

The model was adapted to the UK situation in two other ways. First, adjustments were made to allow for the possibility that another medication, clopidogrel, could become widely used in the UK. Therefore, this was included in the model as a fifth strategy, in a sensitivity analysis.

Second, the data from the trials were short term (typically 6 months) but decision-makers in the UK required the estimation of long-term effects in the form of QALYs. Therefore, a long-term Markov model was developed and populated with UK-specific

Table 10.3 Summary of the limitations of the glycoprotein 11b/111a antagonist trials for a cost-effectiveness model for the UK, and approaches taken to overcome these

Limitation with trial data	Methods used to overcome limitations	Additional data source used
Use of GPAs in the trials does not reflect their range of possible uses in the UK	Four strategies relating to how GPAs are being used in the UK were identified with clinical collaborators	
Baseline event rates in trials unlikely to reflect UK practice due to differences in management of ischaemic heart disease	Separate out baseline event rates in trial control groups from relative treatment effects. Apply latter to UK-specific baseline event rates taken from another sources	UK-specific baseline event rates taken from the Prospective Registry of Acute Ischaemic Syndromes in the UK (PRAIS-UK), and a specific survey of patients undergoing acute PCI at Leeds General Infirmary
The relative treatment effect may also vary by location. In particular, the relative risk may be related to the baseline risk in a location	Undertake a meta-regression to relate the baseline (control group) risks with those in the experimental (GPA) groups. If a clear relationship is identified, this can be used to adjust the relative risks used for a UK analysis to a level commensurate with UK baseline event rates	
Recent changes in clinical practice in the UK include the increased use of PCI and use of clopidogrel as part of standard management. However, the UK data sources may not reflect these changes, and their implications for the cost effectiveness of GPAs is unclear	Use of sensitivity analysis to assess the effect, on the model's results, of using baseline event rates from the trials instead of the UK observational study. Also modelling a strategy of using clopidogrel as a fifth strategy in the model	
No data from the trials (UK specific or otherwise) to extrapolate short-term clinical results to long-term QALYs	Use of a long-term Markov model populated using UK-specific observational data	Transition probability and longer-term resource use data taken from Nottingham Heart Attack Register (NHAR)

GPA, glycoprotein 11b/111a antagonist; PCI, percutaneous coronary intervention; QALY, quality-adjusted life-year.

observational data (a summary of all the limitations in the data and the methods used to overcome these is given in Table 10.3).

5. *Adapting economic data collected alongside a clinical trial.* An example of this approach is the work by Menzin *et al.* (1996) on rhDNase for improvement of pulmonary function in patients with cystic fibrosis. A phase III clinical trial was undertaken in the USA comparing two different doses of rhDNase with vehicle (placebo). Patients were treated for 24 weeks and the outcome measures included change in pulmonary function (FEV_1) and incidence of respiratory tract infections (RTI) requiring parenteral antibiotic therapy.

Because the treatment of infections requires health care resources, one of the arguments for rhDNase was that a reduction in infections reduces costs. (These cost reductions may partly offset the cost of adding the drug, notwithstanding any improvements to patients' quality of life.) Therefore, the trial included prospective data collection for hospital admissions, in-patient days, and days of oral and intravenous antibiotic therapy.

Apart from the addition of rhDNase or placebo, the trial was fairly naturalistic in that clinical care was given according to normal practice. The trial showed that rhDNase once a day did reduce RTI-related hospital admissions (0.41 versus 0.56 for placebo, $P < 0.05$) and days of RTI-related out-patient intravenous antibiotic therapy (2.9 versus 4.4, $P < 0.05$). The results of the economic evaluation undertaken in the USA are shown in Fig. 10.1. Compared with placebo, the cost of treating RTIs over 24 weeks was $1682 less among patients receiving rhDNase once daily, primarily due to reductions in the cost of hospitalization (Oster *et al.* 1995).

In addition, there was interest in conducting the same economic evaluation in France, Germany, Italy, and the UK. One approach would be to take the reductions in resource use observed in the trial and to price these in local currency. Table 10.4 shows the results. It can be seen that the savings range from £434 ($711) in the UK to 7011FF ($1064) in France, all being less than the corresponding figure in the USA, presumably reflecting relative price levels.

However, it could be argued that, because of variations in local practice patterns, these *trial-based* estimates for other countries might be misleading. For example, few

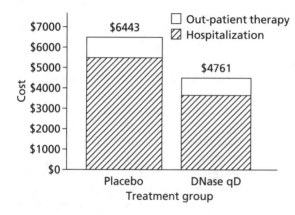

Fig. 10.1 Economic evaluation of DNase therapy in the USA. Mean total costs of care related to respiratory tract infection over 24 weeks by treatment group. From Oster *et al.* (1995).

Table 10.4 Difference in mean cost of respiratory tract infections-related care (placebo minus rhDNase) excluding cost of study medication, over 24 weeks in local currencies and US dollars, by country

Component of cost	France (FF)	Germany (DM)	Italy (L)	UK (£)
		Costs in local currency		
In-patient care				
Days in hospital	4540	711	982 000	300
Antibiotic therapy	806	1259*	122 000	50
Out-patient care	1665	*	181 000	84
Total	7011	1970	1 285 000	434
		Costs in US$†		
In-patient care				
Days in hospital	693	337	660	477
Antibiotic therapy	123	607*	82	79
Out-patient care	254	*	122	134
Total	1070	934	864	690

* A detailed breakdown of in-patient and out-patient antibiotic costs was not available.

† Calculated using 1990 purchasing power parities (Organization for Economic Cooperation and Development Health Data File, OECD, Paris 1992).

From Menzin et al. (1996).

patients may be admitted to hospital for treatment of RTI in Italy, as there is extensive use of injectable antibiotics in ambulatory care. Also, length of stay in hospital could differ from that in the USA, as the hospitals may be operating under different financial incentives, or have a greater or lesser pressure on beds. Therefore, the analysts in the four other countries were asked to consider whether a *practice-adjusted* estimate of resource use and cost should be presented alongside the trial-based estimates. The adjustments were made by

(1) seeking expert opinion on likely treatment patterns for RTI;

(2) analysing a series of patient case notes (charts) to estimate length of hospital stay and resource use for treatment of RTI.

The outcome of this exercise was that in the UK no adjustments (to the trial-based estimates) were considered necessary. However, in Germany, length of stay was considered to be, on average, 14.4 days rather than 12.3 days. In France and Italy, both the rate of hospitalization and the length of stay were adjusted. The overall effect was to reduce slightly the estimates of savings in Italy (from $908 to $607) and in France (from $1064 to $850). In Germany, there was a very small increase in the savings from treating RTI.

The problem with this approach is in justifying the adjustments made. One might argue that the savings observed in the trial, whilst not very generalizable, are relatively free of bias. This is an example of the conflict between internal and external validity mentioned in Chapter 8. In this case the main saving grace was that, in general, the adjustments made were conservative (that is, reduced the estimates of the savings from rhDNase). If the results had gone the other way there might have been more criticism of the adjustments made. Therefore, analysts wishing to make adjustments to trial-based data might be advised to state these up front in the analysis plan for the study, prior to seeing the data. Any adjustments should also be based on empirical data rather than guesswork.

6. *Analysing economic data from multinational trials.* One response to the problem over the lack of transferability of cost-effectiveness data would be to undertake clinical trials with economic data collection in all relevant countries and settings. In part, this is achieved by undertaking multinational trials, except that often relatively small numbers of patients are included from some countries. Indeed, one of the motivations on the clinical side for undertaking multinational trials is to enroll sufficient numbers of patients within a relatively short period of time. Because the intention is usually to pool the clinical data, it is likely that the trial will be underpowered for analysing differences between treatment groups in any single country or centre. Although ultimately an empirical question, it is likely that a multinational trial will also be underpowered for the analysis of resource data at the individual country level.

Currently there are few examples of multinational economic clinical trials in the published literature and there has been little discussion of how the data from these studies should be analysed. One option would be to approach the problem in the same way as it is handled in the analysis of clinical data. Namely, statistical tests could be performed to check for the existence of an interaction between treatment effect and country (or centre).

Normally, these tests turn out to be negative, although they themselves may be short of statistical power. However, a negative test on the resource data may be sufficient grounds to pool them. Economic analyses could then be undertaken by using the overall resource use data set and by applying prices for each individual country. This was the approach used by Cook *et al.* (2003), illustrated by an analysis of the resource use data from the Scandinavian Simvastatin Survival Study (4S), conducted in five Nordic countries. They found that tests of interaction applied to economic endpoints, including cost-effectiveness ratios and net health benefits, were negative. Therefore the pooled estimate of the economic endpoint was considered to be representative of the participating countries. One potential criticism of this approach is that, if the statistical test is negative, there is assumed to be no variability in cost-effectiveness by country. However, zero variability is very unlikely for the reasons outlined in Section 10.4.1 and any differences could be important for local (country-level) decision-making.

If the tests for an interaction between the effect on resources and country (or centre) turn out to be positive, or if such tests are considered inappropriate, the analyst would then have to explore two options. First, country-specific resource data could be used to calculate the cost-effectiveness ratios using the overall clinical data set. The main argument for this approach is that the clinical data are more likely to be generalizable across countries than resource use data. Alternatively, country-specific resource use data could be used to calculate cost-effectiveness ratios with country-specific clinical data. The main argument for this approach would be that impacts on resource use in a given country are likely to be driven, at least in part, by the clinical differences between the therapies. Therefore, country-specific data should form both the numerator and denominator of the ratio.

This was the logic behind the approach used by Willke *et al.* (1998). They considered that, because costs and outcomes of medical treatments may vary from country to

Table 10.5 Cost-effectiveness ratios, overall and by country

	Cost per death averted, with own-country cost and mortality effects ($)	Cost per death averted, with trial-wide mortality effect* ($)	Cost per death averted, own-country prices, trial-wide utilization and mortality effect* ($)
Country 1	11 450	5921	46 818
Country 2	60 358	91 906	57 636
Country 3	244 133	90 487	53 891
Country 4	181 259	93 326	69 145
Country 5	†	†	65 800
Whole sample	45 892	45 892	45 892

* Standard mortality effect = 0.055, based on probit estimate.

† Treatment is cost saving.

country in important ways, decision-makers are increasingly interested in having data based on their own country's health care situations. Therefore they use multiple regression to estimate country-specific cost-effectiveness ratios from a multinational economic clinical trial conducted in five countries. They examine how clinical and economic outcomes interact when estimating treatment effects on cost and propose empirical methods for capturing these interactions and incorporating them when making country-specific estimates.

Table 10.5 shows the implications of allowing more factors to vary when estimating country-specific cost-effectiveness ratios. In the first column all three factors (effectiveness, resource utilization, and prices) are allowed to vary. It can be seen that there is wide variation, by country, around the overall estimate of cost per death averted. By contrast, in the third column only prices are allowed to vary by country, with trial-wide effectiveness and resource utilization data being pooled. It can be seen that the country-specific cost-effectiveness ratios are more similar to each other and to the overall estimate.

Finally, more recent work uses multilevel modelling (MLM) (Manca *et al.* 2005; Grieve *et al.* in press; Willan *et al.* in press). This approach formally accounts for the hierarchical structure of the data in a multinational trial. That is, individual patients are 'clustered' within centres and centres 'clustered' within country. Because of differences in practice patterns, resource availability, and other factors varying from place to place, we might expect patients within a cluster to be more similar, in terms of costs and outcomes, than those in different clusters. By seeking to capture these relationships, MLM allows an estimation of overall cost-effectiveness across countries that allows for the correlations within cluster; this would be expected to change the estimated standard error compared to an analysis that ignores clustering.

Multilevel modelling also facilitates country-specific estimates of cost-effectiveness, which are a combination of the data collected in the specific country of interest and of data from other countries that participated in the trial. In its simplest form, the process of 'shrinkage' estimation effectively makes an estimate of a country's cost-effectiveness a weighted sum of the mean cost-effectiveness in that country and of the overall mean cost-effectiveness across all countries. The weights are determined by the sample size in the country of interest relative to the overall trial sample size, and the proportion of overall variability in cost-effectiveness between patients that takes place within the country of interest compared to that between countries. The key

---

Box 10.3 Location-specific cost-effectiveness using shrinkage estimation in multilevel models

One of the features of multicentre or multinational clinical trials is that different numbers of patients will be recruited by centre, or by country. Manca *et al.* (2005) used multilevel modelling to estimate location-specific cost-effectiveness for 25 centres participating in the EVALUATE Trial (which compared abdominal and laparoscopic hysterectomy). Cost-effectiveness results were expressed as net monetary benefits (NMBs), using a ceiling ratio of £30 000 for a QALY.

The figure illustrates the effect of shrinkage on centre-specific estimates of NMBs for the abdominal (control) arm of the trial. The naïve centre effects are represented as circles, the shrunken effects as triangles. Also, the relative size of the symbols give a guide to the number of observations within each centre. It can be seen that the naïve centre-specific estimates of mean NMB are always further from the overall mean (the horizontal line) than the corresponding shrunken estimates.

Furthermore, the smaller the number of patients within a centre the greater the discrepancy between the naïve and shrunken estimates. This is to be expected as the smaller the number of patients the less information is available from which to derive the centre-specific estimate. Accordingly, one would have less confidence in the resulting estimate and this is reflected by applying greater weight to the shrinkage factor that pulls the naïve estimate to the overall mean.

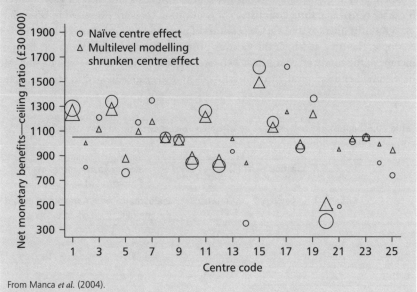

From Manca *et al.* (2004).

advantage of this approach is that it affords a gain in statistical efficiency by 'borrowing' information from all countries in the estimation of cost-effectiveness for individual countries (Willan *et al.* in press) (see Box 10.3).

The analysis of multilocation (multicentre and/or multinational) trials is an active area of research currently. As yet, no single method can be considered unequivocally superior to others, but the use of regression-based methods for this type of analysis is likely to increase in the future. Of particular interest is the possibility that co-variates representing relevant characteristics of centres and countries could be included in such models (Grieve *et al.* in press; Drummond *et al.* in press).

10.4.3. **Exercise: undertaking an economic evaluation of non-steroidal anti-inflammatory drugs in three countries**

Objectives

1 To illustrate how decision trees can be useful in modelling the cost-effectiveness of therapies and in transferring results from one setting to another.

2 To illustrate how differences between clinical trials and clinical practice, and between countries, can affect cost-effectiveness estimates.

Problem

One of the critical differences between NSAIDs is their gastric side-effects. These can affect both the level of tolerability of the drug and its economic impact. (For example, gastric side-effects may have resource consequences if treatment is required.) Whereas there may be little to choose between NSAIDs in terms of their relative efficacy, exploration of the impact of gastric side-effects could be important. In particular, it may mean that a choice of therapy based on acquisition cost alone could be inappropriate.

Data

Data are presented in Table 10.6 on the acquisition costs and rates of gastric ulcers for three NSAIDs in three countries. The acquisition costs are expressed in US dollars for 6 months' therapy and vary by country. This could be for historical reasons (for example, the time at which the various products were launched) and the level of income in the countries concerned. Two rates of gastric ulcers are presented—the rate determined endoscopically in clinical trials and the rate adjusted to exclude silent

Table 10.6 Acquisition costs and rates of gastric ulcers with three non-steroidal anti-inflammatory drugs

	Acquisition costs ($)			Rate of gastric ulcers over 6 months (%)	
	Country 1	**Country 2**	**Country 3**	**Endoscopically determined**	**Adjusted to exclude silent ulcers**
Mobifren	225	75	121	23.9	14.3
Osteotec	294	100	134	17.8	10.7
Voldene	300	136	126	10.2	6.1

Table 10.7 Data on treatment for gastric ulcers in three countries

	Country 1	Country 2	Country 3
Probabilities			
Patients with ulcers treated in hospital	0.086	0.053	0.050
Patients hospitalized for ulcers requiring surgery	0.12	0.43	0.20
Unit costs ($)			
Ambulatory care for ulcer	901	540	87
Medical hospital care for ulcer	3450	1548	133
Surgical hospital care for ulcer	15 700	2533	555

ulcers. (The latter rate reflects the fact that around 40% of the lesions discovered by endoscope may not result in treatment because they are asymptomatic.)

Table 10.7 gives data on the treatment of gastric ulcers in the three countries. This contains data on treatment practices and unit costs. Country 3 is obviously one with a less well-developed economy, where price levels are lower. Finally, Fig. 10.2 provides a decision tree that can be used to combine the data on probabilities and costs to calculate the expected cost of 6 months' therapy.

Tasks

The decision tree shown in Fig. 10.2 can be used to calculate the expected cost (C^*) of 6 months of therapy.

1 Calculate the expected cost of 6 months of therapy for each of the three NSAIDs in each of the three countries.

2 Explain why the relative cost of therapy varies by country.

3 Imagine that you are an economist working for the company that produces Voldene, the NSAID with the lowest rate of gastric side-effects. In a country where this therapy does not give the lowest expected cost, what other economic analyses would you consider?

Solutions

1 To calculate the expected cost of 6 months' therapy, the decision tree model is completed using the data in Tables 10.6 and 10.7. This is done for Country 1 below. Note that the rate of ulcers adjusted to exclude silent ulcers is used because it is more likely to reflect what would happen in regular practice.

The probabilities at each node sum to 1 and the expected cost calculations are made by rolling back the tree from *right to left*. For example, the expected cost at node X is

$$\$((0.12 \times 15\,700) + (0.88 \times 3450)) = \$4920$$

Then, at node Y it is

$$\$((0.914 \times 901) + (0.086 \times 4920)) = \$1247$$

Thus, the expected total cost C^* for treatment with mobifren, which includes acquisition and care costs, is

$$\$((0.143 \times 1442) + (0.857 \times 225)) = \$399$$

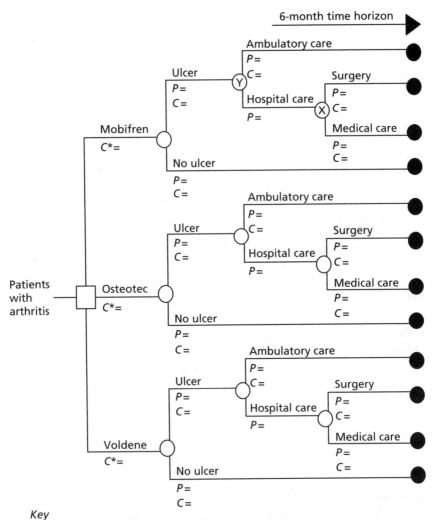

Fig. 10.2 Decision tree for assessing the cost-effectiveness of non-steroidal anti-inflammatory drugs. * Patients developing an ulcer are assumed to incur half of the 6-month cost of therapy.

The equivalent figures for osteotec and voldene in Country 1 are $242 and $374 respectively. (Figures are approximate and subject to rounding.)

2 The relative cost of therapy is influenced both by the acquisition costs of the drugs and the costs of caring for ulcers. The costs of ulcer care have the biggest impact on total cost in Country 1 because these are relatively large in relation to

drug costs. In fact, the rankings of the three drugs by acquisition cost and total cost are completely different in Country 1. The rankings are unchanged in Countries 2 and 3, although in Country 2 the effect of considering the costs of ulcer care is to reduce the difference in total cost between the three therapies.

3 Although voldene is the most expensive drug in Countries 1 and 2, the relative cost of therapy is only highest in Country 2. In this case additional arguments that might be considered are that

(1) a reduction in the rate of ulceration is worthwhile in terms of avoided pain and distress;

(2) there is a small case fatality associated with treatment for ulcers.

10.5. Problems and potential for using economic evaluation in decision-making

Although this book is primarily about the methods of economic evaluation, it is important to address the potential for using study results. If the problems of using economic evaluation are not understood, it may not be worthwhile investing resources in undertaking the studies in the first place. Much of the potential for using economic evaluation and the related problems are situation specific, but it is possible to make a few general observations.

10.5.1. In what situations could economic evaluation be used?

Haan and Rutten (1987) provide a taxonomy of decision-making situations where economic evaluation could be used to encourage a rational diffusion and use of health technology (see Box 10.4). They divide these into situations where regulation (of the health care system) is by directive and those where regulation is by incentive. The extent to which these apply is likely to vary by health care systems. For example, in some socialized health care systems where central control over the finance and planning of the system is possible, it may be feasible to regulate by directive, for example, deciding on the number and location of specialist facilities like heart transplant centres. Clearly, economic evaluation can inform such decisions (see Buxton *et al.* 1985).

One of the other forms of regulation by directive, exclusion of technologies from reimbursement, could apply in all health care systems but might vary in its implementation. For example, in socialized health care systems economic evaluation could inform decisions about the inclusion of new health technologies on a national approved list (for example, national formulary in the case of drugs).

In a more decentralized, market-based, health care system, the relevant decisions are more likely to relate to whether certain technologies are included in the 'benefit package' offered by insurers, or to the level of patient co-payment required for drugs listed on the insurance plan's formulary. The latter example moves us towards

> ## Box 10.4 **Taxonomy of decision-making situations where economic evaluation could be used to influence the diffusion and use of health technology**
>
> | Regulation by directive (central/ regional government) | Regulation by incentive |
> | --- | --- |
> | Pre-market controls for drugs and devices | Reforming payment schemes for health care institutions (e.g. hospitals) |
> | (Conditional) exclusion from public reimbursement | Budgetary reform within institutions |
> | Planning of specialist facilities or specific technologies | Changing payment systems for health care providers |
> | | Cost-sharing arrangements |
> | | Encouraging competition in the health care system |
> | | Medical audit and utilization review systems |
>
> There are many health care decision-making situations where economic evaluation could potentially be used. The range of possibilities depends on the health care system operating in a given country. National, socialized health care systems have a greater potential for using regulation by directive. Liberal, market-based health care systems are more likely to rely on regulation by incentive in order to encourage a rational diffusion and use of health technologies.
> From Haan and Rutten (1987).

regulation by incentive. In principle, economic evaluation could inform these decisions also. Because the worldwide trend is probably towards managed competition in health care, regulation by incentive is likely to be a much more fruitful way of encouraging a rational diffusion and use of health technology in the future.

10.5.2. **Where has economic evaluation actually been used?**

Drummond (1994b) discusses a number of examples where economic evaluation has been used to inform some of the decisions outlined in Haan and Rutten's taxonomy. In general, the actual use of economic evaluation is quite limited in relation to the potential. Coyle (1993) suggests a number of reasons why this would be the case. These include lack of dissemination of findings, lack of recognition (by decision-makers) of their importance, lack of understanding of study results, and a lack of mechanisms to use them in decision-making. In a recent paper discussing the situation in the USA, Neumann (2004) suggests that the main factors explaining the resistance to the use of CEA are a lack of understanding about the conceptual approach, a mistrust of methods and motives, regulatory and legal barriers, and US people's general distaste of limits.

Two of the most widely publicized uses of economic evaluation are in the Oregon Medicaid Plan (Eddy 1991) and in decisions about the reimbursement of pharmaceuticals in Australia (Commonwealth of Australia 1995) and Canada (Ontario Ministry of Health 1994; Anis and Gagnon 2000). Both instances illustrate that the application of economic evaluation is not just a technical issue. In Oregon, a cost-per-QALY league table was constructed in order to inform the public debate about which treatments to include in the state's Medicaid package. Although there were undoubtedly imperfections in the economic analyses carried out, the main problem was that the league table became a focus of political debate. Therefore, the arguments focused not on the role of economic evaluation, but on whether it was right to ration and, if so, the best way of rationing.

In Australia the provision of data on the cost-effectiveness of pharmaceuticals has been mandatory since 1993. Pharmaceutical companies applying for public subsidy of their product, through inclusion on the governments Pharmaceutical Benefits Schedule, must make a submission comparing the costs and consequences of their drug with a relevant alternative (comparator). A similar procedure is followed in the province of Ontario in Canada. Glasziou and Mitchell (1996) have reported on the first 2 years of operation of the scheme in Australia. It has proved workable although there have been disagreements about the choice of comparator, the valuation of productivity changes, and the level of feedback that should be given to applicant companies. The ultimate test of economic evaluation will be whether it improves the quality of decision-making about the pricing and reimbursement of medicines in Australia and other countries. As mentioned above, one of the most recent examples is the use of economic evaluation by NICE in England and Wales (National Institute for Clinical Excellence 2004).

10.5.3. **Do decision-makers apply a cost-effectiveness threshold?**

One of the main topics of interest, in studies of NICE and other public decision-making bodies, is whether they apply a threshold cost-effectiveness ratio (R_T in Chapter 5) in their decision-making and, if so, what the ratio is. Raftery (2001) argues that, by specifying carefully the conditions for use of health technologies (for example, stage of disease, level of patient risk), NICE has generally enabled to keep the incremental cost per QALY below £30 000. The Institute's own guide to the methods of technology appraisal states that

> below a most plausible incremental cost-effectiveness ratio (ICER) of £20,000/QALY, judgements about the acceptability of a technology as an effective use of NHS resources are based primarily on the cost-effectiveness estimate. Above a most plausible ICER of £20,000/QALY, judgements about the acceptability of the technology as an effective use of NHS resources are more likely to make more explicit reference to factors including:
> —the degree of uncertainty surrounding the calculation of ICERs;
> —the innovative nature of the technology;

—the particular features of the condition and population receiving the technology;

—where appropriate, the wider societal costs and benefits. (National Institute for Clinical Excellence 2004, p. 33)

In a study of the decisions made by the Pharmaceutical Benefits Advisory Committee in Australia, George *et al.* (2001) concluded that the Committee 'appears to be unlikely to recommend a drug for listing if the additional cost per life-year exceeded \$AU76 000 (1998/99 values) and unlikely to reject a drug for which the additional cost per life-year was less than \$AU42 000.' However, the cost-effectiveness ratio was not the only factor determining the reimbursement decision. Other factors include the scientific rigour and relevance of the evidence for comparative safety, efficacy, and cost-effectiveness, the lack, or inadequacy of alternative treatments currently in use, the perceived need in the community, whether the drug is likely only to be used in a hospital setting and the seriousness of the intended indication (health condition).

In an econometric analysis of decisions made by NICE, Devlin and Parkin (2004) also found that their results supported the broad notion of a threshold, where the probability of rejection of the technology increases as the cost per QALY increases. However, cost-effectiveness, together with uncertainty and the burden of disease, explained NICE decisions better than cost-effectiveness alone. They also pointed out that there could be different notions of what a cost-effectiveness threshold might be (see Box 10.5).

10.5.4. Could other factors be incorporated more formally?

As it is clear that decision-makers may wish to consider factors such as equity or burden of disease, can these factors be incorporated more formally into economic evaluations? With respect to equity, it is worth noting that all forms of economic evaluation embody some form of equity consideration. This is most obvious in CBA, as discussed in Chapter 7, where individuals' WTP for improvements in health may be

---

Box 10.5 Different notions of the cost-effectiveness threshold in health care decision-making

Devlin and Parkin (2004) point out that the cost-effectiveness threshold for the acceptance or rejection of a health technology can be conceived of in several different ways.

The simplest case is illustrated in Fig. 1. Here the threshold is a precise, 'knife-edge' value for a marginal QALY against which evidence from an economic evaluation is compared. However, in practice the threshold is likely to be less clearly defined, as other factors are likely to enter into the decision. These include equity and the overall burden of the disease. Therefore there may be a threshold range, as illustrated in Fig. 2.

Furthermore, there may be different thresholds for investments and disinvestments in health care. O'Brien *et al.* (2002) provide evidence that the WTA values for

Box 10.5 Different notions of the cost-effectiveness threshold in health care decision-making (*continued*)

giving up QALYs, by reducing or removing services, are higher than the willingness-to-pay (WTP) to obtain QALYs from new services. Therefore, the cost-effectiveness thresholds might look like those in Fig. 3.

Finally, the decision-maker may have views about the uncertainty surrounding the cost-effectiveness evidence. Although some argue that such uncertainty should not influence the decision to approve or reject the technology (Claxton 1999), a risk-averse decision-maker would have a higher probability of rejection for a given base case cost per QALY gained than a risk lowering decision-maker. This is illustrated by Fig. 4.

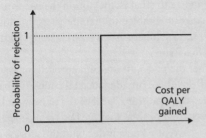

Fig. 1 The cost-effectiveness threshold as a point.

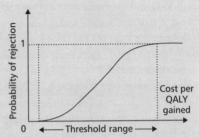

Fig. 2 The cost-effectiveness threshold as a range, reflecting trade-offs against efficiency.

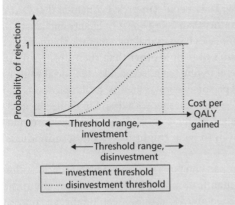

Fig. 3 The cost-effectiveness threshold for investments and disinvestments.

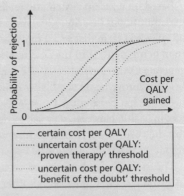

Fig. 4 The cost-effectiveness threshold under uncertainty.

All this illustrates that, even if it made sense to think in terms of a cost-effectiveness threshold, it is difficult to specify what it is!

constrained by their ability to pay. Other elements of the cost–benefit calculation, such as the value placed on individuals' work and leisure time, can also introduce inequalities (Russell 2004). This was discussed in Chapter 4.

Cost-effectiveness analysis and CUA, as normally practised, also embody equity assumptions in that the value of a life-year or QALY is considered the same no matter who receives it. Whilst on the face of it, this may appear to be egalitarian, there are equally plausible equity propositions. For example, as a society we may prefer to give a QALY to someone who is in very poor health compared with someone who is close to full health. Alternatively, we may prefer to give a QALY to someone who has not experienced much good health during their lifetime, compared with someone who has experienced a 'fair innings' (Williams 1997).

This being the case, some analysts have proposed incorporating equity weights in QALY calculations, in order to allow for societal concerns about the severity of health conditions and the realization of potential in health (that is, the notion that we would not want to discriminate against the permanently disabled in that life-years provided to them bring less QALYs) (Nord et al. 1999). (See Johannesson (2001), Nord (2001), and Williams (2001) for a lively debate on this issue.)

The other area of debate concerns whether the person trade-off approach for valuing health states (see Chapter 6) better reflects these broader societal concerns than does the time trade-off or standard gamble. The intuitive appeal of the person trade-off approach is that it mirrors the priority-setting process that QALYs are ultimately intended for. The main drawback is that we currently know little about the process of preference formation that individuals go through in responding to the questions. More research is required in this field, but some studies do indicate that there is more to social value than health gain, even if the findings of studies are not totally consistent (Dolan and Green 1998; Dolan and Tsuchiya 2003).

Based on a recent systematic review, Dolan et al. (in press) conclude that QALY maximization is descriptively flawed. Rather than being linear in quality and length of life, it would seem that social value diminishes in marginal increments of both. Rather than being neutral to the characteristics of people other than their propensity to generate QALYs, members of the general public seem to consider the social value of health improvement to be higher if the person has worse lifetime health prospects and higher if that person has dependents. In addition there is a desire to reduce inequalities in health. However, they acknowledge that there are some uncertainties surrounding the results, particularly in relation to what might be affecting individuals' responses to survey questions.

The issue of overall burden of disease can enter as a decision-making consideration in two ways. First, it can be another manifestation of societal concerns about the severity of health conditions, as discussed above. Second, it could reflect a concern about overall budgetary impact. Namely, a decision-maker would not be indifferent between two programmes with the same cost-effectiveness ratio if one involved treating many more patients than the other. The logic is that, with a larger budgetary impact, the opportunity cost at the margin is likely to be greater. The literature in this area is not so well developed, and concentrates on the methods of calculating budgetary impact, or on discussing how consideration of budgetary impact may be at odds with consideration of cost-effectiveness (Nuijten and Rutten 2002; Trueman et al.

2001). There is no doubt that assessment of budgetary impact is a major concern of decision-makers. Whether it should be a methodological interest of those involved in economic evaluation is less clear.

In a recent paper Al *et al.* (2004) surveyed decision-makers' views on health care objectives and budget constraints. The interviewees were involved in decisions at the macro level (government), the meso level (health care insurers in total, hospitals in total), and the micro level (clinical guidelines, individual hospitals, individual insurers). They found that interviewees were willing to rank and rate the optimality criteria presented to them, although there were considerable variations in rankings. The decision-makers also proposed additional criteria, but some of these were difficult to describe in a formal objective function (for example, political pressure).

The responses to the various budget constraints indicated that most of these were relevant. However, the standard assumption in economic evaluations, of one limited budget, seemed to bear little relation to reality. It would therefore be interesting to study what the effect of different budget constraints is on optimal budget allocation. Clearly more research is required into what health care decision-makers are seeking to optimize and into their attitudes to budgetary and other constraints.

10.5.5. In what ways could economic evaluation be used?

We tend to think of economic evaluation as a basis for undertaking studies and this is what the book has been mainly concerned with. However, from the discussion in Section 10.5.2 above, it is clear that the formal use of economic evaluation in health care decision-making is still quite limited.

Clearly, it is not possible to undertake a formal economic evaluation for every conceivable decision. Sometimes the time horizon for making the decision is very short and this would preclude a study. (However, Schoenbaum *et al.* (1976) did undertake a study within 3 weeks in order to help the US government decide whether or not to launch an immunization campaign for swine influenza.)

On other occasions a formal study may be inappropriate because the cost of the study may be large in relation to the importance of the decision. There is no point in spending $100 000 on a study to decide how to spend $50 000, although this has probably been done somewhere! Therefore, it is worthwhile recognizing two other possible ways of using economic evaluation. First, it could be used as *a way of assessing proposals* for the use of resources. Box 10.6 contains a checklist of questions similar to the methodological checklist outlined in Chapter 3. However, the questions have been re-formulated as a management checklist to be used by someone considering a proposal being made (for exampe, by a clinician wishing to expand a service). Probably, this is the way that many decision-makers use economic evaluation, because it is unlikely that a published study exists, or could be commissioned, to inform a given decision directly. To date there has been little study of how decision-makers actually use economic evaluation. The special journal issues edited by Drummond *et al.* (1994) and Sloan and Grabowski (1997) are a useful starting point for anyone wishing to pursue this further. Second, decision-makers may use economic evaluation more generally as a *systematic way of thinking*, or as a way of structuring problems. Understandably there are few published data dealing with this potential way of using economic evaluation, because the processes for arriving at particular decisions are rarely documented.

Box 10.6 **Questions to ask of anyone making a proposal for the use of resources**

Consideration of alternatives

What is the main justification for the proposed service; what would be the consequence of doing nothing at all?

Does the proposal contain an explicit comparison of alternative treatments or programmes, or is the implicit alternative the existing service provision?

If a completely new alternative treatment or programme is proposed,

- is it adequately described?
- why was this particular option chosen?
- were other options rejected, if so why?

Assessment of cost and benefits

In evaluating the proposed service against alternatives, what range of costs is considered? Does this include

- capital as well as operating costs?
- costs other than those resulting in money expenditure (for example, the opportunity cost of space denied other uses)?
- costs outside the immediate department where the service will be provided?
- costs on other parties (for example, patients, other public or private agencies)?

What is known about the effectiveness of the health treatments or programmes discussed in the proposal?

- Have these been evaluated by a randomized controlled trial or similar method?
- Are there plans to monitor the effectiveness of any new procedures; if so, how?
- Have all relevant dimensions of outcome been considered and will any attempts be made to assign preferences or values to them?

Would costs and benefits be substantially different if the proposed service provision were of a different scale? That is,

- if the service provision could be larger, what would be added and what would be the additional costs and benefits?
- if the service provision had to be smaller, what aspects of it would be cut and what would be the reductions in costs and benefits?

Is it claimed that the proposal will be partly self-funding, in that savings will be generated? If so, what specific actions need to be taken to realize such savings (for example, closing hospital wards or other institutions) and what are the likely resource costs associated with taking these actions?

Other important issues

Does the proposal acknowledge any differences in the *timing* of costs and benefits between the alternatives assessed? If so, how is this dealt with in the proposal?

> **Box 10.6 Questions to ask of anyone making a proposal for the use of resources** *(continued)*
>
> What are the main sources of uncertainty surrounding the proposal (for example, in the effectiveness of new medical procedures, or in expected revenue costs or savings)?
>
> - What happens to costs and benefits if the analysis is re-worked using more pessimistic assumptions?
> - What could be done, perhaps at a slight increase in cost, to reduce uncertainty (for example, by additional information gathering)?
>
> The above checklist does not comprise a comprehensive range of questions. It is the intention that the questions themselves, and the responses they solicit, will suggest further questions pertinent to the evaluation of choices in the use of health service resources.

10.5.6. Overall, has economic evaluation proved useful?

In recent years economic evaluation has been used in a much wider range of jurisdictions. Drummond (2004) reviews the evidence on its use and usefulness both at the central level, where a single agency or organization makes decisions for the whole health care system, and at the local level, where decisions are made by various actors within the health care system. He concludes that the evidence of use and usefulness are currently stronger at the local level, because the conditions likely to foster the use of economic evaluation are more often present. These include a clear decision-making process, clear policy objectives, reasonable timelines and resources to undertake the evaluations, and appropriate incentives to implement the findings of studies.

The most detailed study of the use of economic evaluation in health care is that by Neumann (2005). He discusses the promise and promotion of CEA, resistance to its use in the USA, the legal, political, and ethical concerns, experience from other countries, and ends by offering advice to CEA practitioners and decision-makers.

10.5.7. What should be our overall philosophy for the use of economic evaluation?

In Chapter 2 we discussed three hypothetical analysts, each having a slightly different perspective on the role of economic evaluation. Two perspectives in particular, those of Analysts A and C, merit more discussion here.

Analyst A was the one who thought that economic evaluation ought to be firmly grounded in the theory of welfare economics. The role of the evaluation is therefore to give decision-makers a 'theoretically correct' answer to their question, at least according to the criterion of economic efficiency. On the other hand, Analyst C saw the role of economic evaluation as identifying, measuring, and where possible, valuing a wide range of costs and consequences. However, the valuations of costs and consequences would not necessarily be consistent with welfare economics theory, as they could come from decision-makers acting on behalf of individual members of society, rather than the individuals themselves.

These two perspectives on the role of economic evaluation have been called respectively the *Paretian* and the *decision-making* approaches (Sugden and Williams 1979). Clearly, the Paretian approach has the theoretical high ground, although even the most committed Paretians acknowledge that distributional issues as well as efficiency issues need to be dealt with. This is particularly important because the criterion for a potential Pareto improvement—that the gainers from a particular project should be able to compensate the losers—does not require the compensation to take place in practice.

Sugden and Williams defend the decision-making approach on the grounds that 'there is a fairly strong argument that, at least in a fairly centralized, public, decision-making system, the objective chosen will normally correspond to that implied by the potential Pareto improvement criterion'. They also argue that, through the control of the tax system, government decision-makers can convert potential Pareto improvements to actual improvements.

Departure from the strict Paretian framework would imply that estimates of individuals' WTP for health care programmes are *just another piece of relevant information* in reaching a decision about the allocation of health care resources, alongside data on effects (in physical units) and health state preference scores. Therefore, one does not have to subscribe to the Paretian value judgement in order to be interested in WTP, although those analysts undertaking these measurements clearly believe that individuals' valuations are important in health care resource allocation decisions.

A related issue concerns whether CEA or CUA and CBA are nearly equivalent (Phelps and Mushlin 1991). The logic is that if, at the end of the day, decision-makers must apply their values in reaching a decision, this suggests that presenting a cost-effectiveness ratio is almost the same as undertaking a CBA, because decision-makers will make their own assessment of the societal WTP for a life-year or a QALY.

It should be clear from the discussion in Chapters 2 and 7 that CEA and CBA are not necessarily equivalent. For example, CBA may include the value of aspects of health programmes that are not related to changes in health status (see Fig. 2.2). Second, the total societal WTP for a given health care programme will include the value placed on it by altruistic individuals whose own health state is not directly affected.

Of course, it would in principle be possible to extend the scope of a CEA or CUA to include the gains in quality of life that altruistic individuals experience from observing others who receive health care. However, most CEAs and CUAs consider only the changes in health state (or preference score) for those directly affected by the programme. Usually this means the patient only, although some studies have considered the QALYs gained by caregivers (Drummond *et al.* 1991). On the other hand, the decision-maker, as society's representative, may consider that, for allocation of public resources for health care, only the value directly related to changes in health state is relevant and that, for equity reasons, a gain of a QALY should be valued the same no matter to whom it falls. (This would be close to the position adopted by Analyst B in Chapter 2.) In this case the decision-maker may be happy to use CEA/CUA and to maximize the gains in health status from the allocation of health care resources.

(Ideally, the consideration of these gains should extend beyond the individual patient if it can be shown that there are externalities in the consumption of health care.)

In reflecting on the work of the NICE in England and Wales, Rawlins and Culyer (2004) make it clear that those responsible for formulating NICE's guidance have to make judgements both about what is good and bad in the available science (scientific value judgements) and about what is good for society (social value judgements). Also, in a recent paper, Sculpher *et al.* (2004) argue that economic evaluation should focus more on tackling the needs of social decision-making than on the underlying principles of welfare economics. They even go so far as to suggest that, for this research to be relevant to policy, it needs to be seen less as *economic* evaluation, and more as 'just evaluation for decision-making'.

We have taken a broadly based view in this book, because we feel that it is important for the reader to become familiar with all the forms of economic evaluation. The objective of economic evaluation is to be an *aid* to decision-making, not a complete basis for making decisions. Therefore, it is important to expose the strengths and weaknesses of all the approaches rather than to suggest that there is but one theoretically correct approach.

10.6. **Conclusions**

In this chapter we have explored a range of issues relating to the presentation and use of economic evaluation results. Some issues are relatively straightforward and would command a broad consensus. For example, it is important for the analysts to present their results in a transparent manner. Also, it is important to explore those factors likely to cause the costs or consequences of treatments to vary from one setting to another.

There is more disagreement about other issues, such as the overall philosophy for the use of economic evaluation. Some analysts (like Analyst A) believe that economic evaluations should only be performed in a manner consistent with the theoretical foundations of welfare economics. Others (like Analyst C) believe that the role of economic evaluation is to encourage systematic thinking about costs and consequences of health care treatments and programmes.

Very little is known about decision-makers' attitudes to these issues and the ways in which the results of economic studies, however performed, are used in decision-making. This is likely to be a priority for research in the future.

References

Al, M. J., Feenstra, T., and Brouwer, W. B. F. (2004). Decision makers' views on health care objectives and budget constraints: results from a pilot study. *Health Policy*, **70**, 33–48.

Anis, A. H. and Gagnon, Y. (2000). Using economic evaluations to make formulary coverage decisions: so much for guidelines. *PharmacoEconomics*, **18**, 55–62.

Arrow, K. J. and Lind, R. C. (1970). Risk and uncertainty: uncertainty and the evaluation of public investment decisions. *American Economic Review*, **60**, 364–78.

Barbieri, M., Drummond, M. F., Willke, R., Chancellor, J., Jolain, B., and Towse, A. (2005). Variability of cost-effectiveness estimates for pharmaceuticals in Western Europe: lessons for inferring generalizability. *Value in Health*, **8**, 10–23.

Birch, S. and Gafni, A. (2002). On being NICE in the UK: guidelines for technology appraisal for the NHS in England and Wales. *Health Economics*, **11**, 185–91.

British Medical Journal Working Party on Economic Evaluation (1996). Guidelines for authors and peer reviewers of economic submissions to the *BMJ*. *British Medical Journal*, **313**, 275–83.

Buxton, M. J., Acheson, R., Caine, N., Gibson, S., and O'Brien, B. (1985). *Costs and benefits of the heart transplant programmes at Harefield and Papworth Hospitals*. Department of Health and Social Security Research Report No. 12. Her Majesty's Stationery Office, London.

Canadian Coordinating Office for Health Technology Assessment (1997). *Guidelines for the economic evaluation of pharmaceuticals: Canada*. Canadian Coordinating Office for Health Technology Assessment, Ottawa.

Centre for Reviews and Dissemination (2004). *NHS Economic Evaluation Database*. Centre for Reviews and Dissemination, University of York, York.

Claxton, K. (1999). The irrelevance of inference: a decision-making approach to the stochastic evaluation of health care technologies. *Journal of Health Economics*, **18**, 341–64.

Claxton, K. and Posnett, J. (1996). An economic approach to clinical trial design and research priority-setting. *Health Economics*, **5**, 513–24.

Collège des Économists de la Santé (2004). *CODECS database*. Collège des Économists de la Santé, Paris.

Collinson, J., Flather, M. D., Fox, K. A. A., *et al.* (2001). Clinical outcomes, risk stratification and practice patterns of unstable angina and myocardial infarction without ST elevation: Prospective Registry of Acute Ischaemic Syndromes in the UK (PRAIS-UK). *European Health Journal*, **21**, 1450–7.

Commonwealth of Australia (1995). *Guidelines for the pharmaceutical industry on preparation of submissions to the Pharmaceutical Benefits Advisory Committee: including economic analyses*. Department of Health and Community Services, Canberra.

Cook, J. R., Drummond, M. F., Glick, H. A., and Heyse, J. F. (2003). Assessing the appropriateness of combining economic data from multinational clinical trials. *Statistics in Medicine*, **22**, 1955–76.

Coyle, D. (1993). *Increasing the impact of economic evaluations on health care decision making*, Discussion Paper 108. Centre for Health Economics, University of York, York.

Devlin, N. and Parkin, D. (2004). Does NICE have a cost-effectiveness threshold and what other factors influence its decisions? A binary choice analysis. *Health Economics*, **13**, 437–52.

Dolan, P. and Green, C. (1998). Using the person trade-off approach to examine differences between individual and social values. *Health Economics*, **7**, 307–12.

Dolan, P. and Tsuchiya, A. (2003). The person trade-off method and the transitivity principle: an example from preferences over age weighting. *Health Economics*, **12**, 505–10.

Dolan, P., Shaw, R., Tsuchiya, A., and Williams, A. (in press). QALY maximisation and people's preferences: a methodological review of the literature. *Health Economics*.

Donaldson, C., Currie, G., and Mitton, C. (2002). Cost-effectiveness analysis in health care: contraindications. *British Medical Journal*, **325**, 891–4.

Drummond, M. F. (1994*a*). Guidelines for pharmacoeconomic studies: the ways forward. *PharmacoEconomics*, **6**, 493–7.

Drummond, M. F. (1994*b*). Evaluation of health technology: economic issues for health policy and policy issues for economic appraisal. *Social Science and Medicine*, **38**, 1593–600.

Drummond, M. F. (2004). Economic evaluation in health care: is it really useful or are we just kidding ourselves? *Australian Economic Review*, **37**, 3–11.

Drummond, M. F. and Pang. F. (2001). Transferability of economic evaluation results. In: *Economic evaluation in health care: merging theory with practice* (ed. M. F. Drummond and A. McGuire), pp. 256–76. Oxford University Press, Oxford.

Drummond, M. F., Mohide, E. A., Tew, M., Streiner, D. L., Pringle, D. M., and Gilbert, J. R. (1991). Economic evaluation of a support programme for caregivers of demented elderly. *International Journal of Technology Assessment in Health Care*, **7**, 209–19.

Drummond, M. F., Bloom, B. S., Carrin, G., *et al.* (1992). Issues in the cross-national assessment of health technology. *International Journal of Technology Assessment in Health Care*, **8**, 671–82.

Drummond, M. F., Torrance, G. W., and Mason, J. M. (1993). Cost-effectiveness league tables: more harm than good? *Social Science and Medicine*, **37**, 33–40.

Drummond, M. F., Davies, L. M., and Rutten, F. F. H. (ed.) (1994). From results to action: the role of economic appraisal in developing policy for health technology. *Social Science and Medicine*, **38**, 1591–688.

Drummond, M. F., Brown, R., Fendrick, A. M., *et al.* (2003). Use of pharmacoeconomics information—report of the ISPOR task force on use of pharmacoeconomic/health economic information in health care decision-making. *Value in Health*, **6**, 407–16.

Drummond, M. F., Manca, A., and Sculpher, M. (2005). Increasing the generalisability of economic evaluations: recommendations for the design, analysis and reporting of studies. *International Journal of Technology Assessment in Health Care*, **21**, 1–7.

Eddy, D. (1991). Oregon's methods: did cost-effectiveness analysis fail? *Journal of the American Medical Association*, **266**, 2135–41.

EPIC Investigators (1994). Use of monoclonal antibody directed against the platelet glycoprotein 11b/111a receptor in high-risk coronary angioplasty. *New England Journal of Medicine*, **330**, 956–61.

Fenwick, E., Claxton, K., and Sculpher, M. (2001). Representing uncertainty: the role of cost-effectiveness acceptability curves. *Health Economics*, **10**, 779–89.

Gafni, A. and Birch, S. (1993). Guidelines for the adoption of new technologies: a prescription for uncontrolled growth in expenditures and how to avoid the problem. *Canadian Medical Association Journal*, **148**, 913–17.

George, B., Harris, A., and Mitchell, A. (2001). Cost-effectiveness analysis and the consistency of decision-making: evidence from Pharmaceutical Reimbursement in Australia (1991 to 1996). *PharmacoEconomics*, **19**, 1103–9.

Glasziou, P. and Mitchell, A. (1996). Use of pharmacoeconomic data by regulatory authorities. In: *Quality of life and pharmacoeconomics in clinical trials* (ed. B. Spilker), pp. 1141–7. Lippincott-Raven, Philadelphia.

Gold, M. R., Siegel, J. E., Russell, L. B., and Weinstein, M. C. (ed.) (1996). *Cost-effectiveness in health and medicine*. Oxford University Press, New York.

Graham, D. Y., Agrawal, N. M., and Roth, S. H. (1988). Prevention of NSAID-induced gastric ulcer with the synthetic prostaglandin misoprostol: a multi-centre, double-blind, placebo-controlled trial. *The Lancet*, **2**, 1277–80.

Grieve, R., Nixon, R., Thompson, S. G., and Normand, C. (in press). Using multilevel models for assessing the variability of multinational resource use and cost data. *Health Economics*.

Haan, G. and Rutten, F. F. H. (1987). Economic appraisal, health service planning, and budgetary management for health technologies. In: *Economic appraisal of health technology in the European Community* (ed. M. F. Drummond), pp. 135–46. Oxford University Press, Oxford.

Harvard School of Public Health (2004). *The HSPH cost-effectiveness registry*, www.hsph. harvard.edu/cearegistry. Harvard University, Cambridge, Massachusetts.

Hjelmgren, J., Berggren, F., and Anderson, F. (2001). Health economic guidelines—similarities, differences and some implications. *Value in Health*, **4**, 225–50.

Hull, R. D., Hirsh, J., Sackett, D. L., and Stoddart, G. L. (1981). Cost-effectiveness of clinical diagnosis, venography and non-invasive testing in patients with symptomatic deep-vein thrombosis. *New England Journal of Medicine*, **304**, 1561–7.

Hutubessy, R., Baltussen, R., Barendregt, J., *et al.* (2003). Stochastic league tables: communicating cost-effectiveness results to decision makers. *Health Economics*, **10**, 473–7.

Jacobs, P., Bachynsky, J., and Baladi, J.-F. (1995). A comparative review of pharmacoeconomic guidelines. *PharmacoEconomics*, **8**, 182–9.

Johannesson, M. (2001). Should we aggregate relative or absolute changes in QALYs? *Health Economics*, **10**, 573–7.

Johnson, J. A., Ohimnaa, A., Murti, B., *et al.* (2000). Comparison of Finnish and US-based visual analog valuations of the EQ-5D measure. *Medical Decision Making*, **20**, 281–9.

Laupacis, A., Feeny, D., Detsky, A. S., and Tugwell, P. X. (1992). How attractive does a new technology have to be to warrant adoption and utilization? Tentative guidelines for using clinical and economic evaluations. *Canadian Medical Association Journal*, **146**, 473–81.

Laupacis, A., Feeny, D., Detsky, A. S., and Tugwell, P. X. (1993). Tentative guidelines for using clinical and economic evaluations revisited. *Canadian Medical Association Journal*, **148**, 927–9.

Le Gales, C., Buron, C., Costet, N., *et al.* (2000). The French Health Utilities Index Mark 3 (abstract). *Value in Health*, **3**, 103.

Manca, A., Rice, N., Sculpher, M. J., and Briggs, A. H. (2005). Assessing generalisability by location in trial-based cost-effectiveness analysis: the use of multilevel models. *Health Economics*, (In press).

Mark, D. B., Hlatky, M. A., Califf, R. M., Naylor, G. D., Lee, K. L., *et al.* (1995). Cost-effectiveness of thrombolytic therapy with tissue plasminogen activator as compared with streptokinase for acute myocardial infarction. *New England Journal of Medicine*, **332**, 1418–24.

Mauskopf, J., Rutten, F., and Schonfeld, W. (2003). Cost-effectiveness league tables: valuable guidance for decision makers? *PharmacoEconomics*, **21**, 991–1000.

Maynard, A. K. (1991). Developing the health care market. *Economic Journal*, **101**, 1277–86.

McPherson, L., Wennberg, J. E., Hovind, O., *et al.* (1982). Small area variation in the use of common surgical procedures: an international comparison of New England, England and Norway. *New England Journal of Medicine*, **307**, 1310–14.

Menzin, J., Oster, G., Davies, L., *et al.* (1996). A multinational economic evaluation of rhDNase in the treatment of cystic fibrosis. *International Journal of Technology Assessment in Health Care*, **12**, 52–61.

National Institute for Clinical Excellence (2004). *Guide to the methods of technology appraisal.* NICE, London.

Naylor, C. D., Williams, I., Basinski, A., and Goel, V. (1993). Technology assessment and cost-effectiveness: misguided guidelines? *Canadian Medical Association Journal,* **148**, 921–4.

Neumann, P. J. (2004). Why don't Americans use cost-effectiveness analysis? *American Journal of Managed Care,* **10**, 308–12.

Neumann, P. J. (2005). *Using cost-effectiveness analysis in health care.* Oxford University Press, New York.

Nixon, J., Ulmann, P., Glanville, J., Boulenger, S., Drummond, M. F., and de Pouvourville, G. (2004). The European Network of Health Economic Databases (EURONHEED) Project. *European Journal of Health Economics,* **5**, 183–7.

Nord, E. (2001). The desirability of a condition versus the well being and worth of a person. *Health Economics,* **10**, 579–81.

Nord, E., Pinto, J. L., Richardson, J., Menzel, P., and Ubel, P. (1999). Incorporating societal concerns for fairness in numerical valuations of health programmes. *Health Economics,* **8**, 25–39.

Nuijten, M. J. C. and Rutten, F. (2002). Combining a budgetary impact analysis and a cost-effectiveness analysis using decision-analytic modelling techniques. *Pharmaco Economics,* **20**, 855–67.

O'Brien, B. and Sculpher, M. (2000). Building uncertainty into cost-effectiveness rankings: portfolio risk-return tradeoffs and implications for decision rules. *Medical Care,* **38**, 460–8.

O'Brien, B. J., Gersten, K., Willan, A. R., and Faulkner, L. A. (2002). Is there a kink in consumers' threshold value for cost-effectiveness in health care? *Health Economics,* **11**, 175–80.

Office of Health Economics (2004). *Health economic evaluations database.* Office of Health Economics-International Federation of Pharmaceutical Manufacturers' Associations, London.

Ontario Ministry of Health (1994). Ontario guidelines for economic analysis of pharmaceutical products. Ministry of Health, Toronto.

Oster, G., Huse, D. M., Lacey, M. J., Regan, M. M., and Fuchs, H. J. (1995). Effects of recombinant human DNase therapy on health care use and costs in patients with cystic fibrosis. *Annals of Pharmacotherapy,* **29**, 459–64.

Palmer, S., Sculpher, M., Philips, Z., *et al.* (2005). Management of non-ST-elevation acute coronary syndromes: how cost-effective are glycoprotein IIb/IIIa antagonists in the UK National Health Service? *International Journal of Cardiology,* (In press).

Phelps, C. E. and Mushlin, A. (1991). On the (near) equivalence of cost-effectiveness and cost–benefit analyses. *International Journal of Technology Assessment in Health Care,* **7**, 12–21.

Pocock, S. J. (1983). *Clinical trials: a practical approach.* Chichester, Wiley.

Raftery, J. (2001). NICE: faster access to modern treatments? Analysis of guidance on health technologies. *British Medical Journal,* **323**, 1300–3.

Rawlins, M. D. and Culyer, A. J. (2004). National Institute for Clinical Excellence and its value judgments. *British Medical Journal,* **329**, 224–7.

Reed Johnson, F., Fries, E. E., and Spencer Banzhaf, H. (1997). Valuing morbidity: an integration of the willingness-to-pay and health-status index literatures. *Journal of Health Economics,* **16**, 641–65.

Russell, L. B. (2004). Is cost-effectiveness analysis unfair? *Medical Decision Making,* **24**, 232–4.

Schoenbaum, S. C., McNeil, B. J., and Kavel, J. (1976) The swine-influenza decision. *New England Journal of Medicine*, **295**, 759–65.

Schulman, K. A., Lynn, L. A., Glick, H. A. and Eisenberg, J. M. (1991). Cost-effectiveness of low-dose zidovudine therapy for asymptomatic patients with HIV infection. *Annals of Internal Medicine*, **114**, 798–802.

Sculpher, M. J., Claxton, K., and Akehurst, R. L. (2004). It's just evaluation for decision making: recent developments in, and challenges for, cost-effectiveness research. In: *Health policy and economics: opportunities and challenges* (ed. P. C. Smith, L. Ginnelly, and M. Sculpher), pp. 8–41. Open University Press, Milton Keynes.

Sculpher, M. J., Pang, F. S., Manca, A., *et al.* (2004). Generalisability in economic evaluation studies in health care: a review and case studies. *Health Technology Assessment*, **8(49)**, 1–206.

Sendi, P., Gafni, A., and Birch, S. (2002). Opportunity costs and uncertainty in the economic evaluation of health care interventions. *Health Economics*, **11**, 23–31.

Sloan, F. A. and Grabowski, H. G. (ed) (1997). The impact of cost-effectivness on public and private policies in health care: an international perspective. *Social science and Medicine*, **45(4)**, 505–648.

Sugden, R. and Williams, A. (1979). *The principles of practical cost-benefit analysis.* Oxford University Press, Oxford.

Tan-Torres Edejer, T., Baltussen, R., Adam, T., *et al.* (2003). *WHO guide to cost-effectiveness analysis.* World Health Organization, Geneva.

Task Force on Principles of Economic Analysis of Health Care Technology (1995). Economic analysis of health care technology: a report on principles. *Annals of Internal Medicine*, **122**, 60–9.

Torrance, G. W. and Zipursky, A. A. (1984). Cost-effectiveness of antepartum prevention of Rh immunization. *Clinics in Perinatology*, **11**, 267–81.

Trueman, P., Drummond, M. F., and Hutton, J. (2001). Developing guidance for budgetary impact analysis. *PharmacoEconomics*, **19**, 609–21.

van Hout, B. A., Al, M. J., Gordon, G. S., and Rutten, F. F. H. (1994). Costs, effects and cost-effectiveness-ratios alongside a clinical trial. *Health Economics*, **3**, 309–19.

Willan, A. R., Pinto, E. M., O'Brien, B. J., *et al.* (in press). Country specific cost comparisons from multinational clinical trials using empirical Bayesian shrinkage estimation: the Canadian ASSENT-3 economic analysis. *Health Economics*.

Williams, A.H. (1985). Economics of coronary artery bypass grafting. *British Medical Journal*, **291**, 326–9.

Williams, A. H. (1997). Intergenerational equity: an exploration of the 'fair innings' argument. *Health Economics*, **6**, 117–32.

Williams, A. H. (2001). The 'fair innings' argument deserves a fairer hearing! Comments by Alan Williams on Nord and Johannesson. *Health Economics*, **10**, 583–5.

Willke, R. J., Glick, H. A., Polsky, D., and Schulman, K. (1998). Estimating country-specific cost-effectiveness from multinational clinical trials. *Health Economics*, **7**, 481–93.

Chapter 11

How to take matters further

11.1. Economic evaluator's survival guide

11.1.1. Introduction

Like most other resources, the resources required to undertake economic evaluations are scarce. Therefore, it is important to ensure that these resources are used efficiently (from the individual evaluator's point of view it is also important to avoid wasting one's time when this could be better spent on other activities).

In this short chapter we present a list of questions the economic evaluators should ask themselves, or another party requesting an evaluation, when embarking on a new study. The object is to minimize the following two difficulties:

(1) evaluators becoming involved in inappropriate or inefficient evaluations;

(2) evaluators spending longer than necessary on any given evaluation.

There is no strong scientific basis for the suggested questions proposed in Section 11.1.2, although some of them mirror quite closely the checklist for critically assessing the literature presented in Chapter 3. Rather, our questions reflect years of experience in participating in economic evaluations and the mistakes we have made. We can make no guarantees of course; disease and infirmity among the evaluation team, changes in government, and world wars can disrupt the best-laid plans! However, we feel that the guidance here at least gives the evaluator a fighting chance.

Here's hoping that you survive and can do better than ourselves in the future!

11.1.2. Some questions to ask yourself when beginning a study

1. Who needs this study and why?

- What viewpoints are legitimate/feasible?
- Is the person requesting the evaluation arguing for an unnecessarily restrictive viewpoint?
- Is anyone serious about the evaluation; that is, are the results likely to change any actions/policies that are being contemplated?
- Will it be possible for someone to act on the results of the evaluation, whatever these turn out to be; that is, are the necessary management procedures or decision-making procedures in place?
- In general, do people have an open mind with respect to the evaluation results?

2. How did we arrive at these alternatives for consideration?

- Is more than one alternative programme proposed, or is the implicit comparison the status quo?

- What would happen if the status quo were maintained?

- Have any important alternatives been omitted?

- Is this particular approach to meeting the given service objectives suggested by previous research, or does it represent someone's pet scheme?

- Would slightly more or slightly less of the proposed programme be preferable; what would we lose if the programme were pruned; what could be gained if extra features were added?

3. What do we know about the effectiveness of the proposed alternatives?

- Have any of the alternative programmes, especially the one(s) now being proposed for economic evaluation, been shown to do more good than harm by one or more controlled studies (especially those involving random allocation of subjects to programmes or treatments)?

- If so, what do we know about the methodological quality of the existing studies and how do we know the same results would be obtained in our setting?

- If several effectiveness studies exist, will they all be included in a systematic review? If not, how credible are the arguments for ignoring some of the studies?

- If only limited data on effectiveness are available, are the sponsors of this economic evaluation serious about undertaking a study of effectiveness of the new programme compared to existing approaches?

- If not, what justification can be given for going ahead with an economic evaluation without generating the effectiveness evidence?

4. What do we know about the likely costs and funding implications of the proposed alternatives?

- What would be your quick estimate (to the nearest $25 000) of the additional resources required to fund the new programme (if found to be effective)?

- Is this sum large in comparison to the likely costs (especially in your time input) of the evaluation? (If not, why are you involved at all?)

- Is there any hope that the extra resources needed to implement the new programme will be found, either through cost savings generated by the programme, resources redeployed from elsewhere, or new funding?

- Would any such redeployment or new funding be hard to achieve?

5. How would we carry out such an evaluation?

- What resources would be needed for the evaluation (for example, personnel, computing)?

- Are these already available or would extra support be required? (If so, has any thought been given as to where support might come from; in particular, are people aware of the methods of obtaining research grants?)

- What kind of moral support can you expect from those requesting the evaluation, especially within your own organization?

- When are the results of the evaluation required? Is everybody clear on what can be achieved (with the evaluation resources at your disposal) within the given time period?

- Whose co-operation do you need to undertake your study? (Will they give it willingly, or only if forced to?)

- Do you like the other people involved well enough to spend extended periods of time with them? (You may have to!)

6. How will the results of the evaluation be disseminated?

- Are there any obstacles to the widespread dissemination of the results?

- Is a publication planned? If so, will you be able to meet generally accepted criteria for reporting the study (for example, those implied by the critical appraisal checklist outlined in Box 3.1) and the ethical principles specified by medical journal editors (International Committee of Medical Journal Editors 1997)?

- Will dissemination of the results be in time to influence the relevant decisions?

11.2. **Additional literature**

A number of references have been given at the end of each chapter. In particular, the reader should consult the books by Gold *et al.* (1996), Johannesson (1996), Sloan (1995), Drummond and McGuire (2001) and Neumann (2005), which all contain a wide range of additional references.

Further examples of economic evaluations can be located by normal literature searches. In addition, there are several economic evaluations databases that offer a rich source of information.

The *Health Economic Evaluations Database (HEED)* is a joint venture between the Office of Health Economics and the International Federation of Pharmaceutical Manufacturers' Associations. It contains structured abstracts of studies, methodological papers, and reviews. Further details can be obtained from

OHE-IFPMA Database Limited
12 Whitehall
London SW1A 2DY
UK
Tel: +44 20 7930 9203
Fax: +44 20 7747 1419

The *NHS Economic Evaluation Databas (NHS EED)* is maintained by the Centre for Reviews and Dissemination at the University of York. It contains detailed structured abstracts and critical reviews of studies, plus citations for methodological papers, cost studies, and reviews. Further details can be obtained from

Centre for Reviews and Dissemination
Alcuin B Block
University of York
Heslington
York YO10 5DD
UK

Also, the database can be accessed on-line by dialling +44 1904 321846, or through the web site, www.york.ac.uk/inst/crd/nhsdhp.htm.

The *European Network of Health Economic Evaluation Databases (EURONHEED)* project is funded by the European Union and is implementing, in seven European centres (based in France, Germany, Italy, The Netherlands, Spain, Sweden, and the UK), databases of all economic evaluations undertaken in 15 European Union member states (it excludes evaluations undertaken in the 10 new countries joining in June 2005). The network builds on two existing databases, the NHS EED (described above) and the Connaissances et Décision en Économie de la Santé (CODECS) database, coordinated by the Collège des Économists de la Santé in France. Further details can be found on the project's web site, www.euronheed.org.

The *Harvard School of Public Health Cost-Effectiveness Registry* is a comprehensive registry of cost-utility analyses, which contains detailed information on cost-utility analyses published in the health and medical literature from 1976 to 2001. Further details can be found on the registry web site, www.hsph.harvard.edu/cearegistry.

11.3. **Looking to the future**

Through three editions of this book, spanning 18 years, we have documented how the field of economic evaluation in health care has advanced, both in terms of methodology and practice. No doubt further advances will be made in the near future. We cannot anticipate these here, nor prevent the book becoming out of date. However, we do hope that, by reading the book, you become quickly conversant with the methods of economic evaluation and make your own contribution to this rapidly developing field.

References

Drummond, M. F. and McGuire, A. (ed.) (2001). *Economic evaluation in health care: merging theory with practice.* Oxford University Press, Oxford.

Gold, M. R., Siegel, J. E., Russell, L. B., and Weinstein, M. C. (ed.) (1996). *Cost-effectiveness in health and medicine.* Oxford University Press, New York.

International Committee of Medical Journal Editors (1997). Uniform requirements for manuscripts submitted to biomedical journals. *Annals of Internal Medicine*, **126**, 36–7.

Johannesson, M. (1996). *Theory and methods of economic evaluation of health care.* Kluwer, Dordrecht.

Neumann, P. J. (2005). *Using cost-effectiveness analysis in health care.* Oxford University Press, New York.

Sloan, F. (ed.) (1995). *Valuing health care.* Cambridge University Press, New York.

Author Index

Subject Index